THE
CRITICALLY
ILL CHILD

Diagnosis and Management

Edited by

CLEMENT A. SMITH, M.D.

Based on articles appearing in PEDIATRICS,
The Journal of the American Academy of Pediatrics

1972   W. B. SAUNDERS COMPANY

Philadelphia • London • Toronto

W. B. Saunders Company: West Washington Square
Philadelphia, Pa. 19105

12 Dyott Street
London, WC1A 1DB

833 Oxford Street
Toronto 18, Ontario

The Critically Ill Child: Diagnosis and Management   ISBN 0-7216-8384-3

Print No.:   9   8   7   6   5   4   3   2

PREFACE

Life is Short and the Art Long
The Occasion Instant
Experiment Perilous
Decision Difficult

Carved in stone on the wall of at least one medical school, the familiar words have given generations of medical students an unforgettable explanation of purpose. Many may have found such instant occasions less common than they expected in subsequent professional life. Some may wish their educations had given them wisdom and fortitude for the chronic situation rather than resourcefulness for the instant occasion. Nevertheless, all of us, if worth our salt, carry through life the hope of responding quickly and correctly to the critical problems that come our way.

Hence, when Dr. Morris Green, whose own writings have illuminated the area of less acute but often more trying disease, suggested to PEDIATRICS these articles on The Critically Ill Child, response was enthusiastic. Few of those asked to contribute did not rise to the challenge. Subscribers welcomed the monthly appearance of at least one article they could call "practical," because useful in the kind of pediatrics they hoped to practice. Now, through the interest of the W. B. Saunders Company, and with the particular assistance of Mr. Robert B. Rowan, these papers are here made available in one volume. May it help to reduce the peril of experiment and the difficulty of decision.

CLEMENT A. SMITH, M.D.
Editor, PEDIATRICS

CONTRIBUTORS

C. WARREN BIERMAN, M.D.

Clinical Professor of Pediatrics; Head, Pediatric Allergy; University of Washington School of Medicine; Children's Orthopedic Hospital and Medical Center; University Hospital; Harborview Hospital, Seattle, Washington.

ALFRED M. BONGIOVANNI, M.D.

Chairman and Professor of Pediatrics, University of Pennsylvania School of Medicine. Physician-in-Chief, Children's Hospital of Philadelphia, Philadelphia, Pennsylvania.

GEORGE W. BRUMLEY, M.D.

Assistant Professor, Pediatrics; Pediatric Co-Director, Division of Perinatal Medicine, Duke University Medical Center, Durham, North Carolina.

SIDNEY CARTER, M.D.

Professor of Neurology, College of Physicians and Surgeons, Columbia University. Attending Neurologist, Presbyterian Hospital, New York, New York.

ROBERT O. CHRISTIANSEN, M.D.

Assistant Professor of Pediatrics and Head, Division of Metabolism and Endocrinology, Stanford University School of Medicine. Attending Endocrinologist, Stanford University Hospitals and Children's Hospital at Stanford, Stanford, California.

JOHN D. CRAWFORD, M.D.

Associate Professor of Pediatrics, Harvard Medical School. Chief Pediatrician, Shriners Burns Institute; Chief, Endocrine-Metabolic Unit, Children's Service, Massachusetts General Hospital, Boston, Massachusetts.

DEAN CROCKER, M.D.

Clinical Associate in Anesthesia, Harvard Medical School. Associate in Anesthesiology, Anesthesia Department; Director, Respiratory Therapy Department, Children's Hospital Medical Center, Boston, Massachusetts.

JOHN B. DAS, M.D., Ph.D.

Lecturer on Surgery, Harvard Medical School. Research Associate, Children's Hospital Medical Center, Boston, Massachusetts.

DARRYL C. DEVIVO, M.D.

Assistant Professor, Departments of Pediatrics and Neurology, Washington University School of Medicine, St. Louis, Missouri. Assistant Pediatrician, Division of Neurology, St. Louis Children's Hospital, St. Louis, Missouri.

LOUIS K. DIAMOND, M.D.

Professor of Pediatrics, University of California, San Francisco Medical Center. Pediatric Hematologist, Moffitt Hospital, San Francisco, California.

ROBERT S. DOBRIN, M.D.

Medical Fellow, Department of Pediatrics, University of Minnesota Hospitals, Minneapolis, Minnesota.

PHILIP R. DODGE, M.D.

Professor of Pediatrics and Neurology, The Edward Mallinckrodt Department of Pediatrics, Washington University School of Medicine, St. Louis, Missouri. Medical Director, St. Louis Children's Hospital, St. Louis, Missouri.

ANGELO J. ERAKLIS, M.D.

Assistant Professor of Surgery, Children's Hospital Medical Center, Harvard Medical School. Associate in Surgery and Director, Surgical Outpatient Department, Children's Hospital Medical Center, Boston, Massachusetts.

ROBERT M. FILLER, M.D.

Associate Professor of Surgery, Children's Hospital Medical Center, Harvard Medical School. Chief of Clinical Surgery, Children's Hospital Medical Center, Boston, Massachusetts.

LAURENCE FINBERG, M.D.

Professor of Pediatrics, Albert Einstein College of Medicine. Chairman, Department of Pediatrics, Montefiore Hospital and Medical Center, Bronx, New York.

ARNOLD P. GOLD, M.D.

Associate Professor of Clinical Neurology (Pediatrics), College of Physicians and Surgeons, Columbia University. Assistant Attending Neurologist and Pediatrician, Columbia-Presbyterian Medical Center, New York, New York.

DAVID GOLDRING, M.D.

Professor of Pediatrics, Washington University School of Medicine. Director of Pediatric Cardiology, St. Louis Children's Hospital, Washington University, St. Louis, Missouri.

STEPHEN I. GOODMAN, M.S., M.D.

Assistant Professor of Pediatrics, University of Colorado Medical Center, Denver, Colorado.

ROBERT E. GREENBERG, M.D.

Professor and Chairman, Department of Pediatrics, Charles R. Drew Post-graduate Medical School. Pediatrician-in-Chief, Martin Luther King, Jr. General Hospital, Los Angeles, California.

ALEXIS F. HARTMANN, JR., M.D.

Associate Professor of Pediatrics, Washington University School of Medicine. Attending Pediatric Cardiologist, Washington University, St. Louis Children's Hospital, St. Louis, Missouri.

WILLIAM E. HATHAWAY, M.D.

Associate Professor, Department of Pediatrics, University of Colorado Medical Center, Denver, Colorado.

ANTONIO HERNANDEZ, M.D.

Assistant Professor of Pediatrics, Washington University School of Medicine. Attending Pediatric Cardiologist, Washington University, St. Louis Children's Hospital, St. Louis, Missouri.

JOHN T. HERRIN, M.B.B.S., M.R.A.C.P.

Instructor in Pediatrics, Harvard Medical School. Assistant Director, Joseph Barr Pediatric Intensive Care Unit, Children's Service, Massachusetts General Hospital. Assistant Pediatrician, Shriners Burns Institute, Boston, Massachusetts.

HORACE L. HODES, M.D.

Professor and Chairman, Department of Pediatrics, Mount Sinai School of Medicine. Pediatrician-in-Chief, Mount Sinai Hospital, New York, New York.

MALCOLM A. HOLLIDAY, M.D.

Professor of Pediatrics, University of California, San Francisco. Chief, Renal Electrolyte Division, University of California Hospital, San Francisco, and San Francisco General Hospital, San Francisco, California.

C. DUANE LARSEN, M.D.

Attending Physician, Primary Children's Hospital, Salt Lake City, Utah.

JOHN M. LEEDOM, M.D.

Associate Professor of Medicine, University of Southern California School of Medicine. Attending Physician, Medical Service and Communicable Disease Service, Los Angeles County—U.S.C. Medical Center, Los Angeles, California.

ALLEN W. MATHIES, Jr., M.D., Ph.D.

Professor of Pediatrics, University of Southern California School of Medicine. Head Physician, Communicable Disease Service, Los Angeles County–U.S.C. Medical Center, Los Angeles, California.

DONOUGH O'BRIEN, M.D., F.R.C.P.

Professor of Pediatrics, University of Colorado School of Medicine, Colorado General Hospital, Denver, Colorado.

HOWARD A. PEARSON, M.D.

Professor of Pediatrics, Yale University School of Medicine. Attending Physician, Yale–New Haven Hospital, New Haven, Connecticut.

ROBERT L. REPLOGLE, M.D.

Associate Professor of Surgery, University of Chicago—Pritzker School of Medicine. Chief, Pediatric Surgery, Wyler Children's Hospital; Consulting Physician, Little Company of Mary Hospital, Chicago, Illinois.

HERNAN M. REYES, M.D.

Assistant Professor of Surgery, University of Chicago—Pritzker School of Medicine. Attending Physician, Pediatric Surgery, Wyler Children's Hospital, Little Company of Mary Hospital, and Christ Community Hospital, Chicago, Illinois.

ROBERT SCHWARTZ, M.D.

Professor of Pediatrics, Case Western Reserve University School of Medicine. Director of Pediatrics, Cleveland Metropolitan General Hospital, Cleveland, Ohio.

WILLIAM E. SEGAR, M.D.

Professor of Pediatrics, University Hospital, University of Wisconsin, Madison, Wisconsin.

ROBERT M. SMITH, M.D.

Director of Anesthesia, Children's Hospital Medical Center, Boston, Massachusetts.

CHARLES TREY, M.B., Ch.B., M.D.

Assistant Professor of Medicine, Harvard Medical School, Director, Gastroenterology and Ambulatory Care, St. Elizabeth's Hospital; Department of Gastroenterology, New England Deaconess Hospital; Visiting Physician, Harvard Medical Unit, Boston City Hospital; Consulting Physician, Children's Hospital Medical Center, Boston, Massachusetts.

PAUL F. WEHRLE, M.D.

Hastings Professor of Pediatrics, University of Southern California, Los Angeles, California. Director of Pediatrics, Los Angeles County–U.S.C. Medical Center, Los Angeles, California. Consultant in Pediatrics and Infectious Disease, Los Angeles Children's Hospital and Huntington Memorial Hospital, Pasadena, California.

CONTENTS

1

MANAGEMENT OF TRAUMA AND SHOCK IN THE PEDIATRIC PATIENT.. 1

Robert L. Replogle, M.D., and Hernan M. Reyes, M.D.

2

ENDOTOXIN SHOCK.. 21

Horace L. Hodes, M.D.

3

ACUTE ADRENAL INSUFFICIENCY.. 41

Alfred M. Bongiovanni, M.D.

4

THE SERIOUSLY BURNED CHILD.. 46

John T. Herrin, M.B.B.S., and John D. Crawford, M.D.

5

DIAGNOSIS AND MANAGEMENT OF HEAD INJURY........................ 62

Darryl C. DeVivo, M.D., and Philip R. Dodge, M.D.

xi

6

STATUS EPILEPTICUS... 76
    Sidney Carter, M.D., and Arnold P. Gold, M.D.

7

ACUTE BACTERIAL MENINGITIS.. 80
    *Paul F. Wehrle, M.D., Allen W. Mathies, Jr., M.D., Ph. D., and
    John M. Leedom, M.D.*

8

THE CARE OF THE INFANT IN CARDIAC FAILURE 92
    *David Goldring, M.D., Antonio Hernandez, M.D., and
    Alexis F. Hartmann, Jr., M.D.*

9

ACUTE HEPATIC FAILURE 104
    Charles Trey, M.D.

10

ACUTE RENAL FAILURE... 113
    *Robert S. Dobrin, M.D., C. Duane Larsen, M.D., and
    Malcolm A. Holliday, M.D.*

11

RESPIRATORY ARREST AND ITS SEQUELAE 124
    Robert M. Smith, M.D.

12

MANAGEMENT OF TRACHEOSTOMY... 139
    Dean Crocker, M.D.

13

THE RESPIRATORY DISTRESS SYNDROME OF THE NEWBORN 152
    George W. Brumley, M.D.

14

DIABETIC KETOACIDOSIS AND COMA.. 168
    Robert Schwartz, M.D.

15

HYPOGLYCEMIA... 180

    Robert E. Greenberg, M.D., and Robert O. Christiansen, M.D.

16

ACUTE METABOLIC DISEASE IN INFANCY AND EARLY CHILDHOOD.. 188

    Donough O'Brien, M.D., and Stephen I. Goodman, M.D.

17

SALICYLATE INTOXICATION 199

    William E. Segar, M.D.

18

DEHYDRATION SECONDARY TO DIARRHEA................................. 208

    Laurence Finberg, M.D.

19

INTRAVENOUS ALIMENTATION.. 220

    Robert M. Filler, M.D., Angelo J. Eraklis, M.D., and John B. Das, M.D., Ph. D.

20

THE PROBLEM OF DISSEMINATED INTRAVASCULAR COAGULATION... 239

    William E. Hathaway, M.D.

21

SICKLE CELL DISEASE CRISES AND THEIR MANAGEMENT............... 249

    Howard A. Pearson, M.D., and Louis K. Diamond, M.D.

22

ANAPHYLAXIS... 260

    C. Warren Bierman, M.D.

INDEX 267

1

Management of Trauma and Shock in the Pediatric Patient

Robert L. Replogle, M.D., and Hernan M. Reyes, M.D.

INTRODUCTION

Trauma has long been known to be the leading single killer of children, but the magnitude of its impact is not generally appreciated. Motor vehicle accidents caused the death of 8500 children under the age of 14 years in 1966 and nontransport accidents were responsible for the death of 9000 more, a total of 17,500 deaths from trauma. Contrast this to asthma which was responsible for 150 deaths in the same age group that year, and pneumonia (7600 deaths), the anemias (360 deaths), malignant neoplasms of all kinds (4200 deaths), heart disease (900 deaths), and congenital malformations of all kinds, which were the cause of 14,000 deaths.[1] With the increasing popularity of the motorcycle and the snowmobile, these figures will probably become even more impressive.[2] The economics of accidental injury are of secondary importance, but it has been estimated that the cost of death and disability from trauma amounts to $17 billion for the 50 million Americans injured each year.[3]

From the Section of Pediatric Surgery and the Department of Surgery, Pritzker School of Medicine of the University of Chicago, Chicago, Illinois.

1

When the severely injured patient is brought into the emergency room, it is desirable that extensive resources be immediately available. Since 50 per cent of traffic accidents occur between 1:00 P.M. on Friday and 9:00 A.M. on Monday, it is essential that emergency medical coverage be available seven days a week, 24 hours a day.[4] The need for methods of transporting trauma victims expeditiously to facilities which have the capability for comprehensive management is emphasized by the study of Waller,[5] who found that the death rate from motor vehicle accidents was substantially higher in rural areas (47 per 100,000 population) than in urban areas (17 per 100,000), even though the extent of the injuries that led to death in the rural accidents were of the same severity as the urban accidents, or even less.

While it is unrealistic to overgeneralize on this kind of study, the implication is that the rural patients remained at the scene of the accident for a longer period and then, perhaps, were taken to a hospital of limited resources. However, rapid and effective ambulance service is not entirely the answer, as is illustrated by the Philadelphia study,[4] which noted that in 794 traffic fatalities 50 per cent died at the scene of the accident and 72 per cent died either at the scene, in transit, or within the first 10 minutes of hospitalization. It seems apparent that efforts at salvage must begin before hospitalization. Well-designed transport vans engineered specifically for children have been described, and experience has demonstrated the value of such a system.[6] The experience with helicopter evacuation in Vietnam has been very favorable and several centers are experimenting with the use of this method for civilian injuries.

A basic requirement for emergency care is to provide trained ambulance crews to transport the injured to the designated hospital. These people should be trained in pulmonary resuscitation, techniques of stopping hemorrhage, splinting of extremities and so on. At least one hospital in a community should be identified as an emergency receiving facility so that its emergency room can be fully prepared and equipped. The widespread custom of transporting patients to the nearest medical facility is not an efficient system, since it means that either every hospital must provide equal resources at the expense of duplication or that some of them have inadequate facilities. The nurses in the emergency room and the house staff in a teaching institution must be instructed in the treatment of shock and trauma; if the number of real emergencies is not adequate to keep the team smoothly coordinated, nursing in-service education and the staff physicians must perform the function of continuing to reeducate the team. Ideally, coverage by pediatricians, surgeons, orthopedic surgeons, anesthesiologists, neurosurgeons, urologists, and vascular surgeons makes the professional care comprehensive. If a small but strategically located hospital cannot support this large complement of specialists, it is not only possible but necessary to obtain prompt consultation using modern communication devices, provided that the organizational groundwork has previously been completed.

EMERGENCY FACILITIES

As in all areas of medical practice, elegant facilities and equipment are no substitute for well-trained, thoughtful professionals, doctors and nurses. The preparedness and competence of the emergency room staff should be continuously under surveillance.

In each emergency area, all the equipment and supplies necessary for resuscitation in trauma must be maintained, and checked each shift for completeness. The make-up of this resuscitation equipment may vary according to local requirements, but it must always be ready. For a guide, the emergency equipment in our unit is as follows:

General Equipment

1. Direct current defibrillator, with a range from 20 to 400 watt-seconds.
2. Infant (3 cm), pediatric (5 cm) and adult (10 cm) external defibrillator paddles.
3. EKG machine.
4. Two venous cutdown trays.
5. One tracheostomy tray.
6. One small general surgical tray with abdominal and thoracic retractors.
7. Sphygmomanometer and arm cuffs of various sizes.
8. Blood pressure measuring device, ultrasonic (see below).

Respiratory Equipment

1. Tracheostomy tubes, sizes 000, 00, 0, 1, 2, 3 and 4—two each, plastic.
2. Oropharyngeal airways, sizes 0, 1, 2, 3 and 4—two each.
3. Endotracheal tubes, with connectors, sizes 10 to 26 French, sterile—two each.
4. Laryngoscope, standard handle, extra batteries and bulbs.
5. Laryngeal blades, small straight for infant, Foregger or Flagg for child, and MacIntosh for adult.
6. Hope or Ambu ventilating bag.
7. Various size face masks for infant or adult.
8. Standard portable suction machine.
9. Oxygen tanks or wall oxygen outlet.

10. Metal tonsil type suction tube. Sterile plastic suction catheters, sizes 5, 8, 10, and 14 French.

Supplies

1. Sterile needles and syringes, including intracardiac needles (22 ga., 6 cm in length).
2. Plastic intravenous catheters (some at least 40 cm in length), 14, 16, 18, and 20 ga.
3. Scalp vein needles.
4. Tongue blades.
5. Gauze sponges, alcohol sponges.
6. Antibiotic ointment.
7. Intravenous connection tubing, with and without blood filter.
8. Blood scale and pressure infusor for blood. Calibrated burettes.
9. Three way stopcocks.
10. Chest tubes, sizes 12, 16, 20, and 24 French (preferably the type with a disposable trocar in the tube).
11. Small tubing for arterial cutdown (size 50 PE (polyethylene) and 90 PE).
12. Needle stub adaptors—12, 18, 20, and 22 ga.
13. Knife blades—sizes 10 and 15.
14. Suture material, synthetic and catgut—some with various sized swaged-on needles.

Drugs

1. Sodium bicarbonate—several vials 1 mEq/ml (usual initial dose 2 to 4 mEq/kg repeated each 10 minutes until arterial pH is measured).
2. Epinephrine—several vials, 1:10,000 conc., 0.1 mg/ml (usual dose 0.1 ml/kg by push).
3. Isoproterenol—0.2 to 0.4 mg/100 ml (usual initial dose 1 to 2 ml, then continuous slow infusion).
4. Calcium chloride—10% conc., 100 mg/ml (usual dose 0.2 ml/kg).
5. Solutions—5% serum albumin, 6% dextran (70,000 mol. wt.), 10% dextran (40,000 mol. wt.), lactated Ringer's solution, normal saline, dextrose and water.

MONITORING TECHNIQUE AND INITIAL TREATMENT

Shock in the child is nearly always the result of blood (or fluid) loss, or infection, and frequently the patient has multiple injuries or more than one likely cause for circulatory or respiratory embarrassment. The first objective of the physician is quickly to sort out the various problems so that priorities for treatment can be established. Usually in the severely injured child, several resuscitative measures may be needed simultaneously and even the most experienced physician should call for help as soon as he recognizes the seriousness of the situation.

If the patient is brought in without heartbeat and is making no resuscitative efforts, an instant decision must be made as to whether to attempt resuscitation at all. Unfortunately, there are no infallible signs of brain death that are instantly applicable and this decision has to be based on "clinical judgment," perhaps by taking a quick history from the parents or ambulance attendants who brought the patient to the hospital. They may be able, for instance, to tell the physician when the child stopped breathing spontaneously, or when the pulse ceased. The stethoscope is a more reliable guide to the presence of a heartbeat in the child than in the adult, but nevertheless an electrocardiographic signal is of utmost importance. If the patient has airway obstruction and still maintains a heartbeat, then either endotracheal intubation or positive pressure ventilation with a mask and oxygen is of primary importance. (It is unwise for the inexperienced physician to spend much time trying to insert an endotracheal tube, since the child can nearly always be well ventilated with the mask and bag.) After respiration has been reestablished, massive hemorrhage should be controlled by the application of manual pressure and unstable fractures splinted.

At the first chance, one nurse should be designated to start a chart on the patient, recording at frequent intervals the vital signs, pupil size and reaction, and the fluids and drugs given. A second nurse should be assigned the task of connecting a monitor or EKG machine to the patient and preparing the drugs that may be required for cardiac resuscitation, *labeling* each syringe. (The coordination of this team effort is vital, and the most experienced member of the team should assume charge, since without direction the whole scene may degenerate into an unbelievable shambles.) In most instances, the rapid infusion of blood, fluids or drugs will be essential, and the physician should quickly establish one or more routes for venous infusion. In the child this is best accomplished by cutdown of the greater saphenous vein at the ankle and insertion of a large bore catheter.[7] (Efforts at introducing a needle or catheter percutaneously into a collapsed peripheral vein in a child will usually be very difficult, and unless it it obvious that success is likely, little time should be wasted making multiple attempts.)

One should remember that direct injection of drugs into the heart is a very useful maneuver when time is critical. A 22 ga 6 cm needle introduced parasternally at the left fifth intercostal space, with the tip of the needle directed toward the posterior right axilla, will enter the right ventricle most of the time. This has been done here on many occasions with no cause, as yet, for discontinuing this technique. If the patient is severely injured, a catheter should be introduced into the bladder and a central venous pressure line inserted.

One needs as much information about the hemodynamic and respiratory status of the patient as it is possible to obtain if a sound evaluation of the effectiveness of treatment is to be made. However, enthusiasm for collecting physiological and biochemical data must be tempered with concern for the clinical progress of the patient, and relatively few measurements are really of practical importance. It is essential to know the arterial blood pressure, but an accurate blood pressure may be difficult to obtain by auscultatory methods in the hypotensive patient. Cohn found that the blood pressure obtained by arm cuff in 39 hypotensive patients averaged 33 mm Hg less than the blood pressure obtained directly by intra-arterial needle puncture, and ranged from 164 mm Hg less to 20 mm Hg more than directly measured pressure.[8] Since it is frequently desirable to have samples of arterial blood for pH, pO_2 and pCO_2 measurements as well as accurate blood pressure measurements, in most severely injured patients an arterial catheter should be introduced into the radial artery by direct cutdown (Fig. 1). In the infant a #50 PE tube will be the proper size for the radial artery, and in the child over one year of age, a #90 PE catheter will fit. With care and frequent irrigations with heparinized lactated Ringer's solution, patency can be maintained for prolonged periods even in the smallest infant. We have performed a great many radial artery catheterizations without a single

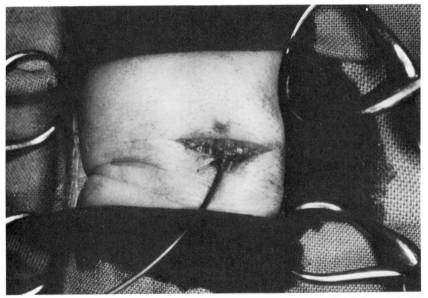

Figure 1.   A radial artery catheter can be inserted in even the smallest infant and will provide really meaningful information on arterial pO_2, pCO_2, pH and blood pressure.

serious complication. A satisfactory substitute for direct intra-arterial blood pressure measurement is provided by either measuring the beginning of blood flow following cuff occlusion, using the transcutaneous Doppler ultrasonic flowmeter,[9] or by Doppler ultrasonic detection of arterial wall motion.[10] Both these techniques give reliable measurements in hypotensive patients of all ages. (It may be redundant to point out that the average systolic pressure during the first week of life is 80 mm Hg, and a systolic pressure of 60 mm Hg during this period may be perfectly normal.[11]). Incidentally, the Doppler flowmeter is extremely valuable in the injured child in whom there is a question of vascular integrity as, for example, in the patient with a fracture-dislocation of the elbow in whom a radial pulse cannot be palpated. We have saved ourselves considerable distress and effort by transcutaneous use of the ultrasonic flowmeter to detect the presence of pulsatile blood flow accurately in distal arteries, even those as small as the digital artery.

Perhaps the most important advance in the management of the injured patient in the past decade has been the appreciation of the usefulness of the central venous pressure as a method of evaluating the adequacy of blood volume replacement and, indirectly, of cardiac function.[12] The blood reservoir function of the venous system is well known and is characterized by the relatively slow increase in venous pressure as the intravascular volume is increased, as compared to the arterial side of the system. When the venous reservoir is filled to capacity, the pressure:volume ratio increases very rapidly, indicating that the vascular system is full (Fig. 2).

When the diastolic filling pressure of the ventricles is increased by means of increasing the central venous pressure or left atrial pressure by volume infusion, a substantial increase in myocardial contractility is achieved through the Frank-Starling effect, and this results in increased

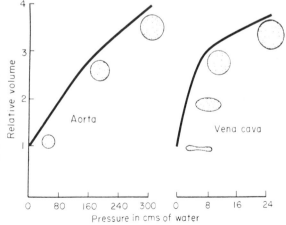

Figure 2. The venous system is more compliant than the arterial circulation, and this is shown in the relatively slow changes in venous pressures, induced by increasing the venous blood volume, until the system is filled. At this point there is a marked increase in venous pressure as volume is further increased.

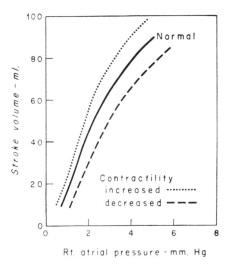

Figure 3. Under normal circumstances ventricular stroke volume and contractility are increased as the diastolic filling pressure is increased, by the Frank-Starling mechanism. When intrinsic myocardial contractility is decreased, a greater filling pressure (right atrial pressure) is required to achieve any given value for stroke volume.

cardiac output (Fig. 3). In the child or young adult in whom coronary artery insufficiency and myocardial dysfunction are of little practical importance, the central venous or right atrial pressure accurately reflects the left atrial pressure (which, to be precise, determines the left ventricular end-diastolic volume and thus the magnitude of the Frank-Starling effect on systemic output). Figure 4 illustrates this point in a group of

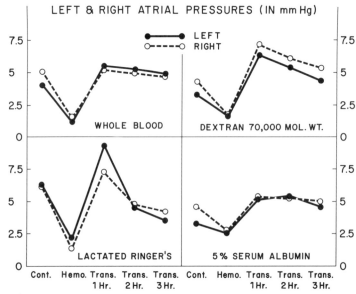

Figure 4. In dogs subjected to hemorrhagic shock and then transfused with blood, colloid or crystalloid fluids, the right atrial and left atrial pressures were virtually identical throughout. (From R. L. Replogle, unpublished data.)

normal dogs subjected to hemorrhage followed by replacement of the volume deficit with a variety of colloid or non-colloid substances. It is quite apparent that left and right atrial pressures vary closely. If ventricular function is compromised, as illustrated, for example, by the dashed lines in Figure 3, then a higher ventricular filling pressure is required to maintain cardiac output. In patients with coronary heart disease, left ventricular function may be more severely compromised than right ventricular function. In such circumstances, the right atrial pressure may be normal at a time when left atrial pressure is elevated; continuing to infuse solutions into these patients may precipitate pulmonary edema.[13] In the patient with compromised right ventricular function (as in a postoperative Fallot's tetralogy) or in pulmonary vascular obstructive disease (as in an asthmatic child) the right atrial pressure may be considerably greater than left atrial pressure and may again confuse the issue. The ultimate usefulness of any physiological measurement depends upon the care with which the data are obtained. The central venous catheter should be positioned at the entrance of the great veins into the right atrium or, preferably, in the right atrium.[14] The routine use of radiopaque tubing will make it easier to delineate the location of the catheter tip. If the saphenous vein at the groin is used in infants it is particularly important to advance the catheter into the thorax, since an artifactually high intra-abdominal pressure may give a falsely high central venous pressure reading.[15] In the newborn, the umbilical veins are convenient, but again the catheter must be advanced into the inferior vena cava, or right atrium, since the pressure in the portal sinus and ductus venosus may be considerably higher than the central venous pressures[16] (Fig. 5). The complications associated with central venous pressure monitoring are largely preventable but can be mortal, and the physician and nursing service should be familiar with the possibilities.[17, 18] Because any cutdown is susceptible to infection, and subsequent septicemia, the local application of antibiotic ointment, frequently reapplied, should be routine, since this technique has demonstrated usefulness.[19]

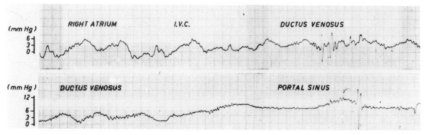

Figure 5. The tracings show the pressures obtained in a newborn infant as an umbilical catheter is pulled back from the right atrium into the inferior vena cava, ductus venosus and portal sinus. The increased pressure in the portal sinus, easily seen, indicates that this is not a good location for monitoring the central venous pressure. (Courtesy of Dr. R. A. Arcilla.)

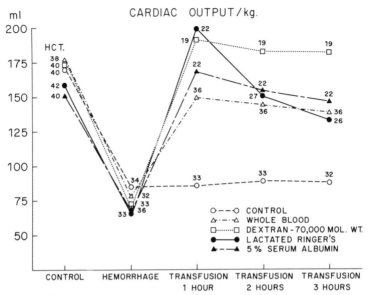

Figure 6. The chart shows changes in cardiac output and hematocrit in dogs subjected to hemorrhagic shock followed by transfusion. The reduced cardiac output associated with hypovolemia was restored by all the fluids, more so with the asanguineous ones than with whole blood. The reduced hematocrit resulted in reduction in systemic vascular resistance as a consequence of reduced blood viscosity. (From R. L. Replogle, unpublished data.)

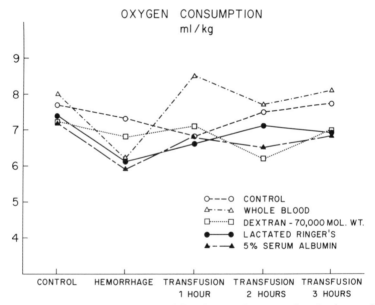

Figure 7. Although the hematocrit fell as low as 19 per cent in animals transfused with asanguineous fluids, there were no significant differences in oxygen consumption between any of the groups. The reduced oxygen-carrying capacity was compensated by increased cardiac output and more efficient oxygen extraction. (From R. L. Replogle, unpublished data.)

The predominant, recurring theme in any discussion of the treatment of shock and trauma in the child should be *volume replacement*. As has been mentioned, following the level of the central venous pressure will provide an excellent guide to fluid replacement in the child, since one can nearly always depend on good myocardial function. Blalock first pointed out that the type of fluid used to replace blood loss is of less importance than giving adequate volume.[20] These observations have been confirmed by many investigators.[21, 22, 23, 24] If asanguineous fluids are used, the reduction in red cell concentration and oxygen-carrying capacity of the blood is compensated by the increased cardiac output or more effective oxygen extraction, so that the oxygen consumption remains constant. This is illustrated in Figure 6, which describes the effects on cardiac output in an animal study in which hemorrhage was followed by volume replacement with a variety of fluids. Oxygen consumption measurements showed no statistically significant differences between any of the groups, even though the hematocrit fell as low as 19 per cent (Fig. 7). If non-colloid fluids are used for volume replacement, the rather rapid loss of solution from the intravascular space into the extravascular space means one must constantly watch for the signs of hypovolemia, as is illustrated in Figure 8. The choice of fluid for volume replacement in the treatment of shock is, to some extent, a matter of personal preference and experience. We believe that colloid agents are preferable, since it is possible to predict the degree of expansion from the amount of fluid infused. There are certain disadvantages to the others which make us regard 5 per cent human serum albumin as the first choice. Despite the widespread enthusiasm for low molecular weight dextran, there is little solid evidence that its usefulness extends beyond a volume replacement effect; since this material of lower weight leaves the vascular space rapidly, as much as 50 per cent may be lost extravascularly within two hours.[25, 26] The larger weight dextran (70,000 mol. wt.) is a more effective plasma expander than the lower molecular weight material, but if it is given in large quantities (over 1000 ml in an adult), it may exert a deleterious effect on blood coagulation.[27] While there is increasing evidence that moderate hemodilution may have a beneficial effect on perfusion during shock,[28] at the present time it is recommended that blood should be given as soon as it is available unless there is evidence of hemoconcentration (hematocrit greater than 40 per cent), in which case a non-sanguineous fluid is preferable. Under no circumstances should the physician wait for blood to be typed and cross-matched before beginning volume replacement, regardless of the hematocrit value, since immediate volume expansion with whatever material is available is much preferable to any kind of delay for whole blood. There is still some controversy about the emergency use of low titer (less than 1:200 anti-A and anti-B saline isoagglutinins) group O Rho (D) positive universal donor blood. The evidence that even a severely diminished hematocrit does not seem to have deleterious effects, the relative scarcity of this type of blood, the

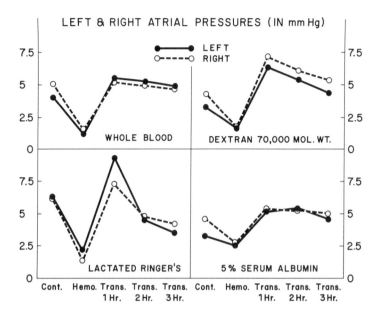

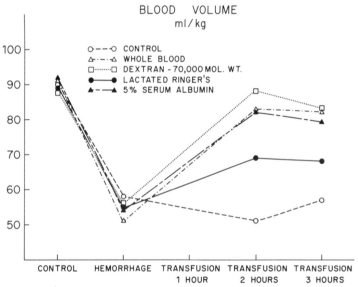

Figure 8. Whole blood and colloid plasma expanders are more effective and longer-lasting agents in maintaining blood volume after infusion than crystalloid solutions such as lactated Ringer's solution. As illustrated here, despite the fact that the volume of lactated Ringer's solution infused was three times that of the colloid fluids, at the end of three hours following transfusion the relative blood volume was 20 per cent less in the lactated Ringer's group. (From R. L. Replogle, unpublished data.)

cost of maintaining a supply, and the fact that when, later, blood of the patient's hereditary type is administered a hemolytic response may be initiated by the reaction between the incompatible isoagglutinins from the transfused O blood and the red cell antigens in donor blood of the patient's type lead us to believe that it is best not to use universal donor blood. If one does give more than the equivalent of 3 units of universal donor blood to an adult, and the patient needs more blood within two weeks, it is best to continue giving universal donor blood and not to switch to transfusions with the patient's hereditary blood type.[29]

There has long existed a "clinical impression" that the massive infusion of stored whole blood is occasionally associated with clinical deterioration even in the absence of tranfusion reactions. Efforts at relating this impression to hypocalcemia (as a result of the chelation of serum calcium by the citrate solution) or acidosis (from the acidity of the bank blood) have not demonstrated a good correlation. Howland,[30] in a large series, observed that the mortality from ventricular fibrillation following the infusion of calcium during massive transfusion was greater than the risk of hypocalcemia in patients not receiving calcium, even when 5 liters of blood and more were transfused. Miller[31] found no correlation between the amount of stored acid-citrate-dextrose blood administered and the magnitude of acidosis in patients given multiple blood transfusions, and recommended that bicarbonate therapy be reserved for patients with severe metabolic acidosis, established by measurement of arterial pH and pCO_2. However, it has recently been established that red cell concentrations of the organic phosphate, 2,3-diphosphoglycerate, fall rapidly during blood storage, and with the loss of this material the affinity of hemoglobin for oxygen increases markedly. As this affinity increases, the position of the oxyhemoglobin dissociation curve shifts to the left and the delivery of oxygen to the tissues may be compromised. When it becomes necessary to transfuse massively, a substantial amount of blood less than five days old should be used, since 75 per cent of the 2,3-diphosphoglycerate is lost after five days of storage.[32] Addition of inosine and a small amount of adenine to banked blood will extend the period of normal erythrocytic concentration of 2,3-diphosphoglycerate to three to five weeks.[33]

It is particularly important to remember that the rapid infusion of cold blood into infants and children will frequently result in ventricular fibrillation or standstill. Blood should be *warmed* before it is given rapidly and there are several convenient methods for doing this.[34]

EVALUATION OF THE TRAUMA PATIENT

The physician should categorize trauma patients rather quickly into those who require *immediate* surgery for massive internal hemorrhage or airway obstruction, those in whom early surgery is probably indicated, and those patients with less obvious major injury.[35] When immediate surgery is required, nothing should be done which will delay the beginning of the operation. The patient should be taken to the operating room at once, and, if possible, intravenous transfusion should be initiated during transportation. The second group of patients consists of those with multiple injuries in whom it would appear that the shock situation can be stabilized and maintained for some time, allowing an interval for certain diagnostic studies. Depending upon the efficiency and experience of the emergency facility and the operating room team, one might better spend a few minutes for treatment in the emergency room rather than risk being caught between floors in an elevator with a patient who has suddenly had a cardiac arrest on the way to the operating room. Finally, there are those patients who have sustained injuries which may not be serious or the seriousness of which may not be readily apparent. In children, this would chiefly mean splenic injury with delayed rupture.

Blood should always be sent for type and cross-match at once and the wise physician asks for at least one more unit than he thinks he may need. In any serious injury an arterial catheter should be inserted and blood sent for pO_2, pH and pCO_2 measurements, and a hematocrit. The Foley catheter and the central venous pressure line complete the basic requirements for monitoring. In the young patient who has sustained trauma, hypotension with a low central venous pressure means hypovolemia, and regardless of one's assessment of the adequacy of volume replacement, transfusion should continue until the blood pressure and signs of improved peripheral perfusion return toward normal, or until the venous pressure begins to climb. The level to which the central venous pressure can be pushed without risk of pulmonary edema varies individually, but certainly in the child or young adult there is little danger until the venous pressure goes above 20 cm H_2O.

If major intra-abdominal bleeding is suspected, confirmation can be quickly obtained with about 80 per cent confidence by aspirating the four abdominal quadrants through an 18 gauge needle.[36] The incidence of false negatives can be reduced still further if a plastic catheter is introduced into the abdominal cavity in the infraumbilical region and 100 to 200 ml of saline are infused and then aspirated. In most instances intra-abdominal bleeding of very low quantity can be detected with this technique.

Hemorrhage into the chest is rarely a critical problem unless there is a laceration of the heart or great vessels. If there is doubt about a patient with diminished breath sounds, a chest tube can be inserted (fifth or sixth intercostal space in the anterior axillary line, well away from the liver and spleen), but ordinarily a chest roentgenogram should be obtained to confirm a suspicion of hemothorax. In most instances bleeding from the lung will cease without the need for thoracotomy and the pneumothorax and hemothorax can be treated with the chest tube alone.[37] When there is damage to the heart or great vessels, extremely fast and well-organized teamwork is required for urgent thoracotomy.

It is unfortunate that the changes in social behavior of our times have provided us with greater experience with stab wounds of the various areas of the body. With this newly acquired information have come some suggestions for modifying the traditional approach to treatment. In the past, stab wounds of the abdomen, because they are penetrating, have been considered to be surgical emergencies, and this attitude has been shown to result in unnecessary laparotomy in over 50 per cent of patients.[38] Currently, many experienced clinicians believe that a more selective approach to exploration reduces the number of unnecessary explorations, at little risk to the patient.[39, 40, 41] The decision for exploration is based on the usual clinical and laboratory criteria (free intra-abdominal air, hematuria, severe hemorrhage, peritonitis, and so on) and in addition radiocontrast injection of the sinus tract to delineate the depth of the wound. With a catheter sewn into the wound, 50 to 75 ml of contrast medium is injected and the patient is x-rayed in several positions to identify contrast in the peritoneal cavity or the bowel. If the radiographic study is negative, the patient is observed clinically for 48 hours and if no signs of peritonitis develop he may be discharged. This protocol has merit and has been very useful and safe.

Stab wounds of the neck are quite different from the abdomen, since there is a plethora of vital structures close beneath the skin. Major injuries to the airway, blood vessels, or esophagus may result from rather innocent-looking wounds, and routine surgical exploration of penetrating neck wounds is the safest course of action.[42]

The patient suffering blunt trauma to the abdomen may be a diagnostic problem. In the absence of intra-abdominal blood from the peritoneal aspiration, and with no evidence of free air in the abdomen, no fractures, and clear urine, the possibility of subcapsular hematoma of the spleen or liver with delayed hemorrhage still gives cause for concern.[43] The abdomen is usually tender from the trauma and difficult to examine. In certain instances liver or splenic radioisotope scans or selective angiography may be very useful in the evaluation of the extent of injury.[44] Even without signs of major intra-abdominal injury after blunt trauma, it is still wise to maintain the child by intravenous rather than oral food and fluids for 24 hours, since the incidence of paralytic ileus (often from a mesenteric hematoma) is high, and vomiting and distention will frequently follow attempts at early oral feeding.

While the discussion of head injury is the subject of another chapter, it is important to emphasize the fact that, except for the neonate, patients with head injury rarely present in shock.[45] If a child with a head injury is seen with hypotension and shock, *look elsewhere* for hemorrhagic blood loss.

SUPPORTIVE TREATMENT OF SHOCK

In the overwhelming majority of cases, rapid restoration of blood volume is all that is necessary for the resuscitation of the child in shock. On occasion, temporary pharmacologic support may be necessary to increase myocardial contractility, reverse metabolic or respiratory acidosis, or simply to maintain arterial pressure until the lost blood can be replaced.

Metabolic acidosis has long been known to accompany reduced tissue perfusion and anaerobic metabolism. Acidosis *per se* has been reported to reduce myocardial contractility, possibly by inhibiting the beta-adrenergic effects of catecholamines on the heart.[46] More recent evidence suggests that this widely held concept may not be entirely correct if it is applied to the patient in shock, since acidosis increases secretion of epinephrine by the adrenal gland, thus enhancing adrenergic activity.[47] Other experimental studies do not support the theory that acidosis, either respiratory or metabolic, has a depressive effect on myocardial function until the pH falls below 6.9[48] In newborn puppies subjected to hemorrhagic shock, the improvement in cardiovascular function that followed correction of metabolic acidosis with sodium bicarbonate was equally good when other hyperosmotic solutions, such as 3 per cent sodium chloride or 25 per cent mannitol, were given, even though the solutions did nothing to correct the acidosis. Nevertheless, one should not conclude from these comments that metabolic acidosis should not be corrected, since, for one thing, the susceptibility of the heart to ventricular fibrillation does appear to be increased by metabolic acidosis.[50] It should be remembered, however, that metabolic acidosis is a "symptom" of the underlying disease, and every effort must be oriented toward treatment of the basic problem.

Occasionally it will be necessary to use sympathomimetic drugs, either on a temporary basis while volume losses are being made up or for more long-term support in the patient with some underlying disorder, such as congenital heart disease or chronic lung disease. Calcium chloride given slowly intravenously, or by intracardiac injection, is extremely useful for improving myocardial function. Isoproterenol has also proved to be of great merit, although some patients have an extreme chronotrophic response, and the tachycardia that develops may be disabling. Epinephrine may be used advantageously in these cases. Children respond very quickly to volume replacement and, over the long term, catecholamines are not usually required. The physician needs a practical working knowledge of these drugs and should develop his personal protocol.[51, 52, 53]

The use of pharmacologic doses of corticosteroids has been advocated in the treatment of shock, some studies indicating a vasodilator effect,[54] others a positive inotropic effect,[55] while still other experimental studies have failed to demonstrate any hemodynamic effects.[56] The role of lysosomal disruption as a consequence of shock, and the apparent stabilizing effect of corticosteroids on the lysosome membrane, may well be of considerable importance.[57] At the present time, although the evidence that large doses of corticosteroids are beneficial in the treatment of shock is not solid, we do have enough experience to know that the very short-term use of this drug is not harmful. Consequently, we frequently use methylprednisolone (25 mg per kg) as an adjunct in the treatment of shock, usually as a single infusion.

The adequacy of urine output remains a very valuable sign of satisfactory circulatory dynamics. The presence of oliguria may simply indicate inadequate volume replacement or may herald the onset of acute renal failure. (See Chapter 10). There is little evidence that the use of osmotic diuresis actually prevents acute tubular necrosis. However, the infusion of hypertonic mannitol is a useful device in permitting one to differentiate between renal shutdown and oliguria secondary to hypovolemia or dehydration.[58] More recently, ethacrynic acid and furosemide are being used for the same purpose without the disadvantages of additional fluid administration.[59] If a diuresis follows the administration of these agents, the likelihood is great (but not certain) that the oliguria is a result of hypovolemia. Measurement of urinary sodium concentration also helps in the differential diagnosis of oliguria, since the possibility of acute tubular necrosis is unlikely if the urine sodium is less than 30 mEq per liter.[60]

While hypovolemia in the older child may be approached in a manner analogous to that useful in the adult, a few special aspects pertinent to the treatment of shock in the newborn require mention. First is the relationship of body temperature to the response to shock. It is well known that the index of surface area to body weight is greater in the infant and that an environmental temperature of 34° C reduces to the lowest level the metabolic activity required to maintain body temperature in the neonate.[61] In the infant with an intact thermoregulatory mechanism, exposure to a cold environment may result in considerable energy expenditure simply to maintain body temperature, and this caloric loss may be detrimental for survival in shock.[62] Therefore, efforts should be made to keep the shocked infant in a warm environment. While the neuroendocrine response of the infant to hemorrhage is the same as in the adult, the degree of hypotension and reduction in cardiac output which accompany moderate (15 per cent of blood volume) blood loss are relatively greater in the infant, and replacement of even apparently moderate amounts of blood lost may be important.[63, 64] The sudden infusion of hypertonic solutions, e.g., 20 per cent mannitol (1400 mOsm/kg), or 7.5 per cent sodium bicarbonate (1465 mOsm/kg), may result in a sudden shift of water out of the central nervous system, and this may cause intra-cranial hemorrhage in the infant. These solutions should be administered slowly.[65] As a matter of fact, anything given intravenously should be given slowly, since an inordinate number of cardiac arrests immediately follow the central intravenous administration of drugs.[66]

If the physician remembers that volume replacement is the name of the game, and that warm feet mean strong heart,[67] he will be well rewarded by the rapid, complete, and gratifying recovery of the child in shock.

References

1. Vital Statistics of the United States, 1966. Department of Health, Education and Welfare, U.S. Public Health Service, National Center for Health Statistics, Washington, D.C., Government Printing Office, 1968.
2. Withington, R. L., and Hall, L. W.: Snowmobile accidents: a review of injuries sustained in the use of snowmobiles in northern New England during the 1968–69 season. J. Trauma, *10*:760, 1970.
3. Schleuter, C. F.: Some economic dimensions of traumatic injuries. J. Trauma, *10*:915, 1970.
4. Spelman, J. W., Bordner, K. R., and Howard, J. M.: Traffic fatalities in Philadelphia. J. Trauma, *10*:885, 1970.
5. Waller, J. A.: Control of accidents in rural areas. J.A.M.A., *201*:176, 1967.
6. Baker, G. L.: Design and operation of a van for the transport of sick infants. Amer. J. Dis. Child., *118*:743, 1968.
7. Randolph, J. G.: Technique for insertion of a plastic catheter into the saphenous vein. Pediatrics, *24*:631, 1959.
8. Cohn, J. H.: Blood pressure measurement in shock. Mechanism of inaccuracy in auscultatory and palpatory methods. J.A.M.A., *199*:118, 1967.
9. Kazamias, T. M., Gander, M. P., Franklin, D. L., and Ross, J., Jr.: Blood pressure measurement with Doppler ultrasonic flowmeter. J. Appl. Physiol., *30*:585, 1971.
10. Kemmerer, W. T., Ware, R. W., Stegall, H. F., Morgan, J. L., and Kirby, R.: Blood pressure measurement by Doppler ultrasonic detection of arterial wall motion. Surg. Gynec. Obstet., *131*:1141, 1970.
11. Contis, G., and Lind, J.: Study of systolic blood pressure, heart rates, and body temperature of normal newborn infants through the first week of life. Acta Paediat. Suppl., *146*:41, 1963.
12. Wilson, J. N., Grow, J. B., Demong, C. V., Prevedel, A. E., and Owens, J. C.: Central venous pressure in optimal blood volume maintenance. Arch. Surg., *85*:563, 1962.
13. Forrester, J. S., Diamond, G., McHugh, T. J., and Swan, H. J. C.: Filling pressures in the right and left sides of the heart in acute myocardial infarction. A reappraisal of central-venous-pressure monitoring. New Eng. J. Med., *285*:190, 1971.
14. Liebert, P. S.: Central venous catheters in children—their placement and care. Clin. Pediat., *10*:218, 1971.
15. Talbert, J. L., and Haller, J. A., Jr.: The optimal site for central venous pressure measurements in newborn infants. J. Surg. Res., *6*:168, 1966.
16. Arcilla, R. A., Oh, W., Lind, J., and Blankenship, W.: Portal and atrial pressures in the newborn period. Acta Paediat. Scand., *55*:615, 1966.
17. Henzel, J. H., and DeWeese, M. S.: Morbid and mortal complications associated with prolonged central venous cannulation. Awareness, recognition and prevention. Amer. J. Surg., *121*:600, 1971.
18. Fitts, C. T., Barnett, L. T., Webb, C. M., Sexton, J., and Yarbrough, D. R., III: Perforating wounds of the heart caused by central venous catheters. J. Trauma, *10*:764, 1970.
19. Moran, J. M., Atwood, R. P., and Rowe, M. I.: A clinical and bacteriologic study of infections associated with venous cutdowns. New Eng. J. Med., *272*:554, 1965.
20. Blalock, A.: Principles of Surgical Care, Shock and Other Problems. St. Louis, C. V. Mosby Co, 1940, p. 158.
21. Moss, G. S., Proctor, H. J., Homer, L. D., Herman, C. M., and Litt, B. D.: A comparison of asanguineous fluids and whole blood in the treatment of hemorrhagic shock. Surg. Gynec. Obstet., *129*:1247, 1969.

22. Rush, B., and Eiseman, B.: Limits of non-colloid solution replacement in experimental hemorrhagic shock. Ann. Surg., *165*:977, 1967.
23. Replogle, R. L., and Merrill, E. W.: Hemodilution: rheologic hemodynamic and metabolic consequences in shock. Surg. Forum, *18*:157, 1967.
24. Takaori, M., and Safar, P.: Treatment of massive hemorrhage with colloid and crystalloid solutions. Studies in dogs. J.A.M.A., *199*:297, 1967.
25. Replogle, R. L., Kundler, H., and Gross, R. E.: Studies on the hemodynamic importance of blood viscosity. J. Thor. Cardiovasc. Surg., *50*:658, 1965.
26. Replogle, R. L., Meiselman, H. J., and Merrill, E. W.: Clinical implications of blood rheology studies. Circulation, *36*:148, 1967.
27. Jacobeus, U.: Studies on the effect of dextran on the coagulation of the blood. Acta Med. Scand., *157* (Suppl. 322): 1957.
28. Replogle, R. L.: Hemodynamic compensation of acute changes of the hemoglobin concentration. *In* Hemodilution: Theoretical Basis and Clinical Application. K. Messmer and H. Schmid-Schonbein, editors. Basel, S. Karger (in press).
29. Barnes, A., Jr., and Allen, T. E.: Transfusions subsequent to administration of universal donor blood in Vietnam. J.A.M.A., *204*:147, 1968.
30. Howland, W. S., Schweitzer, O., and Boyan, C. P.: Massive blood replacement without calcium administration. Surg. Gynec. Obstet., *118*:814, 1964.
31. Miller, R. D., Tong, M. J., and Robbins, T. O.: Effects of massive transfusion of blood on acid-base balance. J.A.M.A., *216*:1762, 1971.
32. Sugerman, J. J., Davidson, D. T., Vibul, S., Delivoria-Papadopoulos, M., Miller, L. D., and Oski, F. A.: The basis of defective oxygen delivery from stored blood. Surg. Gynec. Obstet., *131*:733, 1970.
33. Dawson, R. B., Edinger, M. C., Ellis, T. J.: Hemoglobin function in stored blood. IV. Red cell adenosine triphosphate and 2,3-diphosphoglycerate in acid-citrate dextrose and citrate-phosphate-dextrose with adenine and inosine. J. Lab. Clin. Med., *77*:46, 1971.
34. Boyan, C. P., and Howland, W. S.: Cardiac arrest and temperature of bank blood. J.A.M.A., *183*:58, 1963.
35. Shires, G. T., and Jones, R. C.: Initial management of the severely injured patient. J.A.M.A., *213*:1872, 1970.
36. Yurko, A. A., and Williams, R. D.: Needle paracentesis in blunt abdominal trauma: A critical analysis. J. Trauma, *6*:194, 1966.
37. Virgilio, R. W.: Intrathoracic wounds in battle casualties. Surg. Gynec. Obstet., *130*:609, 1970.
38. Haddad, G. H., Pizzi, W. F., Fleischmann, E. P., and Moynahan, J. M.: Abdominal signs and sinograms as dependable criteria for the selective management of the abdomen. Ann. Surg., *172*:61, 1970.
39. Nance, F. C., and Cohn, I.: Surgical judgement in the management of stab wounds of the abdomen: A retrospective and prospective analysis based on a study of 600 stabbed patients. Ann. Surg., *170*:569, 1969.
40. Wilder, J. R., Haberman, E. T., and Schachner, S. J.: Selective surgical intervention for stab wounds of the abdomen. Surgery, *61*:231, 1967.
41. Steichen, F. M., Efron, G., Pearlman, D. M., and Weil, P. H.: Radiographic diagnosis versus selective management in penetrating wounds of the abdomen. Ann. Surg., *170*:978, 1969.
42. Fitchett, V. H., Pomerantz, M., Butsch, D. W., Simon, R., and Eiseman, B.: Penetrating wounds of the neck. A military and civilian experience. Arch. Surg., *99*:307, 1969.
43. Slate, R. W., Getzen, L. C., and Laning, R. C.: One hundred cases of traumatic rupture of the spleen. Arch. Surg., *99*:498, 1969.
44. Redman, H. C., Reuter, S. R., and Bookstein, J. J.: Angiography in abdominal trauma. Ann. Surg., *169*:57, 1969.
45. Hendrick, E. B., Harwood-Hash, D. C. F., and Hudson, A. R.: Head injuries in children: A survey of 4465 consecutive cases at the Hospital for Sick Children, Toronto, Canada. Clin. Neurosurg., *11*:46, 1964.
46. Darby, T. D., Aldinger, E. E., Gradsden, R. H., and Thrower, W. B.: Effects of metabolic acidosis on ventricular isometric systolic tension and the response to epinephrine and levarterenol. Circ. Res., *8*:1242, 1960.
47. Darby, T. D., and Watts, D. T.: Acidosis and blood epinephrine levels in hemorrhagic hypotension. Am. J. Physiol., *206*:1281, 1964.

48. Andersen, M. N., Border, J. R., and Mouritzen, C. V.: Acidosis, catecholamines and cardiovascular dynamics: When does acidosis require correction? Ann. Surg., 166:344, 1967.
49. Rowe, M. I., and Arango, A.: The role of buffering, osmolality and sodium in neonatal hemorrhagic shock. Surg. Forum, 21:34, 1970.
50. Gerst, P. H., Fleming, W. H., and Malm, J. R.: Increased susceptibility of the heart to ventricular fibrillation during metabolic acidosis. Circ. Res., 19:63, 1966.
51. Moran, N. C.: Evaluation of the pharmacologic basis for the therapy of circulatory shock. Amer. J. Cardiol., 26:570, 1970.
52. MacCannell, K. L., McNay, J. L., Meyer, M. B., and Goldberg, L. I.: Dopamine in the treatment of hypotension and shock. New Eng. J. Med., 275:1389, 1966.
53. Udhoji, V. N., and Weil, M. H.: Circulatory effects of angiotensin, levarterenol and metaraminol in the treatment of shock. New Eng. J. Med., 270:501, 1964.
54. Lillehei, R. C.: Longerbeam, J. K., Bloch, J. H., and Manax, W. G.: Nature of irreversible shock: Experimental and clinical observations. Ann. Surg., 160:682, 1964.
55. Sambhi, M. P., Weil, M. H., and Udhoji, V. N.: Acute pharmacological effects of glucocorticoids. Circulation, 31:523, 1965.
56. Replogle, R. L., Kundler, H., Schottenfeld, M., and Spear, S.: Hemodynamic effects of dexamethasone in experimental hemorrhagic shock — negative results. Ann. Surg., 174:126, 1971.
57. Janoff, A.: Alterations in lysosomes (intracellular enzymes) during shock; Effects of preconditioning (tolerance) and protective drugs. In Shock, edited by S. G. Hershey. Boston, Little Brown and Company, 1964, p. 93.
58. Stremple, J. F., Ellison, E. H., and Carey, L. C.: Osmolar diuresis: success and/or failure. A collective review. Surgery, 60:924, 1966.
59. Stone, A. M., and Stahl, W. M.: Effect of ethacrynic acid and furosemide on renal function in hypovolemia. Ann. Surg., 174:1, 1971.
60. Merrill, J. P.: Acute renal failure. J.A.M.A., 211:289, 1970.
61. Brücke, K.: Temperature regulation in the newborn infant. Biol. Neonat., 3:65, 1961.
62. Rowe, M. I., and Arcilla, R. A.: Body temperature and the neonatal response to hemorrhage. Ann. Surg., 172:76, 1970.
63. Wallgren, G., Barr, M., and Rudhe, U.: Hemodynamic studies of induced hypo- and hypervolemia in the newborn infant. Acta Paediat., 53:1, 1964.
64. Rowe, M. I., and Arcilla, R. A.: Hemodynamic adaptation of the newborn to hemorrhage. J. Pediat. Surg., 3:278, 1968.
65. Kravath, R. E., Aharan, A. S., Abal, G., and Finberg, L.: Clinically significant physiologic changes from rapidly administered hypertonic solutions: Acute osmol poisoning. Pediatrics, 40:267, 1970.
66. Camarata, S. J., Weil, M. H., Hanashiro, P. K., and Shubin, H.: Cardiac arrest in the critically ill. 1. A study of predisposing causes in 132 patients. Circulation, 44:688, 1971.
67. Joly, H. R., and Weil, M. H.: Temperature of the toe as an indication of the severity of shock. Circulation, 39:131, 1969.

2

Endotoxin Shock

Horace L. Hodes, M.D.

For practical purposes we may consider that endotoxins of gram-negative bacteria are the cause of endotoxic shock. In general, endotoxins are produced by bacteria which form smooth colonies. However, it should be mentioned that small quantities of endotoxin have been found in colonially rough, gram-negative rods and in some gram-positive bacteria.

Endotoxins are found in the outer layers of the bacterial cell wall. They are so closely associated with other constituents of this structure that their isolation requires strong chemical treatment.[1] Endotoxins are macromolecules which readily form complexes with each other and with other macromolecules. The two major constituents of endotoxins are lipids and polysaccharides. Endotoxins also contain a small percentage of peptides, so we may consider that endotoxins are lipid-polysaccharide-peptide macromolecules. All endotoxins contain phosphorus also. The polysaccharide moiety is composed of a number of different carbohydrates, such as glucose, galactose, and mannose, as well as pentoses, heptoses, and hexosamines.[2] Also present are di-deoxy hexoses, which are found only in endotoxins.

The lipid moiety contains even-numbered saturated and unsaturated fatty acids. The chemical constituents of endotoxins are arranged

From the Department of Pediatrics, The Mount Sinai School of Medicine of the City University of New York, New York.

in three major zones in the macromolecule: the polysaccharide, the lipid-rich, and the amino acid-rich moieties. The backbone of the molecule is polysaccharide, to which are attached amino acids. The fatty acids are also attached to the carbohydrate backbone; these are ester bound to OH groups or amide bound to NH_2 groups of the carbohydrate, probably through such compounds as glucosamine.[2] The endotoxin molecule is unique in its fatty acid-carbohydrate linkages, which have not been found in any other natural substance.[3] Phosphoric acid is found in both the lipid and carbohydrate moieties.

Endotoxins elicit, directly or indirectly, a large number of reactions affecting many organ systems of the host. It seems very likely that most of these toxic reactions are caused by the presence of the lipid moiety, particularly the long chain fatty acids. Rough mutant, gram-negative bacteria (which contain no polysaccharide moiety) have been shown to contain endotoxins which have full endotoxic action. The polysaccharide moiety probably corresponds to the O antigen of the gram-negative bacilli. This portion of the macromolecule determines the serologic specificity of the organism. The peptide moiety appears to have little, if any, endotoxic activity, since removal of this portion of the molecule does not decrease its endotoxic potency.

Although endotoxins have a basic general structure, it should be noted that there is no single type of endotoxin molecule. Several fully active, chemically different molecular complexes may be found in endotoxins prepared from one bacterial culture.[4] Whether or not these different molecules act in exactly the same manner is not known. The greater the heterogeneity of the endotoxin preparation, the greater is its toxicity. It is probable that a number of organs and more than one kind of organelle may be targets for endotoxin. Different endotoxin molecules may injure different cells or different subcellular elements simultaneously, or they may act in sequence. If the latter is the case, a chain reaction might result.[3]

Endotoxin is found soon after its injection into animals in the cells of the reticuloendothelial system. About 90 per cent of the endotoxin appears in the liver and spleen, but endotoxin also accumulates in the endothelium of blood vessels and in the alveoli of the lungs.[5] Endotoxin is adsorbed to the surface of polymorphonuclear leukocytes (or it is actually present in the cytoplasm of these cells) within 10 minutes after it has been injected intravenously.[6] Endotoxin quickly becomes adsorbed to platelets but not to erythrocytes.

BIOLOGIC EFFECTS OF ENDOTOXINS

Endotoxins elicit many of the reactions which we sum up in the term inflammation. These include local vasodilatation, increased vascular permeability which permits plasma and leukocytes to leave the capillaries, enhanced phagocytosis, and stimulation of host resistance. However, many of the reactions caused by endotoxins are not related to inflammation. These include the following:

1. Mobilization of interferon by endotoxin.
2. Induction of local and generalized Shwartzman reactions.
3. Endotoxin, by a number of mechanisms, causes alterations in the systemic blood pressure which may lead to fatal shock. These actions include the release of kallikreins from leukocytes with the consequent production of kinins, the alteration of the action of epinephrine and norepinephrine on blood vessels, and the release of histamine from mast cells.
4. Endotoxin causes a biphasic febrile reaction; the second peak is probably due to release of an "endogenous pyrogen" from leukocytes.
5. Endotoxin induces leukopenia followed by leukocytosis.
6. Endotoxin causes a fall in number of circulating platelets.
7. Endotoxin causes injury to endothelium of blood vessels.
8. Endotoxin may cause widespread intravascular clotting, with fibrin formation. In this condition there occurs a decrease in circulating platelets, prothrombin, fibrinogen, and intrinsic clotting factors V and VIII. Intravascular clotting may be initiated by activation of Hageman factor (XII) by endotoxin injury of endothelium of blood vessels.
9. Endotoxin causes deleterious changes in carbohydrate and protein metabolism.
10. Endotoxin causes hemorrhagic necrosis in tumors, probably by injury to blood vessels.
11. Mice are protected from a lethal dose of radiation by preceding injection of endotoxin.

It is clear from the very extensive literature on the subject that endotoxins are directly responsible for the shock which occurs during the course of infection with gram-negative bacteria. Changes in the cardiovascular system due in part at least to altered response of the blood vessels to vasoactive substances play an important part in the fatalities which occur in such infections. In addition, extensive intravascular clotting is obvious in some instances, and it is quite possible that some degree of intravascular clotting occurs in all instances. It is also certain that deleterious changes in metabolism occur in many instances, and there is evidence that these alterations are accompanied by cell and organelle injury.

EFFECTS OF ENDOTOXIN ON CARDIOVASCULAR SYSTEM

We shall consider first the circulatory changes which are induced by endotoxin. Some confusion has resulted from the fact that endotoxin affects the circulatory system somewhat differently in different animal species. For example, endotoxin brings about the pooling of a large volume of blood in the portal system of the dog, but this does not occur in the monkey.[7] Another factor which has produced conflicting data is the use of anesthesia in some experiments and not in others. This variance may be due to the fact that anesthetics alter the normal circulatory reflexes and may alter the effects of endotoxin. Also, the sequence of the events observed is dependent on the dose of endotoxin used. Finally, the circulatory changes which occur early in the course of endotoxic poisoning may be different from those which are observed later.

It is clear from experiments conducted on unanesthetized rhesus monkeys that the initial response to endotoxin is a decrease in systemic blood pressure which is due to a decrease in peripheral arterial resistance. The decrease in arterial resistance is accompanied by an increase in venous tone. Arterial resistance is decreased in all organs except the spleen, indicating that the microcirculation in the monkey does not undergo selective constriction on exposure to endotoxin. This suggests that the entire microcirculation is involved in potential pooling of blood in the early phase of shock.[8]

Coincident with the peripheral vascular changes, an increase in heart rate and a decrease in cardiac output occur. The decrease in cardiac output reverts in 2 to 3 hours to normal or rises to above normal values.

Wilson and his colleagues have presented evidence which suggests that the early phase of shock in patients with bacteremia caused by gram-negative organisms is very similar to that seen in endotoxin shock in the rhesus monkey.[9]

Presence of Kinins

It has been shown that the early phase cardiovascular changes induced by endotoxin in monkeys are accompanied or slightly preceded by the appearance of kinins in the plasma.[10] Recent findings support the belief that kinins may have an essential role in the early phase of endotoxin shock. These include the observation that infusion of kinins in man is followed by all the changes seen in the early phase of endotoxin shock.[11] The fall in blood pressure observed in the early phase of endotoxin shock is due almost entirely to a decrease in peripheral vascular resistance. Kinins are the most potent endogenous vasodilating agents known. The concentration of kinins in the plasma of monkeys injected with endotoxin is sufficient to cause the vasodilation and fall in blood pressure observed in them.

Nies and his co-workers[10] made serial measurements of plasma kinin concentration in the early phase of endotoxin shock in the unanesthetized monkey. Kinin concentration rose from the normal state, in which no kinin is detectable, to concentrations which were as high as 29 ng/ml. The kinins appeared in less than 15 minutes after intravenous infusion of endotoxin was begun (the infusion was conducted over a period of 40 minutes). The appearance of kinins in the plasma preceded or coincided with the beginning of the fall in blood pressure and the decreased peripheral resistance which were observed. The peak concentration of plasma kinin was reached in 1 to 2 hours, and it returned to undetectable levels in the monkeys which survived the dose of endotoxin. Plasma kinin concentration remained slightly elevated for 24 hours in the monkeys which did not survive. As might be expected, plasma concentration of kininogen (the globulin precursor of kinin) fell as the kinin level rose, and returned toward normal values as kinin disappeared from the plasma. Kinins have a short survival time in plasma; they have a half life of about 30 seconds. They are destroyed by a kininase (carboxypeptidase-N). In the experiments of Nies et al.[10] described here, kininase remained elevated for at least 24 hours in the monkeys killed by the endotoxin, but very little rise was seen in animals which survived.

In the later (second) phase of endotoxin shock in the unanesthetized monkey, peripheral resistance is elevated rather than greatly reduced, as it is in the first phase.

Also, unlike the earlier phase, cardiac output is decreased in the second phase of shock. Kinin concentration is not elevated in the second phase. Therefore, other vasoactive substances must be involved in the later stages of endotoxin shock. It is probable that epinephrine and norepinephrine are involved in the later stages of shock, while it is clear that kinins and possibly histamine play a key role in the cardiovascular changes in the early phase.[12] Kinins have been shown to have a number of interesting interrelationships with epinephrine, norepinephrine, and histamine, which we shall describe later in this discussion. It is possible that the effect of kinins in the first phase of endotoxin shock determines the occurrence and severity of the later stages of shock.[10] For this reason, a brief discussion of kinins may be useful.

Characteristics of Kinins

Kinins are linear polypeptides, having from nine to 11 amino acids and molecular weight a little over 1000. The two best studied kinins are bradykinin, which is made up of nine peptides, and kallidin, which has the same nine amino acids in the same order as bradykinin, as well as a tenth amino acid-lysine. The structure of these two kinins is shown in Figure 1.

```
          Arg-Pro-Pro-Gly-Phe-Ser-Pro-Phe-Arg
(N-terminal)                                          Bradykinin
                                     (C-terminal)

          Lys-Arg-Pro-Gly-Phe-Ser-Pro-Phe-Arg        Kallidin
```

Figure 1.

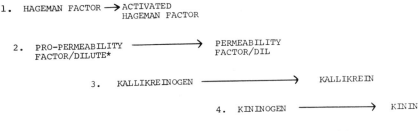

1. HAGEMAN FACTOR ⟶ ACTIVATED
                         HAGEMAN FACTOR

2. PRO-PERMEABILITY   ⟶   PERMEABILITY
   FACTOR/DILUTE*   FACTOR/DIL

3. KALLIKREINOGEN   ⟶   KALLIKREIN

4. KININOGEN   ⟶   KININ

* Permeability factor/dilute is a protein found in serum which causes
increased vascular permeability at site of injection into the skin.

Figure 2.

The precursor of kinins are kininogens, which are alpha-2-globulins present in plasma. Kinins are split from kininogens by the action of enzymes called kallikreins, which are present in an inactive form (kallikreinogens) in the plasma, in urine, and in the exocrine glands. Kallikrein, or an activator of kallikreinogen, is present in granulocytes also. One of the biochemical pathways which has been proposed for the *in vivo* generation of kinin is the sequence of interdependent reactions, with the product of each one activating the subsequent reaction,[12] shown in Figure 2.

Hageman factor may be activated as a consequence of injury to vascular endothelium. The sequence of reactions outlined here may be set off by the injury endotoxin causes to endothelial cells of blood vessels. Furthermore, there is no doubt that kinins are produced by the action of endotoxin on granulocytes.[10, 13] This is probably brought about by the release of kallikrein (or a kallikrein activator), which is present in granulocytes.

Kinins in nanogram quantities cause vasodilatation of the arterioles of the systemic circulation, including cerebral and coronary vessels. They very probably, at least in part, cause the systemic vascular dilatation and the fall in blood pressure which occurs in the early phase of endotoxin shock. However, kinins are not found in the plasma for more than a few hours. They are not detectable in the plasma in the later stages of shock when there is an increase in peripheral resistance, decreased venous return to the heart, and greatly decreased cardiac output.

Vasoactive Agents: Epinephrine, Norepinephrine, and Histamine

Kinins may play an indirect part in the later phases of shock by setting in motion chemical changes which lead to the formation of other potent vasoactive agents. These include epinephrine, norepinephrine, and histamine. It is very probable that the first two compounds play a very important role in the vascular changes of endotoxin shock; the importance of histamine is not clear. Large doses of kinins release catecholamines by direct action on the medulla of the adrenal.

A reciprocal relationship between catecholamines and kinins is suggested by the fact that norepinephrine and epinephrine have been shown to cause the formation of kallikrein from tissues. Norepinephrine causes the excretion of kallikrein from salivary glands, and epinephrine infusion of carcinoid tumors also brings about the production of kallikrein. Conversely, epinephrine enhances the action of kininase, thus increasing the destruction of kinin. It is possible that this is one mechanism which serves to control the plasma kinin production.[12, 14, 15]

It is of interest also that kinins cause the release of histamine from mast cells. It has been shown by Hinshaw, Jordan, and Vick[14] that histamine rises in the blood of monkeys given endotoxin. This rise accompanies the fall of blood pressure in the early stage of shock, beginning within 30 minutes after the injection of the endotoxin. In fatally poisoned monkeys, histamine remains in higher than normal concentration in the plasma for at least 10 hours. There is no direct proof that the serum histamine rise is brought about by the action of kinins, but this possibility cannot be excluded. That interactions exist between kinins and the vasoactive amines (histamine, epinephrine, norepinephrine, serotonin) has been well established by experiments on man and laboratory animals. These relationships are shown in Figure 3, which is modified from a paper by Melmon and Cline.[15]

It is probable that all these compounds play a part in the circulatory changes which are induced by endotoxin. Present knowledge indicates that kinins, epinephrine, and norepinephrine may be of more importance than histamine or serotonin.

It has shown by Thomas[16] in 1956 that epinephrine caused hemorrhagic necrosis of the skin in rabbits which had previously been given an intravenous injection of endotoxin. Mixtures of epinephrine and endotoxin injected into the skin caused similar lesions. These observations led to the examination of the possibility that some of the harmful effects of endotoxin might be due to the fact that it altered the reaction of peripheral blood vessels to epinephrine and norepinephrine. Zweifach, Nagler, and Thomas[17] demonstrated that endotoxin does change the normal vasoconstricting action of epinephrine on blood vessels. Small doses of endotoxin cause epinephrine to exert a greatly increased degree of vasoconstriction. In the presence of endotoxin, prolonged and intense

Figure 3.

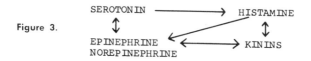

vasoconstriction is caused by a quantity of epinephrine which will normally have no effect on blood vessels. A large dose of endotoxin produces a reversal of this effect. With large doses of endotoxin, blood vessels fail to constrict, or actually dilate when they are exposed to epinephrine. Similar results were obtained with norepinephrine.

Zweifach and his co-workers[17] showed that, in the rat, application of threshold doses of epinephrine (0.2 to 0.4 nanogram per milliliter) induced transient constriction of terminal arterioles and capillaries, with brief stoppage of capillary blood flow. After 10 to 20 seconds the blood vessels resumed their normal caliber, and blood flow became normal. When endotoxin was given intravenously in small sublethal doses, the application of the same threshold dose of epinephrine caused intense, widespread constriction of arteries, arterioles, venules, and small veins and complete ischemia of the capillary bed. The venules and veins proved to be more reactive to the combination of endotoxin and epinephrine than were the terminal arterioles. The venous outflow from the capillary bed was completely stopped by quantities of epinephrine which had no effect on the arterioles.

When larger (lethal) doses of endotoxin were given, terminal arterioles and venules became totally unresponsive to epinephrine and norepinephrine, while the arteries and veins continued to be hyperreactive to these amines and remained greatly constricted. As a result, blood became pooled in all the distended capillaries and venules, while the arteries and veins were contracted to threadlike diameter. The distension of the capillaries and venules was followed by the appearance of petechiae.

We shall now consider in more detail the hemodynamic effects which the vasoactive compounds bring about. The changes which are observed probably depend upon which of these compounds (or which combination of them) is acting on the circulatory system at a given time. The amount of time which has elapsed after the beginning of exposure to endotoxin is also of great importance. The dose of endotoxin given, the species of animal studied, and the use of anesthesia all have an influence on the data which are obtained. When these factors are taken into account, we find that there is general agreement regarding many of the changes which have been observed following administration of endotoxin.

There is a high degree of agreement among investigators concerning the alterations which occur soon after endotoxin is given to the experimental animal. In the anesthetized dog and the anesthetized and unanesthetized monkey, the injection of endotoxin is very quickly followed by a fall in blood pressure. In the dog this is accompanied by a decrease in responsiveness of the precapillary vessels to vasoconstricting substances and an increase of responsiveness of the postcapillary vessels, which become greatly constricted. There is a marked rise in the total peripheral resistance. Blood becomes pooled in the mesenteric and portal venous systems, and venous return to the heart decreases. Cardiac output decreases, and blood pressure falls. This pooling phenomenon is always observed in dogs.[7]

In the unanesthetized monkey, injection of endotoxin is also followed by a prompt fall in blood pressure. Heart rate increases and cardiac output falls, but these return to normal or even to above normal values within 3 hours.[10] In sharp contrast to the dog, the monkey experiences a fall in total peripheral resistance. This decline is roughly parallel to the decrease in blood pressure. No pooling of blood in portal, splanchnic, or other large areas is found in the unanesthetized monkey.

The decrease in venous return, which probably accounts for the lowering of cardiac output, is believed by some authors[18] to be due to a net increase in the volume of blood in the small veins throughout the circulatory system. This would amount to a uniform pooling of blood, in contrast with the hepatosplanchnic pooling seen in the dog.

As shock progresses in the dog, dilatation of the arterioles and capillaries progresses while constriction of the veins continues. Blood enters the capillary beds in increasing amounts but is unable to leave them because of the venous constriction. Hydrostatic pressure is increased in the capillary beds, forcing fluid and blood cells out of the circulatory system and into the tissues. Circulating blood volume is decreased and perfusion of the organs is diminished. Hemorrhagic necrosis of the viscera occurs, with the intestinal mucosa suffering the most severe damage. Venous return to the heart falls further, causing more marked decrease of cardiac output and blood pressure.[19, 20]

Late in the course of endotoxic shock in the unanesthetized monkey, circulatory changes occur which are different from those encountered soon after endotoxin has been injected. In this second phase, which may begin a short time before death, the total peripheral resistance is somewhat increased and cardiac output is decreased. Even at this point, however, no localized pooling of blood is found in the monkey.[10]

Cardiovascular Effects in Man

In man, endotoxin induces circulatory changes which in many ways resemble those it causes in the unanesthetized monkey. The effects on the human circulation are quite different from those suffered by the dog.

It is apparent that endotoxin causes a decrease in the total peripheral resistance (TPR)* in the septic patient. Wilson and colleagues[9] stud-

---

*TPR is calculated from mean arterial blood pressure (MBP), central venous pressure (CVP), and cardiac output (CO) by the following formula:

$$\text{TPR (dyne-sec/cm}^5) = \frac{\text{MBP (mm Hg)} - \text{CVP (mm Hg)}}{\text{CO (liters/min)}} \times 80.$$

TABLE 1 DISTINCTIONS BETWEEN TYPES OF SHOCK

Findings	Endotoxic Shock	Hypovolemic Shock	Cardiac Shock
Total peripheral resistance	Low	High	High
Cardiac output	Low, normal, high	Low	Low
Central venous pressure	Normal range	Low	High

ied the TPR in 12 patients with septic shock uncomplicated by hypovolemia due to massive blood or fluid loss (hypovolemic shock) or by myocardial infarction (cardiac shock). Eleven of these patients with "pure" septic shock had a TPR which was lower than the normal value of 1000 to 1300 dyne-sec/cm⁵, one patient had a normal value, and none had an elevated TPR. Similar results are reported by others.[21]

The patients with endotoxic shock studied by Wilson and co-workers[9] had central venous pressure recordings in the normal range. This is in very sharp contrast to the findings in dogs.

Cardiac output has been described as showing a steady decline in patients with endotoxic shock.[21] However, Wilson et al.[9] reported that this is not a uniform finding. Three of their patients had a normal cardiac output together with decreased TPR, five had an increased cardiac output, and four had a decreased cardiac output. The cardiac output appeared to be related to survival. Only a small percentage of patients with a cardiac index of 2.0 l/minute/square meter survived. The cardiac index is the cardiac output per square meter of body surface; the normal cardiac index is 2.5 to 3.75 l/minute/square meter.

Wilson et al.[9] showed that endotoxic shock differed from the shock caused by hemorrhage or other large-volume fluid loss (hypovolemic shock) and from the cardiac shock of myocardial infarction. This is summarized in Table 1.

Every physician knows that the distinctions among the three types of shock made here often are not very sharp. In a significant number of patients, shock is caused by combinations of endotoxemia, blood and fluid loss, and cardiac disease. Such patients present clinical findings of great complexity. For example, when hypovolemic and endotoxic factors coexist, TPR may be either elevated (as it is in hypovolemic shock), decreased (as it is in endotoxic shock), or normal. Similarly, when myocardial infarction complicates endotoxemia, TPR may be elevated, cardiac output may be decreased, and central venous pressure may be high.

INTRAVASCULAR COAGULATION

Thrombi have been found in the blood vessels of many organs in animals which have been injected with endotoxin. There are also many well-documented examples of widespread intravascular clotting in patients with sepsis due to gram-negative bacteria, other bacteria, viruses, and rickettsial infections. Perhaps the bacterial infection which most often causes extensive intravascular coagulation is meningococcemia.

It has been demonstrated that endotoxin acts to disturb the intravascular clotting mechanism in a number of ways. Some of these effects we shall consider here. It has been shown by McGrath and Stewart[22] that endotoxin injures the vascular endothelium of rabbits. Within 1 hour after these animals are given one dose of endotoxin intracardially, histologic changes are seen in the endothelium of systemic arteries. The normally elliptical nuclei of the endothelial cells become spindle-shaped and stain irregularly. In some areas the endothelial cell nuclei show vacuolization, and a few red and white blood cells are stuck to the cell surface. Twenty-four hours later the damage is more severe; some of the nuclei are almost unrecognizable. In some parts of the arteries, all cellular structure is destroyed. Clumps of red cells and platelets are adherent to the surface of the injured endothelial cells.

The clear-cut evidence of almost immediate injury of the vascular endothelium is of interest in several ways. First, it is of importance in that it is probable that some injury to the endothelium is necessary for the formation of fibrin clots. Second, it is believed that injury to the endothelium may bring about activation of Hageman factor (coagulation factor XII), which begins the chain of reactions that culminates in the action of thrombin on fibrinogen to form fibrin.

After injection of endotoxin in animals, platelets decrease, probably owing to formation of platelet thrombi. According to Hardaway,[23] intravenous injection of endotoxin into the dog brings about the same widespread intravascular coagulation as does the injection of thrombin. However, thrombin causes clotting by direct action on fibrinogen, while endotoxin does not affect fibrinogen directly. Thrombin removes negatively charged peptides from fibrinogen, and the removal of these repelling charges permits the fibrinogen molecules to aggregate and form a fibrin network. Endotoxin probably starts coagulation by activating Hageman factor. Both agents bring about widespread coagulation in the microcirculation, which causes severe obstruction to blood flow. Hardaway has shown that, within 5 minutes after intravenous injection of endotoxin, the plasma of the dog has undergone a severe decrease in fibrinogen, prothrombin, and coagulation factors V, VII, VIII, IX, X, XI, and XII.

Similar decrease in the components of the intravascular clotting mechanism occurs in man in endotoxemic conditions. Decreases in circulating platelets, coagulation factors V and VIII, prothrombin, and fibrinogen have been demonstrated. Blockage of the circulation may be widespread, causing necrosis of large areas of the skin. Occlusion of vessels large enough to require amputation of extremities may occur.

As soon as fibrin is formed, fibrinolysis begins. This is carried out by a proteolytic enzyme system—the plasminogen-plasmin system. Plasminogen is present in all body fluids, but the highest concentration is in the plasma. Plasminogen is always incorporated into fibrin deposits as they form. Plasminogen activators, which are also present in many body fluids, convert plasminogen to plasmin. Plasmin hydrolyzes fibrin into two large components which are antigenically distinct.

In many instances, soon after intravascular coagulation occurs, plasma fibrinogen is restored to normal or to higher than normal levels, and the platelets in the blood reach or exceed their precoagulation number. However, in some instances fibrinogen and platelets are not restored in proper quantity while fibrinolysis continues, and compounds are formed which interfere with the polymerization of fibrin. In this situation intravascular coagulation may be followed by severe bleeding into the skin, mucous membranes, and internal organs.

EFFECT OF ENDOTOXIN ON METABOLISM

Endotoxin has an adverse effect on carbohydrate and protein metabolism. In addition, animals and patients with endotoxemia are usually in metabolic acidosis. These effects probably are in part the result of cell injury which is secondary to interference with the microcirculation. However, there is reason to believe that endotoxin causes direct injury to cells and cellular organelles. For example, the plasma concentration of the lysosomal enzyme alpha glucosidase rises within 2 hours after the unanesthetized monkey is given an injection of endotoxin.[10] This indicates that the membrane of the lysosome has been injured sufficiently to allow the escape of an enzyme when changes in the microcirculation of the animal are not yet profound.

There is convincing evidence from animal experiments that endotoxin causes derangement of carbohydrate metabolism. It was shown by Berry and co-workers[24] that mice given a large dose of endotoxin suffer severe depletion of blood glucose liver glycogen and total body carbohydrate. Endotoxin prevents the conversion of injected glucose into liver glycogen, but no effect on muscle glycogen is produced.

It has been shown that endotoxin interferes directly or indirectly with essential molecular reactions in carbohydrate metabolism. For example, endotoxin inhibits the oxidative decarboxylation of pyruvate. This was demonstrated in animals given salmonella or meningococcus endotoxins.[25] Pyruvic acid ($CH_3 \cdot CO \cdot COOH$) normally is converted to acetaldehyde by the enzyme carboxylase and the coenzyme cocarboxylase (thiamine pyrophosphate or TPP). Then, by a series of reactions involving lipoic acid, flavin adenine dinucleotide (FAD), nicotinamide adenine dinucleotide (NAD), and coenzyme A (CoA · SH), it is converted to acetyl-coenzyme A. In this form ("active" acetate) it enters the citric acid cycle (Krebs cycle). The conversion of pyruvic acid to ace-

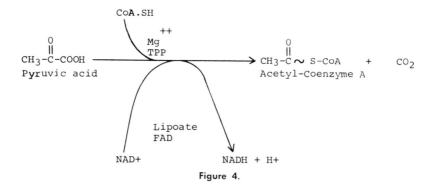

Figure 4.

tyl-coenzyme A may be summarized as shown in Figure 4. Endotoxin blocks this reaction. As a result, no pyruvate enters the Krebs cycle in the form of acetyl-coenzyme A, and further carbohydrate metabolism is greatly diminished. Since pyruvate cannot enter the Krebs cycle to be metabolized to ketoglutarate, it is metabolized to lactic acid to a greater extent than is normal. Lactic acid thus becomes the end product of the glycolytic glucose cycle. Accumulation of lactic acid may contribute to the acidemia seen in endotoxin shock. Furthermore, because of the decreased function of the Krebs cycle, fewer energy molecules pass through the cycle, and production of adenosine triphosphate (ATP) is reduced. Endotoxin may interfere with the pyruvate/acetyl-coenzyme A reaction indirectly – by its effect on the microcirculation, an effect which might injure cell mitochondria. If this is the case, the reaction may be blocked by the breakdown of the cytochrome enzyme system, which normally accomplishes the final step in the removal of the hydrogen produced. Or, endotoxin may interfere with enzymes by directly injuring mitochondria.

There is in fact evidence that endotoxin does damage liver mitochondria. Endotoxin causes a decrease in the oxygen uptake of rat liver mitochondria, and it uncouples oxidative phosphorylation in these organelles.[26]

Endotoxin has also been shown to have effects on protein metabolism. It inhibits the induction of the enzyme tryptophan pyrrolase in liver cells. This enzyme, which is an oxygenase, catalyzes the first step in the metabolism of tryptophan.[27]

There is also evidence that endotoxin interferes with the energy production which is required for cell metabolism. Adenosine triphosphate (ATP) production appears to be decreased in cells of animals poisoned by endotoxin. This effect also would result from injury to mitochondria. Takeda and co-workers[28] reported that mice could be completely protected from the effects of a lethal quantity of salmonella endotoxin by intravenous injection of ATP if a dose of 1 mg per 20 gm of body weight was used.

Schumer and Sperling[29] have recently proposed that we should consider shock as a disorder of the molecules of cells. They believe that the defects in the microcirculation which occur in shock cause damage to cellular function. They imply that the block at the pyruvate/coenzyme A step is due to alteration of cell metabolism, which is caused by the anoxic effect of the decreased microcirculation. Because of this block, lactic acid accumulates. The anaerobic glucose pathway is reversed, with the reaction proceeding from pyruvate to glyceraldehyde to dihydroxyacetone to glucose-6-phosphate. Glucose (which cannot be made into glycogen since endotoxin prevents this process) leaves the cell. Amino acids, which normally enter the glycolytic pathway at the step which produces pyruvate, now leave the cell as the pathway is reversed. A similar course is taken by fatty acids which normally enter the glycolytic cycle at the pyruvate/coenzyme A step. Because of injury to the mitochondria and the decreased activity of the Krebs cycle, less energy and less than the normal amount of ATP is formed. This causes the accumulation of phosphates. Thus, the blockage in anaerobic glucose metabolism leads to the accumulation of lactic acid, phosphates, fatty acids, and amino acids in the plasma, and produces acidemia. With increasing injury to the cell (caused directly by endotoxin or by the microcirculatory deficiency), lysosomal membranes rupture, and phosphatases and hydrolases escape into the plasma.

LABORATORY DIAGNOSIS OF ENDOTOXEMIA

It would be of great assistance to the clinician if there were available a laboratory method for the detection of endotoxin in the blood. A number of such methods have been published, but until recently none has been clinically useful. In 1964, and in subsequent reports, Bang and Levin[30] described a method which may be of clinical value, since it can be performed in any laboratory and gives results within three or four hours. The method is extremely sensitive; it detects as little as 0.1 to 1.0 nanograms of endotoxin per milliliter of serum. As will be shown below, it is probable that even this method has limitations, since it fails to detect endotoxin in every patient with endotoxemia. The method is based on the discovery that there can be obtained from the amebocytes of the horseshoe crab (Limulus polyphemus) a water clear lysate which gels in the presence of very minute quantities of endotoxin. In brief, the method of Bang and Levin is carried out in the following manner:

Blood from patients is collected in endotoxin-free glassware containing 5000 units of heparin. The plasma is separated by centrifugation and 0.1 ml of it is added to 0.1 ml of the amebocyte lysate. The mixtures are kept at 37°C for 1 hour and then read for gel formation. The degree of gelation is compared to that which is produced by known quantities of endotoxin.

There is a globulin substance in serum which binds endotoxin. If all the endotoxin in a serum is bound by this globulin, the test described above will be negative. Treatment with chloroform releases the endotoxin from the globulin, enabling one to determine the presence of bound endotoxin also. Specimens of plasma which are negative when tested directly with limulus lysate may be shown to be positive when the chloroform extract is tested. For this reason we perform the limulus test with untreated plasma and with a chloroform extract of plasma.

Recently Levin has recorded his experience with the limulus test. Levin and co-workers[31] performed the limulus test on the plasma of 98 patients suspected of having bacteremia due to gram-negative bacteria. Seventeen of these patients had endotoxemia as determined by the limulus test. Twelve of these patients had gram-negative rod bacteremia. In contrast, 77 normal controls and 27 patients with pneumococcal pneumonia or with pneumococcal, streptococcal or staphylococcal bacteremia all gave a negative test for endotoxemia. Levin's results indicate that the limulus test is not invariably positive in gram-negative bacterial infections. Three of his patients who had enterobacter bacteremia gave a negative test.

We have used the limulus test in a number of patients with gram-negative rod infections. Our results, in general, agree with those of Levin. Also, we have recently had the opportunity to test the blood of one infant with meningococcus septicemia and meningitis and one baby with *H. influenzae* septicemia and meningitis. The plasma of both these infants gave a strongly positive limulus test for endotoxin. On the other hand, no endotoxin was detected in the cerebrospinal fluid of either child.

We have stated previously that there is a globulin in normal human plasma which binds endotoxin. This binding is probably the first step in the degradation and detoxification of endotoxin. In studying this globulin, Ainbender[32] in our laboratory has found that the blood of the newborn infant contains only one tenth of the concentration of the endotoxin-binding globulin as that which is present in the blood of his mother.

Although more extensive study of the limulus test is needed, it now seems likely that this method will have clinical usefulness in the treatment of patients with endotoxemia. We believe that treatment of patients with endotoxin shock can be successful only if treatment is begun early. If we are able to determine in a patient who shows no clinical evidence of shock that endotoxemia is present, we might be able to begin anti-shock treatment earlier than it is possible for us to do at the present time.

TREATMENT OF ENDOTOXIN SHOCK

There is little doubt that, if endotoxin shock is permitted to go untreated for a long period, its effects may become irreversible. The best chance for successful treatment is present at the onset of shock. It is of the utmost importance that careful and continuous observation be afforded the patient who is suffering from an infection which may induce endotoxin shock. Such infections include meningococcemia and neonatal sepsis, which is very often caused by gram-negative enteric bacilli. Children with leukemia, lymphoma, and other malignant diseases who are suffering from any bacterial infection are liable to go into shock. Such patients also require special attention.

At the onset of endotoxin shock, there may be changes in the patient's mental state. There may be a loss of alertness or even brief lapses into a torpid or semistuporous state. Often, with the onset of shock, the pulse rate and respiratory rate rise abruptly. The blood pressure should be recorded at regular intervals, since it may drop precipitously. A fall in diastolic pressure may precede a systolic drop. It is our practice to record the blood pressure every hour during the first 8 hours after beginning treatment of patients with meningococcic meningitis; after this period blood pressure is taken every 3 hours for the next 24 hours.

Endotoxin shock is a multiple system disease which exerts a harmful effect on the circulation, on many organs, and on a number of metabolic processes of the patient. These deleterious effects vary with the amount of endotoxemia and with duration of the exposure to the toxin. Furthermore, patients with septic shock are often suffering from other conditions, such as coronary artery disease, malignancy, and surgical trauma. These conditions often complicate or obscure the symptoms caused by endotoxic poisoning. It is not surprising, therefore, that no single drug and no prearranged protocol will be useful for the treatment of all patients with endotoxic shock. Every patient must be treated individually, with careful consideration of all the clinical findings and of all the available laboratory data. In many instances decisions about treatment must be made almost entirely on clinical grounds. The patient may be too sick to undergo laboratory studies, or his condition may be too grave to permit the physician to wait for the results of laboratory studies before he begins therapy. Therapy should be altered promptly if laboratory data provide information which shows that such a change is needed.

With these reservations, we may outline certain principles of treatment which we believe may be useful.

1. Start treatment as soon as the diagnosis of endotoxic shock is made. To delay is to jeopardize the patient's life. In the neonate with gram-negative bacterial sepsis or the patient with meningococcemia, the appearance of any of the clinical symptoms of shock described here warrants institution of anti-shock therapy.

2. Restore blood volume. In many instances there is no doubt that hypovolemia is present. This is the case in septic infants with diarrhea and vomiting. Children who have undergone surgical operation and show signs of infection with gram-negative bacteria following this are often hypovolemic. Glucose and electrolyte solutions may be given as ini-

tial therapy, but blood or plasma are usually required to maintain blood volume.

3. Treat with antibiotics the bacterial infection which is the source of endotoxin.

4. Give intravenously a "pharmacologic" dose of hydrocortisone. Thirty-five to 50 mg per kilogram of body weight is recommended. This may be given in a 10-minute period. It may be repeated at 30- to 60-minute intervals for four doses if necessary. Cortisone is recommended because, in the doses recommended here, it exerts many anti-shock effects, which include actions on blood vessels and on molecular reactions. Cortisone acts as an adrenergic blocking agent, relieving the vascular spasm caused by the abnormal action which epinephrine and norepinephrine exert in the presence of endotoxin. Cortisone exerts a favorable action on carbohydrate metabolism. It counteracts the depletion of glycogen which endotoxin causes. It decreases lactic acid formation by stimulating the pathways which lead to the eventual conversion of lactic acid into glycogen. Cortisone induces the entrance of amino acids into the pyruvate cycle and the entrance of fat into the Krebs cycle; both these actions favor production of ATP.[29] Cortisone has a protective action on lysosomes, preventing their rupture. Cortisone prevents kallikrein from forming kinin from kininogen. It should be noted that the concentration of corticosteroids in the plasma is not decreased in patients with endotoxemia. In fact, in some instances, the corticosteroid level is somewhat elevated. The effects of cortisone described here are obtained only with very large, "pharmacologic" doses of cortisone, which raise the plasma level far above those normally found.

It should be noted that the published data indicate that there is no need for "replacement" therapy with adrenal corticosteroids. The concentration of these steroids in the blood may be normal, high, or low in patients with endotoxin shock. Furthermore, several controlled series in which corticosteroids have been used in "physiologic" dosage have given negative results.

There is no controlled series which proves the value of "pharmacologic" doses of corticosteroids in endotoxin shock. However, the results of animal experiments, and the proved favorable effects of large doses of cortisone in reversing some of the effects of endotoxin warrant its clinical use. A controlled, large-scale study of this problem is urgently needed.

Many authors have advised against the use of cortisone in the presence of endotoxin-producing bateria. This recommendation is based on the fear that a generalized Shwartzman reaction might occur if cortisone is used in these circumstances. In fact, in 1952 Thomas and Good[33] reported that a single injection of endotoxin in cortisone-treated rabbits produced a generalized Shwartzman reaction. However, more recently (in 1967), Corrigan and co-workers[34] were unable to produce a Shwartzman reaction with endotoxin in cortisone-treated rabbits, even when they used extremely large doses of cortisone and endotoxin. We do not believe there is convincing evidence that a generalized Shwartzman reaction has been evoked in endotoxemic patients treated with cortisone. We have never observed such a reaction, although we have used cortisone in the treatment of endotoxic shock since 1952.[35]

5. Vasodilators such as isoproterenol and phenoxybenzamine are recommended by some authors. Their value in endotoxin shock is not clearly established. Lillehei[20] was unable to increase the survival of dogs in endotoxin shock by treating them with phenoxybenzamine. Hydrocortisone was much more effective. We believe that the vasodilating effect which can be obtained with phenoxybenzamine and isoproterenol may be more effectively obtained with "pharmacologic" doses of cortisone.

6. Correct the metabolic acidemia if it is present. Many patients in endotoxic shock are in severe acidemia. This should be corrected by administration of bicarbonate.

7. Intravascular coagulation—when it is extensive—should be treated at once with heparin. Heparin should also be used when the clotting threatens the loss of a limb or of toes or fingers. When there is evidence of less severe intravascular clotting—such as scattered petechiae—it seems best at this time to look for laboratory evidence of coagulopathy before using anticoagulation therapy. If such evidence is found in the presence of symptoms of endotoxic shock or impending shock, heparin therapy should be started. For example, if a low platelet count is found, heparin should be administered; the same is true if there is a decreased concentration of plasma fibrinogen. Abildgaard[36] recommends the use of rapidly obtained screening tests, including observation of the whole blood clot, platelet count, fibrinogen concentration by the semiquantitative heat precipitation method, thrombin time, and partial thromboplastin time.

If a decreased value is obtained by these methods, we may assume that intravascular coagulation has occurred. However, the finding of normal values does not exclude the existence of intravascular coagulation, because, after coagulation has occurred, the clotting factors may be rapidly restored. Thus, we often must make a decision which is based on clinical judgment alone.

When heparin is used, it is given intravenously in a dose of 1 mg per kilogram of body weight every 4 hours. The whole-blood clotting time should be kept at 20 to 30 minutes prior to each succeeding dose of heparin.[36] The laboratory screening tests referred to here should be carried out at regular intervals; and, if possible, several more time-consuming laboratory measurements should be made. These include assay of factors V and VIII. Heparin treatment should be continued until coagulation values have returned to normal or until the patient has recovered from the infection which has caused shock.

On occasion, patients under heparin treatment for intravascular clotting may have a hemorrhage from mucous membranes. When this occurs, the action of heparin may be rapidly counteracted by injection of protamine sulfate.

References

1. Carey, W. F., and Baron, L. S.: Comparative immunologic studies of cell structure isolated from *Salmonella typhosa*. J. Immunol., *83*:17, 1959.
2. Nowotny, A. M.: Molecular aspects of endotoxic reactions. Bacteriol. Rev., *33*:72, 1969.
3. Nowotny, A. M.: Chemical structure of a phosphomucolipid and its occurrence in some strains of Salmonella. J. Amer. Chem. Soc., *83*:501, 1961.
4. Nowotny, A. M.: Heterogeneity of endotoxic bacterial lipopolysaccharides revealed by ion-exchange column chromatography. Nature, *210*:278, 1966.
5. Levy, E., Path, F. C., and Ruebner, B. H.: Hepatic changes produced by a single dose of endotoxin in the mouse. Amer. J. Pathol., *51*:269, 1967.
6. Rubenstein, H. S., Fine, J., and Coons, A. H.: Localization of endotoxin in the walls of the peripheral vascular system during lethal endotoxemia. Proc. Soc. Exp. Biol. Med., *3*:458, 1962.
7. Hinshaw, L. B.: *In* Overwhelming Bacterial Infections in Childhood. Report of the Fifty-fifth Ross Conference on Pediatric Research. Columbus, Ohio, Ross Laboratories, 1966, pp. 53–57.
8. Forsyth, R., Nies, A. S., Wyler, F., Neutze, J., and Melmon, K. L.: Endotoxin induced microcirculatory changes in the unanesthetized primate. Clin. Res., *16*:107, 1968.
9. Wilson, R. F., Thal, A. P., Kindling, P. H., Grifka, T., and Ackerman, E.: Hemodynamic measurements in septic shock. Arch. Surg., *91*:121, 1965.
10. Nies, A. S., Forsyth, R. P., Williams, E. H., and Melmon, K. L.: Contribution of kinins to endotoxin shock in unanesthetized rhesus monkeys. Circ. Res., *22*: 155, 1968.
11. Mason, D. T., and Melmon, K. L.: Abnormal forearm vascular responses in the carcinoid syndrome: The role of kinins and kinin-generating system. J. Clin. Invest., *45*:1685, 1966.
12. Kellermeyer, R. W., and Graham, R. C., Jr.: Kinins – possible physiologic and pathologic roles in man. New Eng. J. Med., *279*:754, 1968.
13. Melmon, K. L., and Cline, M. J.: Interaction of plasma kinins and granulocytes. Nature, *213*:90, 1967.
14. Hinshaw, L. B., Jordan, M. M., and Vick, J. A.: Histamine release and endotoxin shock in the primate. J. Clin. Invest., *40*:1631, 1961.
15. Melmon, K. L., and Cline, M. J.: Kinins. Amer. J. Med., *43*:153, 1967.
16. Thomas, L.: The role of epinephrine in the reactions produced by the endotoxins of gram-negative bacteria. J. Exp. Med., *104*:865, 1956.
17. Zweifach, B. W., Nagler, A. L., and Thomas, L.: The role of endotoxin in the reactions produced by the endotoxins of gram-negative bacteria. J. Exp. Med., *104*: 881, 1956.
18. Hinshaw, L. B., Emerson, E. T., Jr., and Reins, D. A.: Cardiovascular responses of the primate in endotoxin shock. Amer. J. Physiol., *210*:335, 1966.
19. Lillehei, R. C., Longerbeam, J. K., Bloch, J. H., and Mannax, W. G.: The nature of irreversible shock. Ann. Surg., *160*:682, 1964.
20. Lillehei, R. C.: *In* Overwhelming Bacterial Infections in Childhood. Report of the Fifty-fifth Ross Conference on Pediatric Research, Columbus, Ohio, Ross Laboratories, 1966, pp. 58–63.
21. Gilbert, R. P.: Mechanisms of the hemodynamic effects of endotoxin. Physiol. Rev., *40*:245, 1960.
22. McGrath, J. M., and Stewart, G. J.: The effects of endotoxin on vascular endothelium. J. Exp. Med., *129*:833, 1969.
23. Hardaway, R. M.: *In* Overwhelming Bacterial Infections in Childhood. Report of the Fifty-fifth Ross Conference on Pediatric Research. Columbus Ohio, Ross Laboratories, 1966, pp. 34–35.
24. Berry, L. J., Smythe, D. S., and Young, L. G.: Effects of bacterial endotoxin on metabolism. I. J. Exp. Med., *110*:389, 1959.

25. Kun, E., and Abood, L. G.: Mechanism of inhibition of glycogen synthesis by endotoxins of Salmonella aertrycke and type 1 meningococcus. Proc. Soc. Exp. Biol. Med., *71*:362, 1949.
26. Mager, J., and Theodor, E.: Inhibition of mitochondrial respiration and uncoupling of oxidative phosphorylation by fractions of the Shigella paradysenteriae type III somatic antigen. Arch. Biochem., *67*:169, 1957.
27. Berry, L. J., and Smythe, D. S.: Effects of bacterial endotoxin on metabolism, VII. J. Exp. Med., *120*:721, 1964.
28. Takeda, Y., Miura, Y., Sazaki, H., and Kasai, N.: The elimination of metabolic disturbances produced by the injection of S. typhi, S. paratyphi B, S. flexneri and the prevention of animals from death through the application of adenosine triphosphate. Jap. J. Exp. Med., *25*:133, 1955.
29. Schumer, W., and Sperling, R.: Shock and its effect on the cell. J.A.M.A., *205*:215, 1968.
30. Levin, J., and Bang, F. B.: The role of endotoxin in the extracellular coagulation of Limulus blood. Bull. Johns Hopkins Hosp., *115*:265, 1964.
31. Levin, J., Poore, T. E., Zauber, N. P., and Oser, R. S.: Detection of endotoxin in the blood of patients with sepsis due to gram-negative bacteria. New Eng. J. Med., *283*:1313, 1970.
32. Ainbender, E.: Unpublished data.
33. Thomas, L., and Good, R. A.: The effect of cortisone on the Shwartzman reaction. J. Exp. Med., *95*:409, 1952.
34. Corrigan, J. J., Abildgaard, C. F., Seeler, R. A., and Schulman, I.: Quantitative aspects of blood coagulation in the generalized Shwartzman reaction. Pediat. Res., *1*:99, 1967.
35. Hodes, H. L., Moloshok, R. E., and Markowitz, M.: Fulminating meningococcemia treated with cortisone. Pediatrics, *10*:138, 1952.
36. Abildgaard, C. F.: Recognition and treatment of intravascular coagulation. J. Pediat., *74*:163, 1969.

3

Acute Adrenal Insufficiency

Alfred M. Bongiovanni, M.D.

Acute adrenal insufficiency in infancy and childhood has several causes. It may be due to primary aplasia of the adrenal gland and may be accompanied by other congenital anomalies such as anencephaly. Hypoplasia of the adrenal with a longer period of survival has also been described.

Bilateral adrenal hemorrhage, usually in the newborn, may be the result of a traumatic delivery. The symptoms occur early and resemble those of overwhelming septicemia. Without immediate recognition and vigorous treatment the condition is fatal. Certainty of such diagnosis in an infant who survives is difficult, although calcification of the adrenal glands may be visible by x-ray in later life.

Temporary hypofunction of the adrenal cortex in early life has also been described and may represent a defect in the biosynthesis of aldosterone. However, the indiscriminate treatment of numerous infants presumed to have this condition, as has been promulgated from time to time, is not endorsed by this writer.

Fulminating infections may be accompanied by acute adrenal insufficiency, as in the Waterhouse-Friderichsen syndrome. The mortality rate is high and postmortem examinations often reveal damage to the

---

From the Department of Pediatrics, School of Medicine, University of Pennsylvania, and Children's Hospital of Philadelphia, Pennsylvania.

adrenal cortex. Although suitable therapy as described herein may be required for adrenal insufficiency per se, there is little to support the notion that empirical employment of large doses of adrenal steroids exerts a beneficial effect in the treatment of a variety of infections.

In about one-fourth of patients with the adrenogenital syndrome (and this incidence varies from clinic to clinic) due to congenital adrenal hyperplasia, the condition is complicated by an electrolyte disturbance attributable to a deficiency of the salt-retaining steroids. Infants affected with this condition fail to thrive and have emesis, dehydration, and shock in the early weeks of life. In contrast to other forms wherein steroid levels in blood and urine are low, there is a rise in urinary 17-ketosteroids as well as other "abnormal" adrenal products.

The sudden withdrawal of adrenal steroids administered for purposes other than primary adrenal disease may be followed by acute adrenal failure. Adrenal crisis may also occur after unilateral adrenalectomy for a tumor causing Cushing's syndrome, since the other gland in such cases is usually atrophic. Finally, acute insufficiency may occur in chronic adrenal disease (Addison's disease) and is often precipitated in this condition by superimposed infection or injury.

TREATMENT

With deficiency of adrenocortical steroidal hormones, there is a loss of extracellular water and sodium into the urine, the intracellular compartment, and possibly bone. There is also loss into the sweat. This leads to extracellular dehydration and hypotension. On the other hand, there is potassium retention. Thus, supplementary potassium in the treatment of this condition is contraindicated unless hypokalemia develops later as a consequence of excessive treatment with adrenal steroids.

The keys to therapy of adrenocortical failure thus include fluid and electrolyte replacement as well as appropriate steroid hormone replacement. Approximately 100 to 120 ml of isotonic saline solution per kilogram of body weight should be administered intravenously within the first 24 hours to children weighing up to 20 kg, and 75 ml per kilogram should be administered when body weight is above 20 kg. These recommendations are based on the special situation applicable to the dehydration of adrenal failure in which extracellular fluid loss predominates. When shock is especially severe, 5 ml of plasma per kilogram of body weight may be substituted, volume for volume, as part of the initial replacement fluid. About 20 to 25 per cent of the total may be given carefully during the first 2 hours. After the first day, maintenance may be continued as half isotonic saline solution in 5 per cent glucose, about one-third to one-half the volume stated here.

When liquids may be taken by mouth, ordinary fluids may be administered as tolerated, with additional sodium chloride, 1 gm per each 10 kg of body weight.

Simultaneously, it is necessary to administer those steroid hormones which are believed to be deficient. This writer strongly urges that the "newer" steroids be avoided, and that cortisone or hydrocortisone always be used in the treatment of acute adrenal insufficiency. Initially, one of the soluble hydrocortisone products, either hemisuccinate or phosphate, should be given intravenously, 1.5 to 2.0 mg per kilogram of body weight. Hydrocortisone phosphate has a longer duration of action, but this is of secondary importance since it is well to administer hydrocortisone (or cortisone acetate) intramuscularly, 2 mg per kilogram, as soon as possible, to be repeated daily for several days. The intramuscular dose is slowly absorbed; the plasma level does not reach its peak for several hours and is then maintained for 24 hours or longer, thus obviating the need for further intravenous steroid. It is also necessary to give one of the salt-retaining steroids, and for this purpose desoxycorticosterone acetate is most often employed intramuscularly in a dose of 2 mg on the first day and 1 mg a day thereafter. This compound restores the electrolyte regulation and diminishes the salt requirements.

Often a vasopressor substance is required. About 25 mg of metaraminol bitartrate may be added to 250 ml of 5 per cent glucose and connected via a Y tube to the system delivering the recommended electrolyte solution. The rate of flow which will support the blood pressure is maintained. In severe adrenal cortical insufficiency, vasopressor drugs may be without effect until after the administration of hydrocortisone. After complete restoration, the steroids may be tapered rapidly in the hospital, by 25 per cent diminution per day, over 4 days. The decision to proceed with such a course depends on the patient's reaction. On the other hand, if chronic adrenocortical insufficiency supervenes, maintenance doses of cortisone (about 20 mg per square meter per day by mouth) and, less often, salt-retaining steroids are required.

Some recommendations are necessary in order to avoid the occurrence of acute adrenal insufficiency in situations well known for their association with this condition. Such situations include the child about to undergo unilateral (or bilateral) adrenalectomy; the child who has been treated for a long time with large doses of steroids and now requires surgery for one reason or another; and the child previously maintained on suitable treatment for chronic adrenocortical insufficiency (including the adrenogenital syndrome), suddenly confronted with the stress of serious illness or injury.

We have advised that some children carry on their person an identification card or tag, which gives, or directs the finder to, instructions in case of sudden need. Under such circumstances adrenal crisis may be averted by the use of cortisone acetate, intramuscularly, 2 mg per kilogram of body weight daily. It is unwise to rely upon continued oral treatment during an emergency and this intramuscular route provides a satisfactory depot for the maintenance of adequate blood levels for 24 hours or longer. In addition 1 mg of desoxycorticosterone acetate in oil may be given daily. Throughout the period of stress the serum electrolytes should be determined daily. Usually within a few days it is possible to return to the previous routine of control.

It is to be recalled that the adrenal steroids exert some of their beneficial influence on the salt-water balance by shifts between the extracellular and intracellular compartments. Thus the sodium requirements must be given careful consideration and excess administration of sodium should be avoided when the adrenal steroids are used, as they should be, concomitantly. Overtreatment may lead to hypertension, edema, cardiac failure, hypernatremia, and hypokalemia with muscle weakness. The child should be observed repeatedly for undue elevation of the blood pressure, pretibial edema, and impending heart failure. The serum electrolytes should be determined daily and frequent electrocardiograms are advisable.

Following the successful management of the acute episode, the commitment of the child with apparent adrenal failure due to unknown causes to indefinite therapy may be unwarranted. As the patient recovers from the crisis, the treatment with steroids should be slowly discontinued and the adrenocortical function carefully evaluated to differentiate between temporary and chronic adrenal deficiency. For example, after unilateral adrenalectomy the contralateral gland, at first atrophic, usually recovers its function and is restored to normal.

SUMMARY

Acute adrenal insufficiency in infancy and childhood must be recognized quickly and treated adequately at once. Both the rapid replacement of fluids and electrolytes and suitable steroid therapy are essential. Because the dehydration is primarily extracellular, isotonic saline is appropriate. Rapid correction is essential and overtreatment must be avoided, particularly when adrenal steroids are employed, since they will counteract the prior loss of sodium and retention of potassium within the extracellular compartment. During recovery the child should be carefully studied in order to determine the rate at which the various therapeutic measures may be withdrawn and in order to distinguish between acute and chronic adrenal insufficiency. The indiscriminate assignment of nonspecific diseases in childhood to the category of acute adrenal insufficiency is decried.

References

1. Bongiovanni, A. M.: Fluid therapy in adrenocortical failure. Pediat. Clin. N. Amer., *11*:971, 1964.
2. Bongiovanni, A. M., and Eberlein, W. R.: Defective steroidal biogenesis in congenital adrenocortical hyperplasia. Pediatrics, *21*:661, 1958.
3. Gardner, L. I.: Review article—adrenocortical metabolism of the fetus, infant and child. Pediatrics, *17*:897, 1956.

4. Geppert, L. J., and Richmond, A. M.: Adrenal insufficiency in infancy. J. Pediat., 37:1, 1950.
5. Hudson, J. B., Chobanian, A. V., and Relman, A. S.: Hypoaldosteronism. New Eng. J. Med., 257:529, 1957.
6. Jaudon, J. C.: Hypofunction of the adrenals in early life. J. Pediat., 29:696, 1946.
7. Jaudon, J. C.: Further observations concerning hypofunctioning of the adrenals during early life. J. Pediat., 32:641, 1948.
8. Kagawa, C. M., Cella, J. A., and Van Arman, C. G.: Action of new steroids in blocking effects of aldosterone and deoxycorticosterone on salt. Science, 126:1015, 1957.
9. Kock, R., and Carson, M. J.: Meningococcal infections in children. New Eng. J. Med., 258:639, 1958.
10. Liddle, G. W.: Sodium diuresis induced by steroidal antagonists of aldosterone. Science, 126:1016, 1957.
11. Migeon, C. J., and Stempfel, R. S., Jr.: Laboratory diagnosis in pediatric endocrinology. Pediat., Clin. N. Amer., 4:959, 1957.
12. Talbot, N. B., Sobel, E. H., McArthur, J. W., and Crawford, J. D.: Functional Endocrinology from Birth through Adolescence. Cambridge, Mass., Harvard University Press, 1952.
13. Thorn, G. W.: The Diagnosis and Treatment of Adrenal Insufficiency. Springfield, Ill., Charles C Thomas, 1951.
14. Ulick, S., Vetter, K. K., Gautier, E., Nicolis, G. L., Markello, J. R., and Lowe, C. U.: An aldosterone biosynthetic defect in a salt-losing disorder of infancy (abstract). J. Clin. Invest., 43:1261, 1964.
15. Wilkins, L.: The Diagnosis and Treatment of Endocrine Disorders in Childhood and Adolescence, 2nd ed. Springfield, Ill., Charles C Thomas, 1957.

4

The Seriously Burned Child

John T. Herrin, M.B.B.S., M.R.A.C.P., and John D. Crawford, M.D.

INCIDENCE AND PREVENTION

Burns are the third most important cause of accidental death in childhood, outranked only by automobile casualties and drownings.[1] In the United States 12,000 deaths occur annually, but over the same period 2,000,000 patients seek medical attention for burns.[2] Among these, a very large number of children must undergo prolonged, painful, and restrictive hospitalization, from which they emerge with scars to both body and personality profoundly affecting their social and emotional development.

The tragedy is that the great majority of burn injuries are preventable.[3, 4, 5, 6, 7] Seventy per cent take place in children under 5 years, generally at times when supervision of activities is minimal. The periods of greatest jeopardy are the early morning hours when parents are still in bed and the interval between the end of school and suppertime. Burns

From the Shriners Hospitals for Crippled Children, Burns Institute, Boston Unit, the Children's Service of the Massachusetts General Hospital, and the Department of Pediatrics, Harvard Medical School, Boston, Massachusetts.

Supported in part by grants from the Shriners Hospitals for Crippled Children and from the National Institute of Child Health and Human Development (5 T1 HD 00033), United States Public Health Service.

in this age group are far more frequent in large than in small families. In the toddler stage the most common accident occurs when the youngster reaches up and pulls on a pot handle at the front of the stove and thereby receives a scald of the extended arm, shoulder, and chest. Another frequent accident at this stage is the mouth burn from chewing on an electric cord.

Burns have a seasonal incidence. House fires are more frequent in cold weather, particularly in rural areas where dwellings are of wooden construction and facilities for heating are apt to be makeshift. These factors result in increased risks in winter in the south, where demands for home heating are only occasional. With the advent of summer, burns from the outdoor barbecue become epidemic. These flash flame burns of face, hands, arms, and chest, usually in boys, follow explosive ignition of the outdoor fire on which the victim has poured gasoline, kerosine, or other highly flammable starter fluid. The pant-leg burn is prevalent during the autumn when the burning of leaves is common. At all seasons one encounters burns of the chest and other areas when the loose, frilly nightdresses of young girls ignite from too close proximity with an open fire, gas range, or candelabrum.

Burns resulting from ignition of clothing carry a significantly higher mortality than those due to scalds or contact with hot solid objects or chemicals. Mandatory treatment of cloth with fire retardants could greatly reduce the incidence of these injuries at a negligible cost.[8] As early as possible children should be taught never to run if their clothing ignites but rather to fall to the ground and smother the fire by rolling. Should they be bystanders, they can help to extinguish the flame rapidly by throwing a coat, a rug, a blanket or a similar immediately available item on the victim.

The frequency of burn injuries, as of other types of childhood accident, is much increased in families wracked by marital discord. Fire-setting by small boys is often to be interpreted as a signal of distress over the dissolution of the family, especially the loss of the father. Conversely, many serious injuries, both scalds and flame burns, prove to be a form of battering. The unwanted child, frequently the product of an extramarital affair, is likely to be the last rescued from a burning house.

TREATMENT

In dealing with an extensive burn, an established routine is helpful to eliminate the possibility of error or oversight. Special measures are required to prevent or treat shock, to control infection, to obtain early skin covering, and to restore both physical function and psychological well-being.

First aid treatment should consist of no more than reassurance and wrapping the involved area in clean cotton or linen until the extent and severity of the burn can be rapidly evaluated at the nearest medical facility. In general, there is a tendency to underestimate the seriousness of the local problem, especially in burns due to scalds or alkali, and to overlook respiratory involvement. Inhalation injury is far more frequent when burns have been sustained in enclosed spaces. No child should be transported until any respiratory difficulties are relieved and control of the airway obtained. If it is necessary to transfer the patient elsewhere, intravenous fluid therapy should be commenced, and a concise record should accompany the patient giving the time and history of the burn including notation as to whether it occurred indoors or out, an account of the vital signs and urine formation, and a record of the drugs and fluids administered. Whenever possible, a qualified nurse or medical attendant involved in the initial care should accompany the patient to supervise and record treatment during transit, observe trends in vital signs, and facilitate assumption of responsibility by the team undertaking definitive treatment.

In the makeup of the team assuming ultimate care, there must always be a captain primarily responsible for therapuetic decisions, but all team members, including nurses, physical therapist, social worker, and dietician, should meet the patient as early as possible. Only in this way can changes in the child's condition be recognized promptly and a well-coordinated treatment program be planned and carried through.

The following is an outline of initial evaluation and treatment measures for a patient with an acute, extensive burn, as carried out at the Shriners Burns Institute of Boston. The order of procedure is only approximate and frequently several of the functions can be carried on simultaneously.

1. Check adequacy of airway and provide oxygen, intubation, tracheotomy, and/or ventilatory assistance as indicated.
2. Sedate patient only if necessary, using the intravenous route.
3. Remove clothing and weigh patient.
4. Establish an intravenous line adequate to deliver fluids at a high rate of flow. A central venous pressure line is desirable in patients with extensive burns.
5. Evaluate extent and depth of burn (See Figure 1).
6. Consider need for escharotomy and/or fasciotomy for circumferential burns of extremities and chest.
7. Cover burns with gauze dressings wet with 0.5 per cent silver nitrate solution. Use Sulfamylon or silver sulfadiazine for facial burns.
8. Splint areas of potential contracture.
9. Obtain blood sample for baseline laboratory studies.
10. Calculate fluid requirements and establish fluid regimen.
11. Insert Foley catheter and obtain urine specimen for analysis.
12. Commence "critical care" type of tabular chart of intake, output, vital signs, and chemical values for blood and urine.
13. Initiate low dosage penicillin prophylaxis.
14. Give appropriate protection against tetanus.
15. Obtain detailed history, including circumstances and time of injury.
16. Consider means of achieving temporary and permanent skin cover.

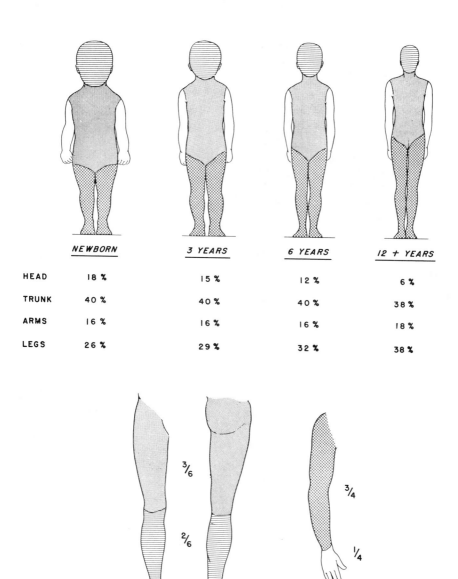

	NEWBORN	3 YEARS	6 YEARS	12 + YEARS
HEAD	18 %	15 %	12 %	6 %
TRUNK	40 %	40 %	40 %	38 %
ARMS	16 %	16 %	16 %	18 %
LEGS	26 %	29 %	32 %	38 %

Figure 1. The percentage figures in the above chart refer to front and back. For example, if an individual suffered a burn of the whole anterior chest, this would comprise 10 per cent of his body surface. (From Talbot, N. B., Richie, R. H., and Crawford, J. D.: Metabolic Homeostasis, Harvard University Press, 1959. After Lund, C. C., and Browder, N. C.: The estimation of areas of burns. Surg. Gynec. Obstet., 79:352, 1944.)

17. Plan nutritional support, treatment of anemia and hypoproteinemia, and rehabilitation, including physiotherapy and emotional support.

It is imperative immediately after a patient arrives at the treatment center to check the adequacy of the airway and to reappraise this periodically, especially in burns that have occurred indoors, when there is involvement of the face, or when prolonged exposure to smoke has occurred. Attention to color, respiratory rate, character of the voice, appearance of the pharynx, and presence or absence of restlessness will usually tell if there is glottic swelling, respiratory "burn," or significant reduction in blood oxygen carrying capacity due to methemoglobinemia. Hemoglobinuria is another sign of pulmonary inhalation injury and should alert one to the need for respiratory care. A decision to intubate the patient at once or to observe while monitoring the arterial blood gas concentrations should be made at this stage.

In cases of respiratory inadequacy requiring control of the airway, the passage of an endotracheal tube, by the nasal route if possible, allows time to evaluate the patient progress over hours or a few days, thus avoiding a hasty or unnecessary tracheotomy. Furthermore, prior intubation provides a secure airway and makes possible the administration of general anesthesia if it is later decided that a tracheotomy is indeed indicated.

In circumferential burns of the chest with formation of a thick, leathery, inelastic surface, escharotomies may be required to permit adequate respiratory excursions.

Corticosteroids in large doses (dexamethasone, 2 to 10 mg per square meter q. 8 hr.)* have been recommended to combat pulmonary inflammatory changes secondary to inhalation of irritating products of combustion. Their efficacy has not been fully established.

Sedation should not be considered a routine part of early treatment. Since restlessness is very often a sign of hypoxia, respiratory depressants are contraindicated. Deep third degree burns are seldom painful in the early hours after injury; paradoxically, morphine (6 mg per square meter) or meperidine (25 mg per square meter) are most often indicated to relieve the pain of extensive first and second degree burns. When given in the early stages of a burn injury, these medications should be administered intravenously because absorption of agents given subcutaneously or intramuscularly is erratic. Most children who have suffered severe burns are fully conscious; anxiety is a major component of their distress and requires constant attendance, interpretation, and reassurance.

Once the respiratory status has been evaluated and the immediate needs provided, all clothing should be removed, and the patient

---

*The estimation of body surface area, a useful parameter for calculation of drug dosage, fluid requirements, and extent of burns, is readily made from weight, or better, height and weight, using tables or nomograms that have been widely reprinted.[9]

weighed. The exact extent and severity of the burn should be mapped and the percentage of the child's total surface area computed by reference to standard charts.

There is little to be gained from an attempt to discriminate deep second from third degree involvement nor should an inordinate period be spent in meticulous débridement. Great care must be taken to evaluate the influence of circumferential burns of the extremities on the vascular supply of distal parts. Prompt escharotomies or fasciotomies may result in preventing loss of fingers and toes through ischemic gangrene (Fig. 2). If there has been mechanical trauma in association with the burn injury, rapid examination for fractures, ruptured spleen, and similar consequences should be conducted.

With all possible dispatch the burned areas should be wrapped without constriction in loose mesh gauze wet with warm 0.5 per cent silver nitrate solution to a thickness of one half inch. Splints or traction should be applied to maintain joints in extension if the burn involves areas such as the antecubital space, popliteal fossa, or axilla. When the

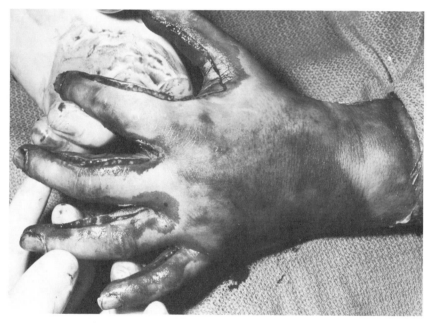

Figure 2. Escharotomies done to prevent ischemic gangrene and loss of digits. A full thickness flame burn involving the wrist circumferentially, the entire dorsum of the hand, portions of the palm, and volar surfaces of the fingers of this 16-year-old girl resulted in swelling under the inelastic eschar. The incisions shown were made approximately 12 hours after injury and resulted in an improved blood supply. Staged excisions of all nonviable skin were carried out at two and five days after injury, with initial application of allografts, later replaced by autografts. The fingers were maintained in a position of function during healing by the use of Zimmerman pins placed through the distal phalanges. The escharotomies were instrumental in preventing the loss of digits and in the final achievement of a fully functional hand.

hands are burned, the wrist should be maintained slightly cocked and the metacarpophalangeal joints moderately flexed. Burns of the anterior neck require that the child be placed on a half mattress extending up to the shoulder so that when he is supine his neck is extended. Skeletal traction to maintain joints in a position of function has been used with a high degree of success.[10] Not only are contractures prevented but elevation of burned extremities is more easily obtained, nursing and grafting procedures are facilitated, and the incidence of osteomyelitis and septic complications has been remarkably low.

There has been a recent trend in fluid therapy toward using balanced saline solutions rather than the large amounts of plasma formerly advocated in the early treatment of burns.[11, 12] Crystalloids, in the large amounts adequate to maintain the circulation, give rise to a much greater degree of early edema, but the interstitial fluid is more rapidly reabsorbed because of lesser entrapment of protein in the extravascular spaces once the normal permeability of capillaries is restored, 36 to 48 hours following the accident. It is our practice to use intravenous fluids in all deep burns involving more than 10 per cent of the body surface, commencing treatment with Ringer's lactate solution and providing 2 ml/per cent burn/kg plus 1500 ml/square meter per 24 hours for maintenance. Since individual requirements vary, this formula is only a rough guide.

The intake is monitored by means of urinary output plus, in larger burns, measurement of central venous pressure. An increase in the rate of infusion of Ringer's lactate is required if the urine output falls below 30 ml/square meter per hour, or if the hematocrit rises above 50 per cent. If, in the early phase of treatment, difficulty is experienced in maintaining blood pressure, central venous pressure, or urine output at adequate levels despite an increase in rate of infusion of the Ringer's lactate to as much as 300 ml/square meter/hr., rapid delivery of plasma (300 ml per square meter) or an equivalent amount of albumin is recommended. Otherwise, enough plasma or albumin is administered to provide 0.5 to 1.0 gm of protein per kg if the serum protein concentration falls to less than 3.0 gm per 100 ml in the acute phase of therapy.

After diuresis the serum total protein should be maintained above 5.5 gm per 100 ml. Similarly, in the acute phase, blood transfusion should be given if the hematocrit falls below 30 per cent; later, values should be maintained between 35 and 40 per cent. If greater than 50 per cent of the body surface is burned, fluid requirements calculated as for a 50 per cent burn provide the maximum volume tolerated and it is usually necessary to supply colloid in addition to the Ringer's lactate. The rate of fluid administration must be decreased if anesthesia or surgery is necessary because these procedures so commonly lead to antidiuresis.[13, 14] Oliguria may also develop as a consequence of pigment nephropathy (vide infra), and this, too, is an indication for slowing the rate of fluid delivery to prevent vascular overload. Our

TABLE 1 DIFFERENTIAL DIAGNOSIS OF OLIGURIA DEVELOPING IN TREATMENT OF PATIENT WITH SEVERE BURNS

Cause	Clinical Findings	Urinary Volume	Urinary Sodium	Urinary Osmolality	Urinary Urea[1]	BUN and Serum Creatinine
Prerenal						
Hypovolemia Dehydration Salt depletion		Low	10–20 <10	Increased >800 mosM/kg (SG > 1.025)	3000	Both increased (Ratio 40:1)
Parenchymal Acute Tubular Necrosis	Hypotensive episode	Low	40	Isotonic ~300 mosM/kg (SG 1.010)	300	Both increased (Ratio 15:1 but may show elevation early)
Cortical necrosis	Hypotensive episode	Very low	20	Often increased (SG 1.015)	800–2000	Both increased (Ratio 15:1)

[1] Mg per 100 milliliters.
[2] The ratio normally is 15:1 but in prerenal oliguria will rise to 40:1 or greater in most cases.

aim through the first 5 to 7 days after injury is to keep urine flow at 40 ml per square meter per hour, the urinary sodium concentration between 20 and 80 mEq/L, the serum sodium between 130 and 140 mEq/L, and the potassium concentration between 3.5 and 5.0 mEq/L.

The requirements for sodium chloride are very much increased by silver nitrate wet dressings. Because endogenous chloride forms an insoluble complex with the silver ion, it is lost to the body with its companion cation at a rate of approximately 3.5 mM per day per 100 square centimeters of deep second or third degree burn.[15]

In the early phase of therapy, if hemoglobinuria is present (often a sign of inhalation of toxic products of combustion and extensive pulmonary involvement), alkalinization of the urine is advantageous because of the insolubility of hematin in acid solution. Alkalinization of the urine can be accomplished by giving sodium bicarbonate (0.5 mM/kg) and maintaining or establishing good urine flow with mannitol (0.5 gm/kg) or furosemide (1 to 2 mg/kg).

In the first few days oliguria is more commonly the result of inadequate fluid replacement than of acute renal failure. However, isotonic urine in volumes of less than 0.5 ml/kg/hr. suggests renal failure and requires examination of the urine for pigment casts and for a combination of high sodium concentration, low osmolality, and low urea concentration (Table 1).[16] Renal failure is uncommon in burns of less than 20 per cent of the body surface; it occurs more frequently after flame burns sustained indoors than after scalds. It is most common with extensive electrical burns in which myoglobinemia often complicates the pigment load to be dealt with by the kidneys. It is ordinarily preventable if oliguria is promptly recognized and appropriately treated. Dialysis is the only resort should anuria supervene.

Half of the estimated first day's fluid requirement should be given in the initial 8 hours after the burn (not 8 hours from commencement of therapy) and one fourth in each of the second and third 8-hour periods. On the second day the requirement for Ringer's lactate is approximately two thirds of the volume required on the first day. Since Ringer's lactate does not contain dextrose, the fluid should be enriched with 2.5 to 5 per cent dextrose if measured blood glucose levels fall below 140 mg per 100 ml. Oral fluids are best withheld in the early shock phase but may be begun after 24 to 48 hours. Oral intake should not be relied upon for support of vascular volume, although it is often adequate to meet the needs for maintenance fluid. After 48 to 72 hours, a diuretic phase is entered. At this stage interstitial fluid is being rapidly returned to the vascular bed, and it is important not to overload the patient's circulation with large amounts of fluid given intravenously.

A skilled, well-coordinated team is necessary for institution of acute therapy. Evaluation of the pulmonary situation and the extent and severity of the burn requires experience and nice judgment. Most children in incipient or full-blown shock will require a venous cutdown, and unless an operator skilled in this procedure or in percutaneous introduction of a large bore intravenous catheter is available, time will be wasted. A centrally placed venous catheter with a suitable manometer attachment may be used both as an intravenous line and as a means to monitor central venous pressure. When appropriate care is taken to avoid dead space dilutional errors, the catheter can also serve for blood sampling.

Experienced nursing help is required for expeditious bandaging and splinting and an additional person should be available to initiate an accurate record of vital signs, medications and fluids administered, urine output, and values for blood pO_2, pCO_2, pH, hematocrit, total protein, and sodium, chloride, and potassium concentration.

Vital signs and urine output are measured at half hour intervals initially and hourly thereafter. Rectal temperature is taken at not greater than 2-hour intervals initially, for hypothermia is frequently a complication not only when the patient is uncovered but also as a response to evaporative heat loss when wrapped in wet dressings.[17] A continuous temperature record using a direct reading probe is advantageous in very severe burns. Urinary sodium content and osmolality, serum electrolyte concentrations and hematocrit, total protein, and blood gases should be monitored and recorded not less often than at intervals of 6 hours in large burns. A skilled technician in a close-at-hand laboratory equipped with modern analytical instruments designed to give rapid answers on small samples can immeasurably improve chances for survival of the extensively burned child.

Because of their susceptibility to rapidly spreading cellulitis from beta hemolytic streptococci, all patients with serious burns are given relatively low doses of parenteral penicillin (200,000 units q. 6 hr.) at entry. If previously immunized they also receive a booster dose of tetanus toxoid (0.5 ml). Penicillin is continued for 10 to 14 days or until the serum IgG immunoglobulin levels are restored. The sharp fall in these levels following a burn usually reaches it nadir at 4 to 5 days.

Continuous topical application of 0.5 per cent silver nitrate solution or Sulfamylon cream has been shown to give a high level and broad spectrum of surface bacterial control.[18, 19, 20] The effectiveness of these agents as well as of gentamicin[20] or silver sulfadiazine creams[21] depends upon close contact with residual, viable tissue. None can penetrate thick eschar. Thus, the wet dressings or cream must be totally removed daily and the burn surface carefully débrided of necrotic tissue easily separable from the granulating bed. Special care must be taken to identify and unroof abscesses forming beneath the leathery eschar resulting from flame or electrical burns. Initial and subsequent daily cultures should be taken from representative areas of the injury to provide constant knowledge of the bacterial flora. If invasive infection is present it should be treated early and vigorously with the appropriate antibiotics.

Continuous fever, tachycardia, an elevated respiratory rate, and leukocytosis with a "left shift" are invariable sequelae of an extensive burn. These are manifestations of an adaptive state of hypermetabolism and will be intensified by superimposed infection, but they are not, per se, indications for a change in the antibacterial regimen. In addition to evidence from cultures and sensitivity tests, a change in systemic antibacterial therapy requires good judgment and perspective. Infection markedly augments surface losses of electrolytes and an appropriate increase in sodium chloride supplementation will be required.[15]

A significant advance in the care of burned patients has been the introduction of the laminar air flow isolation units, one of which is shown in Figure 3. Bacteria-free air is introduced through ceiling panels which distribute it in a uniform "shower" descending over the patient. The air pressure is maintained slightly positive in respect to the external environment to exclude entry of air-borne organisms from outside and the unit is exhausted through floor panels on either side of the bed. Humidity and air temperature are individually controlled. With use of silver nitrate wet dressings, humidity is maintained at 80 per cent to reduce evaporation and, for patient comfort, the temperature is set at approximately 84°. In combination with the new topical antiseptics, these units have resulted in a sharp drop in septic complications.

In children, another frequent complication of burns, both large and small, is central nervous system dysfunction.[22] The clinical manifestations range from hallucination, personality change, and delirium to seizures and coma. "Burn encephalopathy" has been thought to have an obscure etiology but in our experience the cause has usually been readily discoverable: in about one third of our patients it has been due to hypoxia, with hypovolemia, hyponatremia, and septicemia each contributing about 15 per cent to the total incidence. Once the cause is determined, treatment is readily provided. Notable has been the fact

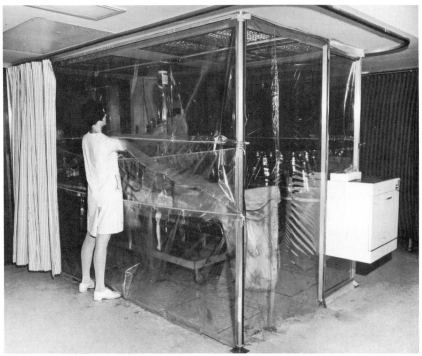

Figure 3. Laminar air flow in a bacteria-free nursing unit. Plastic curtains permit child to maintain contact with nurses, parents, and other children. The need for use of masks and gowns by attendants is obviated. The nurse shown wears thin, plastic gauntlets extending to her shoulders. The white box at the foot of the bed is a pass-through for trays and equipment which subjects all items to ultraviolet sterilization.

that, in spite of prolonged and serious manifestations, full neurological recovery has been the rule.

The amount of scarring and contracture following a major burn depends, in general, upon the rapidity of achievement of skin coverage. Early excision of small but sharply demarcated full thickness burns much reduces the time required for healing. It has become increasingly evident that excision is advantageous in large burns also, especially since the introduction of allografting[23, 24] (and xenografting[25]) as a highly effective method of hastening preparation of the burned areas for autografting. The development of a method for preservation of cadaver skin by freezing allows flexibility in such therapy and, in the future, tissue matching may increase the survival time of allografts (Fig. 4). Nonetheless, whatever are the means employed of dealing with the local injury, the condition of the patient will remain precarious until the majority of the burn surface is reepithelialized.

It is during the period preceding reepithelialization, generally beginning within 48 hours of the injury and frequently lasting for many weeks, that nutrition is of paramount importance. A high caloric intake

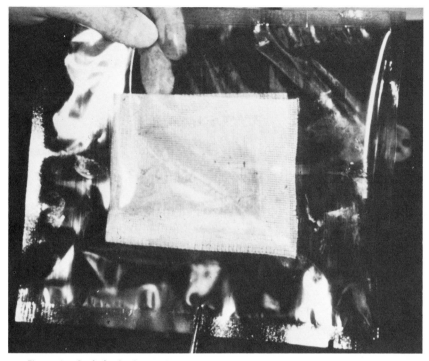

Figure 4. Sealed, plastic envelope of frozen skin for use in allografting. These packets of glycerolized tissue spread on gauze are maintained in liquid nitrogen until used. Supplies of the patient's own skin may be similarly preserved for primary autografting delayed to allow time for better preparation of the graft site or for secondary repair of areas of graft loss. This results in a lesser need for repeated anesthesia because application of such grafts can be accomplished at the bedside.

is essential to sustain the adaptive hypermetabolism mentioned earlier, to replace the protein lost by exudation, and to support synthesis of immunoglobulins and structural protein.[26, 27] It is not sufficient simply to write in the order book "high caloric intake." Great ingenuity is required to devise the kind of diet which will appeal to the often anorexic and frequently manipulative child. In the early phase after the burn, a liquid diet is often better tolerated than solids. Enormous patience, understanding and explanation, and a consistent firmness of approach are necessary to insure that the food is taken. Success in use of a nasogastric tube to supplement what the child can take by mouth is largely dependent upon the attitude of the staff. In general, an intake of at least 3000 calories per square meter or, differently expressed, 60 calories per kg, plus 30 per 100 square centimeters of burn, is required daily to meet the needs for energy metabolism and healing. This will almost automatically supply sufficient protein (3 to 5 gm/kg/day). Higher protein intakes are apt to be distasteful and it is well to recall that the availability of ingested protein for synthetic processes varies directly with the number of calories provided from fat and carbohydrate.

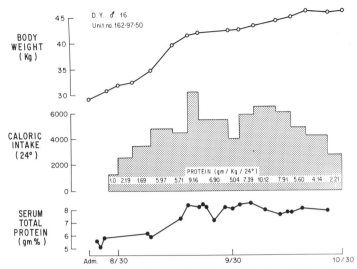

Figure 5. Realimentation in syndrome of postburn malnutrition. The patient had incurred a 55-pound weight loss in the two months following an injury originally involving only 26 per cent of the body surface. The restoration of his weight was accomplished by steady advancement of his food intake. A nasogastric tube was used to supplement what he could take by mouth during the first three weeks. The average daily caloric intake between weighings (*top*) is shown by the height of the columns in the center portion of the figure. Average daily protein intakes are shown by the numbers in the clear zone of the stippled columns. The serum total protein values are shown at the bottom of the figure.

Figure 5 gives information concerning the realimentation of a 16-year-old boy admitted 2 months after a 26 per cent full thickness burn injury. During the interval between the injury and his transfer to this hospital there had been a failure to recognize and to meet adequately his caloric needs. The result had been no progress in the healing of his original wounds while his donor sites had been converted to full thickness skin losses. He had lost 55 pounds from his preinjury weight of 116 pounds. This malnutrition syndrome, which can be prevented if adequate attention is paid to the principles stated in the foregoing paragraph, has been seen so often as to deserve special attention.

In this instance, the patient was encouraged to take all he could by mouth. The importance to his healing of a high caloric intake was carefully explained and the use of a nasogastric tube presented as a means to help him achieve the requisite food intake. The constituents of normal, appetizing meals were blended to an appropriate consistency to pass easily through the nasogastric tube using milk or water as a diluent. This practice may have nutritional advantages over use of some of the commercially prepared mixtures and has significant psychological merit. To avoid overloading the bowel and the development of diarrhea the initial prescription was for 1200 calories daily. As seen in Figure 5, this was advanced stepwise to reach ultimately an intake in excess of 6000 calories per day. Use of the nasogastric tube was discontinued after approximately 3 weeks. The figure shows the response in terms of weight gain and the rise in serum total protein. Equally dramatic was the rapid healing of the original burn injuries and the donor sites.

In very large burns, temporary use of intravenous "hyperalimentation" is under exploration. The very high carbohydrate contents of the preparations currently available carry the disadvantage of requiring delivery into a large central vein[28] and the low-insulin pseudodiabetes which many of these seriously burned patients develop may necessitate concurrent use of insulin.[29] Nevertheless, impressive results in terms of reduction of body protein losses have been obtained and further advances in the preparation of more suitable fluids and techniques of administration are anticipated. In patients so treated, particular attention needs be paid to the level of red cell 2,3-diphosphoglycerate.[30] Deficiency of this compound, which plays such an important role in the release of hemoglobin-bound oxygen to the tissues, may develop as a result of a markedly depressed serum inorganic phosphate, massive transfusion of depleted bank blood, or other as yet not fully defined circumstances. The consequence of 2,3-DPG deficiency is tissue hypoxia due to an increase in the affinity of hemoglobin for oxygen, shifting the oxygen saturation curve to the left. The patient will be found exhibiting the anxiety and hyperventilation of oxygen starvation despite normal arterial pO_2 values, with a tendency to low pCO_2 tension and elevated arterial pH.

During treatment with silver nitrate, extra sodium chloride (350 mM per square meter of burn per day) must be supplied to counterbalance the losses resulting from silver nitrate treatment. Once the period of mandatory intravenous therapy is passed, the salt supplement can be given by mouth, along with other food to avoid gastrointestinal irritation. Adequacy of salt replacement can be conveniently judged by monitoring urine sodium concentration. The latter should be maintained in the range 20 to 80 mEq/L; lower values suggest a maximal effort to conserve, and higher levels can indicate substantial salt or vascular volume surfeit, with the attendant risk of hypokalemia. Use of Sulfamylon over significantly large body surface areas (30 per cent) may be associated with an acidosis and hyperventilation which can be confused with respiratory disease.[31] This results from the carbonic anhydrase inhibitory activity of degradation products of Sulfamylon and may require sodium bicarbonate supplementation. Maintenance of a large urine output will help to minimize metabolic effects by ensuring adequate clearance of such products.

After the acute phase of edema and diuresis has passed, repeated transfusions of albumin to keep total serum protein above 5.5 gm per 100 ml and packed erythrocytes to maintain the hematocrit between 35 and 40 per cent are often necessary. Spontaneous reepithelialization and graft acceptance are never optimal unless the granulations are relatively sterile, nonedematous, and richly oxygenated.

Children with severe burns commonly exhibit retrogressive behavior beginning soon after the injury and persisting until skin coverage is all but complete. This behavior is aggravated by the requisite, but nonetheless painful, daily débridement and dressings, the physical therapy to prevent joint contractures, the fixation to restrict motion following grafting, and the increasingly distorted body image conjured up by the children as they view their wounds. This change in personality makes care emotionally traumatic to physicians, nurses, physical therapists, dieticians—indeed, all with whom patients have contact, including their parents.

Dressings and other painful procedures should not be scheduled immediately before mealtimes. Analgesics and brief-acting anesthetics have their role but the pain threshhold is principally lowered by apprehension; thus, reassurance, efficient workmanship, and encouragement of participation by the child are often of more value. Members of the team caring for the child must be judicious in their word choice during all "professional" discussions. By and large, these should be carried on away from the child, and conversations at the bedside should be primarily with the child. One must at all times strive to furnish a cheerful environment and encourage visits from parents and relatives. Visitors as well as nurses and other attendants will need to be counseled in techniques to provide diversion and to promote constructive thinking in the child and to reestablish channels of communication between the child and the world, which so many fear to reenter.

In the years intervening between the Cocoanut Grove tragedy in 1942, that great stimulus to burns research at this hospital, and the present time, enormous advances in lifesaving and rehabilitation have been made. Nonetheless, few illnesses still pose so great a problem as the severe burn. Even with physical survival and accomplishment of full skin coverage, scarring, contractures, and distortion of the self image (often unwarranted from the objective viewpoint) all too frequently culminate in "social death."[32] Much research is still required on every facet of the care described here, and the efforts of every member of the team—pediatrician, surgeon, anesthesiologist, orthopedist, psychiatrist, pharmacologist, nurse, nutritionist, social worker, biochemist, immunologist, and epidemiologist—are needed.

References

1. American Public Health Association, Technical Development Board, Program Area Committee on Accident Prevention: Accident Prevention. New York, McGraw-Hill, 1961, p. 51.
2. Fox, C. C.: Early treatment of severe burns. Opening remarks. Ann. N.Y. Acad. Sci., *150* (Art. 3):473, 1968.
3. Smith, E. I.: The epidemiology of burns. The cause and control of burns in children. Pediatrics, *44*:821, 1969.
4. Iskrant, A. P.: Statistics and epidemiology of burns. Bull. N.Y. Acad. Med., *43*:636, 1967.
5. Caudle, P. R. K., and Potter, J.: Characteristics of burned children and the after effects of the injury. Brit. J. Plast. Surg., *23*:63, 1970.
6. Borland, B. L.: Prevention of childhood burns: conclusions drawn from an epidemiologic study. Clin. Pediat., *6*:693, 1967.

7. Biggs, J. S. G., and Clarke, A. M.: Burns in children: a five year survey of a burns unit. Med. J. Aust., *1*:787, 1964.
8. Oglesby, F. B.: The flammable fabrics problem. Pediatrics, *44*:827, 1969.
9. Shirkey, H. C.: The dose of drugs. *In* Textbook of Pediatrics, 9th ed. W. E. Nelson, V. C. Vaughan, III, and R. J. McKay, editors. Philadelphia, W. B. Saunders Company, 1969, p. 236.
10. Evans, E. B., Larson, D. L., and Yares, S.: Preservation and restoration of joint functions in patients with severe burns. J.A.M.A., *204*:843, 1968.
11. Blocker, T. G., Jr., Lewis, S. R., Lynch, J. B., and Blocker, V.: Early treatment of severe burns. Part IV: Fluid therapy. Trends away from blood and plasma in the early treatment of severe burns. Ann. N.Y. Acad. Sci., *150* (Art. 3):912, 1968.
12. Davies, J. W. L., Jackson, D. M., and Cason, J. S.: Early treatment of severe burns. Part IV: Fluid therapy. A comparison of the efficacy of plasma and sodium salts. Ann. N.Y. Acad. Sci., *150* (Art. 3):852, 1968.
13. Aprahamian, H. A., Vanderveen, J. L., Bunker, J. P., Murphy, A. J., and Crawford, J. D.: The influence of general anesthetics on water and solute excretion in man. Ann. Surg., *150*:122, 1959.
14. Moran, W. H., Jr., and Zimmermann, B.: Mechanisms of antidiuretic hormone (ADH) control of importance to the surgical patient. Surgery, *62*:639, 1967.
15. Burke, J. F., Bondoc, C. C., and Morris, P. J.: Early treatment of severe burns. Part II: Metabolism. Metabolic effects of topical silver nitrate therapy in burns covering more than fifteen percent of the body surface. Ann. N.Y. Acad. Sci., *150* (Art. 3):674, 1968.
16. Cameron, J. S.: Disturbances of renal function in burn patients. Proc. Roy. Soc. Med., *62*:49, 1968.
17. Roe, C. F., Kinney, J. M., and Blair, C.: Water and heat exchange in third degree burns. Surgery, *56*:212, 1964.
18. Monafo, W. W., and Moyer, C. A.: Effectiveness of dilute aqueous silver nitrate in the treatment of major burns. Arch. Surg., *91*:200, 1965.
19. Moncrief, J. A., Linberg, R. B., Switzer, W. E., and Pruitt, B. A.: The use of a topical sulfonamide in the control burn wound sepsis. J. Trauma, *6*:407, 1966.
20. Altemeier, W. A., and MacMillan, B. G.: Comparative studies of topical silver nitrate, sulfamylon and gentamicin. Ann. N.Y. Acad. Sci., *150*:966, 1968.
21. Stanford, W., Rappole, B. W., and Fox, C. L., Jr.: Clinical experience with silver sulfadiazine, a new topical agent for control of Pseudomonas infections in burns. J. Trauma, *9*:377, 1969.
22. Warlow, C. P., and Hinton, P.: Early neurological disturbances following relatively minor burns in children. Lancet, *2*:978, 1969.
23. Brown, J. B., and Freyer, M. P.: Postmortem homografts to reduce mortality in extensive burns. Early "biological" closure and saving of patients for permanent healing; use in mass casualties and national disasters. J.A.M.A., *156*:1163, 1954.
24. Burke, J. F., and Bondoc, C. C.: Combined burn therapy utilizing immediate skin allografts and 0.5% silver nitrate. Arch. Surg., *97*:716, 1969.
25. Bromberg, B. E., Song, E. C., and Mohn, M. P.: The use of pig skin as a temporary biological dressing. Plast. Reconstr. Surg., *36*:80, 1965.
26. Blocker, T. G., Levin, S. L., Nowinski, W. W., Lewis, S. R., and Blocker, V.: Nutrition studies in the severely burned. Ann. Surg., *141*:589, 1955.
27. Becker, J. M., and Artz, C. P.: The treatment of burns in children. Report No. 5, Surgical Research Unit, Brooke Army Hospital, Fort Sam Houston, Texas, 1956.
28. Filler, R. M., and Eraklis, A. J.: Care of the critically ill child: intravenous alimentation. Pediatrics, *46*:456, 1970.
29. Hinton, P., Littlejohn, S., Allison, S. P., and Lloyd, J.: Insulin and glucose to reduce catabolic response to injury in burned patients. Lancet, *1*:767, 1971.
30. Benesch, R.: How do small molecules do great things? New Eng. J. Med., *280*:1179, 1969.
31. White, M. G., and Asch, M.: Acid-base effects of topical mafenide acetate in the burned patient. New Eng. J. Med., *284*:1281, 1971.
32. Macgregor, F. C.: Facial Disfigurement and Problems of Employment: Some Social and Cultural Considerations. Chapter 10, in Facial Disfigurement: A Rehabilitation Problem. B.O. Rogers, Ed. Proceedings of a Conference of the Institute of Reconstructive Plastic Surgery of the New York University Medical Center, March 21–22, 1963, New York. Washington, D.C., U.S. Government Printing Office, 1966, pp. 123–133.

5

Diagnosis and Management of Head Injury

Darryl C. DeVivo, M.D., and Philip R. Dodge, M.D.

Head injury ranks high among the causes of death and disability in childhood. And it is the rare child who attains adulthood without ever having sustained a significant bump or blow to the head. Although accurate statistics are not available, the majority of children who suffer such injury do not require hospitalization, and probably only a fraction of them are seen by the family doctor or pediatrician. Yet it has been estimated that 200,000 children are hospitalized each year for evaluation and treatment of a head injury and perhaps 5 to 10 per cent of this number exhibit neurological signs.[1] Some indication of the scope of the problem in a pediatric setting is indicated by the fact that during the year 1967 approximately 500 children were evaluated for head injury in the Emergency Room of St. Louis Children's Hospital, and that 187 of this group were hospitalized for further observation and treatment.

From the Edward Mallinckrodt Department of Pediatrics and the Department of Neurology, Washington University School of Medicine, and the Division of Neurology, St. Louis Children's Hospital, St. Louis, Missouri.

This work supported in part by the Allen P. and Josephine B. Green Foundation of Mexico, Missouri, and Grant #TO 1-NS 5633 from the National Institute of Neurological Diseases and Stroke.

Over the past 30 years many investigators have attempted to quantitate the effects of closed head injury. Denny-Brown and Russell, in developing an experimental model to study concussion, demonstrated that a much greater force is necessary to render an animal unconscious when the skull is held firmly in place as compared to the situation in which the skull is free to move after impact.[2] They termed these two circumstances compression concussion and acceleration concussion.

In the majority of human situations, acceleration-deceleration is more descriptive of the circumstances surrounding head injury. Thus, the rate of change in head position after impact and the associated deformation of the skull at the time of impact have become the major factors used in evaluating the effects of experimentally induced head injury. The force transmitted to the intracranial contents which produces acceleration and deformation of the skull gives rise to significant distortion and cavitation of the brain. There is little or no change in the volume of brain substance at the time of injury, but there is substantial change in its shape. This distortion causes bruising or laceration of brain which may occur at the site of injury (coup) or at a distance (contrecoup).

A shearing force may tear small arteries and veins and produce parenchymatous bleeding, or subdural hemorrhages in the case of those bridging vessels which are coursing from the cerebral surface through the meninges to enter the dural sinuses. Less well recognized stretching or shearing effects can be transmitted to ascending and descending fiber tracts as they pass through the brain stem, separating these long processes from their cell bodies.[3] An appreciation of these several effects of a blow to the head leads to an understanding of various clinical syndromes which follow an acute head injury.

CLINICAL SYNDROMES AND PATHOLOGY

Concussion

The term concussion refers to the reversible neuronal dysfunction associated with loss of awareness and responsiveness (unconsciousness) which follows immediately upon a head injury and which persists for a brief period of time, usually measured in terms of minutes or hours. If the patient is observed carefully during this period, the duration of impaired consciousness can be precisely noted; but if one must rely on the history given by the patient at a later date, a false impression as to the duration of unconsciousness will be obtained. The reason for this is that the patient will be amnesic not only for the period of unconsciousness but also for events immediately before and after this. This loss of memory surrounding a concussion, termed post-traumatic amnesia (PTA), is considered by many investigators the single most important clinical phenomenon reflecting the extent and severity of injury to the brain following blunt trauma.

Post-traumatic amnesia is composed of two parts: retrograde amnesia or that period of time before impact for which the patient has no memory; and anterograde amnesia or the period of memory loss after injury. Both periods tend to shrink with time but the patient is always left with some permanent amnesia. It is usually said that concussion has no significant pathological counterpart if the brain is examined by light microscopy. It should be mentioned here that concussion and PTA may not occur in injuries by sharp objects striking the head at high velocity and penetrating the skull (and even the brain) without producing significant deformities of the skull or acceleration-deceleration of the head. Under these circumstances severe focal damage to cerebral tissue and consequent neurologic defects can occur.[4]

Experimentally, concussion in animals is characterized by loss of consciousness, respiration, postural tone, and corneal and pinnal reflexes, associated with a rapid rise in blood pressure, and followed by recovery. These findings relate to autonomic functions in the lower brain stem; and certain investigators believe the primary lesion is damage to the large fibers in the ventral surface of the upper cervical cord from cervical extension and consequent stretching of the cord around the odontoid process.[5, 6] Preliminary physiological and pharmacological studies of experimental concussion have demonstrated interruption in the sensory evoked responses in the reticular activating system and the liberation of large quantities of free acetyl choline into the cerebrospinal fluid.[7] Although the significance of these observations at present remains unclear, such investigations may lead ultimately to a better understanding of the mechanism underlying concussion.

Contusion and Laceration

If visible injury to the brain exists, the terms contusion and laceration are used to describe respectively the bruising or tearing of cerebral tissue, frequently accompanied by parenchymatous hemorrhage. The contusion or laceration is characteristically directly beneath the site of impact but, as noted earlier, the lesion may be remote from the site of direct trauma. Often in serious accidents there may be multiple sites of injury. The poles and undersurfaces of frontal and temporal lobes are most frequently injured.

Focal disturbances in strength, sensation, or visual awareness may result from such injury unless the damage involves so-called silent areas. Such disturbances on examination need not, however, always imply this type of cerebral injury. Focal signs may also follow seizures (Todd's paresis), but in these cases are quite transient, usually resolving within two or three days after the cessation of seizure activity. Rapidly clearing focal findings in the absence of seizure activity may represent localized disturbances in neuronal function, referred to as "local concussion."[4] We have proposed that such a mechanism might underlie the transient loss of vision seen after mild head injury.[8] In some instances development of such focal signs is delayed, suggesting that local edema and ischemia may be responsible.

Epidural and Subdural Hemorrhages

Hemorrhages developing between the calvarium and cerebral surfaces will compress the underlying brain. If the hemorrhage results from arterial bleeding, the temporal course of the resulting neurologic syndromes will be more rapid than if the bleeding is from veins.

Epidural bleeding is usually accompanied by roentgenographic evidence of skull fracture; however, in children a fracture may be absent radiographically and at surgery in more than a quarter of the cases.[1] This fact presumably is attributable to the reactive plasticity of the child's skull and the looseness with which the dura mater is attached to the overlying calvarium. For similar reasons, the hematoma may derive from diploic veins or dural sinuses rather than from an arterial source. Consequently, even in the absence of radiographic evidence of skull fracture, one must be alert to the possibility that an epidural hemorrhage can supervene.

Symptoms and signs of cerebral compression from acute subdural hemorrhage usually evolve within hours or days of injury. Or the hemorrhage may develop more slowly, the clot undergo dissolution, and a chronic subdural effusion result. It is taught that symptoms and signs of epidural or subdural hemorrhage develop after a transient period of normalcy (lucid period) following concussion or other immediate effects of head injury. Clinically, however, this sequence of events is seldom recognized. More often in serious head injury the effects of a developing mass lesion appear before recovery from the immediate effects of the trauma has occurred.

Skull Fracture

Breaks in the calvarium may be associated with any of the aforementioned clinical syndromes. The location and nature of the fracture may suggest additional complications. For example, if the fracture line extends through the squamous portion of the temporal bone, the possibility of an epidural hemorrhage from laceration of the middle meningeal artery is increased.

Fractures extending through the base of the skull may be associated with leakage of cerebrospinal fluid into either the auditory or nasal passages, resulting in otorrhea or rhinorrhea, and presence of either implies a break in the skull bone even though the fracture cannot be demonstrated radiographically. The observation of intracranial air on x-ray films after trauma always means anatomic continuity between nasal or ear cavities and the interior of the skull. This finding may exist even in the absence of obvious otorrhea or rhinorrhea. Rarely, such basal fractures also injure the pituitary stalk and cause transient or, less often, permanent diabetes insipidus. If the fracture line involves the rim of the foramen magnum, acute respiratory failure may occur secondary to direct injury of the lower brain stem or to subsequent compression of this region by a blood clot. Cranial nerve signs may also reflect direct injuries to these nerves captured in the line of fracture as they course through various bony canals.

The likelihood of a complicating intracranial infection is increased when there is a fracture, particularly when it extends through the base of the skull. Nuchal rigidity and peripheral leukocytosis frequently accompany head injury, particularly if there has been bleeding into the subarachnoid space. Even though a low grade fever may also follow severe head injury as a direct consequence of the injury itself, its occurrence always should raise the possibility of a complicating meningitis or parameningeal infection; this is especially so when there is evidence of disruption of the natural anatomic barriers to entrance of bacteria from the outside. In the face of any of these findings, diagnostic lumbar puncture is indicated, although this test should not be performed routinely following every head injury. The potential risk of neurological deterioration developing in the patient with increased intracranial pressure after a lumbar puncture must be remembered; but this perhaps overemphasized potential hazard should not countermand the use of such a test to evaluate the possible existence of an intracranial infection suggested by the clinical circumstances.

HISTORY AND EXAMINATION

Even though the diagnosis of head injury seems obvious, a detailed present and past history is essential. That it is important in management to know that the unconscious child also may suffer from drug allergies, hemophilia, diabetes mellitus, or epilepsy is obvious, but it is surprising how frequently historical data germane to the problem are missed on the initial assessment of the patient.

Similarly, a precise knowledge of the details immediately surrounding the injury may help the examiner to interpret the significance of the injury. For example, if the child stumbles while running and strikes his head on the pavement, it is reasonable to assume that the resulting neurologic syndrome is the direct result of the injury. On the other hand, if a child crumples to the ground and, in doing so, strikes his head on the pavement, one would have to consider seriously why he fell and search for predisposing factors, which could include a seizure or an intracranial hemorrhage. Similarly, if the injury is minor and the neurological deficit profound, aggravation by the trauma of a preexisting, clinically compensated intracranial disease process, such as a tumor, should be considered. Over the years, numerous examples of each of these several combinations have been witnessed.

Finally, a precise understanding of the circumstances surrounding the accident often will suggest to the physician sites of additional injury which could prove to be important if shock or sepsis develop. It is axiomatic that multiple sites of trauma, as well as the presence of coexisting disease, demand consideration in every seriously injured child. The vigilant pediatrician can serve the vital function of coordinating the efforts of several other specialists, each focusing upon a particular facet of a complex problem. Unfortunately this rarely obtains. The average pediatrician in our experience fails to assume this role.

Following a minor head injury, such as might occur in a fall from the bed, the child will commonly exhibit a transient period of lethargy usually associated with one or more episodes of vomiting. To the inexperienced parent or physician, this sequence of events may evoke great concern and bring immediately to mind the question of an evolving intracranial catastrophe. In the majority of such cases, however, this concern is unrealistic, particularly when consciousness has been preserved during the acute period, best assessed by determining that the baby cried immediately after injury. Nevertheless, careful evaluation of the infant or child is mandatory before one can justifiably return him to the care of his parents who must continue to observe him until recovery is complete. The vast majority of children who sustain minor trauma with or without a brief period of unconsciousness can be managed with the expectation that they will recover uneventfully.

With severe head injury, as may occur following a fall from a significant height or as associated with a vehicular accident, prompt evaluation and recognition of developing complications and treatment are essential if the outcome is to be favorable. These patients constitute true emergencies demanding a thorough understanding of the nature of the problem requiring medical or surgical therapy.

Awareness of the rapidity with which complications of acute head injury can evolve may lead to fear and uncertainty and impede the methodical evaluation of the patient by the pediatrician. All too frequently, recently injured patients will be sent for such tests as skull radiographs before an adequate clinical evaluation has been completed. Without accurate baseline clinical information, subsequent examinations of the patient are rendered more difficult and early recognition of developing complications may be delayed. Whenever possible, serial examinations by a single observer are strongly recommended. Only in this way can subtle worsening in the neurologic status over time be appreciated. Alterations in mental status, including increased difficulty in arousing the patient and mounting agitation, almost invariably imply an extension of the basic pathological process. Developing focal or lateralizing neurological findings or alarming changes in the vital signs, including those detailed in the succeeding paragraphs, should alert the examiner to the presence of a progressive lesion. It should be noted, however, that careful serial examinations of the child's level of alertness are fatiguing not only for the examiner but also for the patient. A desire to fall asleep under these circumstances is not unreasonable and should not be confused with depression of consciousness due to progressing cerebral dysfunction.

The child's level of consciousness, heart rate, blood pressure, and breathing should be assessed rapidly, with primary attention to those vital circulatory and ventilatory functions upon which life depends; also, impaired circulation, hypoxia, and hypercapnea, if not life-threatening, will all compromise cerebral functions and tend to elevate intracranial pressure further by increasing cerebral edema and vascular volume. Rising systemic blood pressure associated with slowing of the pulse rate and irregularity of breathing usually implies increasing intracranial pressure. Rapid pulse with marked hypotension and irregularity of respiration may reflect disturbed brain stem function, as occurs with occipital fractures involving the foramen magnum; these alterations may lead to fulminant pulmonary edema. But the same combination of findings in an injured child always should raise the question of occult hemorrhage, ruptured viscus, aspiration, sepsis, or massive fat embolization.

In the young infant, bleeding into the subdural space may be of such magnitude as to lower the hematocrit significantly; in such circumstances the associated increase in intracranial pressure should produce obvious evidence of the probable site of bleeding. The signs of acute subdural hemorrhage may include vomiting, enlarging head size, full fontanelle, squint, and retinal hemorrhage. In older children, the volume of blood lost into the cranial cavity is usually insignificant.

Although the relative fixation of the cranial bones at the suture lines precludes a significant increase in head size, other signs of increased intracranial pressure should be evident. In the absence of significant intracranial hemorrhage, the prompt increase in intracranial pressure which all too frequently follows head trauma in children has been related to rapidly developing cerebral swelling ("flash edema").[9] Careful assessment of responsiveness and of pupillary size can give important additional signs of such an increase in pressure. Surprisingly, perhaps, the significance of pupillary changes, always stressed in the evaluation of raised intracranial pressure, is incompletely understood by physicians. A dilated pupil, poorly reactive or unreactive to light, most often indicates compression of the third nerve on that side by the herniating mesial portion of the temporal lobe through the incisura of the tentorium, caused by increased pressure. While this may be due to cerebral edema as well as to intracranial hematoma, the latter surgically remediable lesion should be kept foremost in mind and appropriate contrast studies performed to verify its presence. This pupillary finding is often accompanied by paresis of the oculomotor nerve on the same side and contralateral, ipsilateral, or bilateral body weakness or intermittent decerebrate posturing.

It is important to be certain that no one has instilled a mydriatic preparation into the conjunctival sac before concluding that the above circumstances apply. In general mydriatic drugs should be avoided; but if administered, a sign should be placed on the patient's bed and in his chart to make this fact clear to all those involved in his care. The dilation of one pupil may also occur during a seizure.[10] Conjugate jerking of the eyes away from the side of the seizure discharge often accompanies the pupillary dilation which may occur on either the contralateral or ipsilateral side. The intravenous administration of an anticonvulsant, such as diazepam (Valium), may result in prompt equalization of pupillary size, cessation of the ocular jerking, and return to consciousness of the patient. Direct injury to the eye, or to the second or third cranial nerve, may also result in a dilated and poorly reactive pupil.

Bleeding into the subarachnoid or subdural spaces may be suggested by retinal or preretinal hemorrhages. These usually develop in the face of a marked increase in intracranial pressure and may be coupled with venous distention and early signs of papilledema. Well-developed papilledema is usually not seen within the first hours or days of injury. When it is, associated but unrelated cerebral lesions, e.g., brain tumor, must be considered. Spontaneous pulsations of the retinal veins usually reflect normal intracranial pressure, particularly if the systemic blood pressure is not elevated, and may be a reassuring finding in the child with head injury.

SPECIAL TESTS

After a thorough clinical evaluation, skull and other roentgenograms are usually indicated, especially if the patient lost consciousness following the injury. If hyperextension or flexion injury to the cervical spine is a consideration, appropriate x-ray films of this region should be obtained. Cervical cord injury is not uncommon following severe, blunt head injury and should be considered even in the absence of recognizable spinal fracture.

In the infant or young child, paracentesis of the subdural spaces through the coronal sutures may establish the presence of an extracerebral clot. Acute epidural or subdural hemorrhages are not associated with increased transillumination; rather there is usually less of a glow about the rim of the light in such circumstances. Only when the subdural hematoma undergoes dissolution and the fluid becomes less turbid, and eventually xanthochromic, is excessive transillumination found.

Electroencephalography is not particularly helpful as an emergency procedure but may become so in the acute period after head injury, to define a focal destructive lesion or seizure activity, thus confirming or supplementing the clinical impression and assisting in the design of appropriate therapy. Echoencephalography (the recording of an ultrasonic echo from the interface of intracerebral structures normally midline), considered by some to be useful in the management of head injury, has been of limited value in our experience. Isotopic scan techniques similarly have contributed relatively little to diagnosis. Lumbar puncture is inadvisable as a routine procedure following craniocerebral injury but may be necessary when the diagnosis is obscure and should be performed if intracranial sepsis, especially meningitis, is a serious diagnostic consideration, as noted earlier. Cerebral angiography may contribute much to the diagnosis and management. In particular, extra- or intracerebral hemorrhages may be outlined by this technique or, equally important, their presence rendered unlikely. It is self-evident that these special tests must be performed by physicians experienced in their use.

MANAGEMENT

The majority of infants and children who have not lost consciousness following head injury can be cared for by their parents, after a careful examination satisfies the physician that no serious intracranial injury exists. Those patients who have focal or diffuse neurological disturbances and all who have been rendered unconscious for a period of time, with or without an associated skull fracture, should be hospitalized until their condition is stable and the neurological signs are abating.

In the obtunded or comatose patient, intravenous fluids may be necessary, particularly if vomiting persists. Maintenance fluids of a balanced electrolyte solution such as 5 per cent dextrose and Isolyte-M should be restricted to 1000 to 1200 cc per square meter of body surface area per day. This solution, although hypotonic after metabolism of the glucose, has proved to be safe if the volume administered is monitored carefully. The primary purpose of restricting fluids is to avoid hypotonicity which will aggravate brain swelling, so common after trauma. Accurate recording of fluid intake and output, daily weights, and serum osmolalities (the serum sodium level in mEq/L × 2 plus 10 approximates the osmolality) should be followed closely. When nonionic solutes such as urea, glucose, or mannitol have been administered, the serum sodium does not reflect accurately the osmolality, and the determination of serum osmolalities is essential. These data are absolutely necessary to avoid weight gain from water retention, excessive dehydration, and states of hypotonicity or hypertonicity. Hypertonicity may also occur when injury to the hypothalamus or pituitary stalk has produced diabetes insipidus. As stated earlier, this is usually a transient disorder. Sedatives and hypnotics should be avoided although persistent vomiting may be treated with an appropriate antiemetic such as trimethobenzamide hydrochloride (Tigan).

Certain problems will require further consideration by the neurosurgeon. With skull fracture, rhinorrhea persists more commonly as a clinical problem than does otorrhea and may require surgical repair of the anatomical defect. Of course, the risk of intracranial infection remains as long as the defect exists. Depressed fractures should be referred to the neurosurgeon for possible elevation. Compound fractures require prompt surgical treatment, with débridement and removal of bone fragments, hair, and other foreign· material which predisposes to intracranial infection.

When serial examinations suggest that the intracranial pressure is increasing significantly, various measures to minimize this complication should be employed. Glucocorticoids, hyperosmolar agents, and assisted ventilation may help forestall herniation of cerebral tissue at either the tentorial opening or foramen magnum.

Dexamethasone (Decadron) and methylprednisolone sodium succinate (Solu-Medrol) are the two glucocorticoids most commonly used; Decadron is administered usually in a dose of 10 to 12 mg and Solu-Medrol in a dose of 40 to 50 mg per square meter of body surface area per day in four divided doses intramuscularly.[11, 12] One half of the first day's dose is usually given in the initial injection. Recent evidence suggests that glucocorticoids act primarily on the normal brain tissue to prevent cellular decompensation and increasing cerebral edema.[13]

Hyperosmolar agents are used to develop a transient osmotic gradient between the blood and the brain which will cause water to move from the brain tissues into the blood. Water moves from other cells as well, and the result is an expanded extracellular (including the vascular) space. Under usual circumstances the solute and water are excreted by the kidneys. Urea, as a smaller molecule, enters cells more rapidly than does mannitol; therefore, if urea is used a higher osmolality must be achieved in the blood to effect comparable shifts of water from the brain. Mannitol, readily available for intravenous infusion as a 20 per cent solution (Osmitrol), contains 1.1 milliosmols per ml. To increase the serum osmolality approximately 10 to 20 milliosmols per liter, it is given in a dosage of 2 to 3 gm per kilogram of body weight. Urea, stored as a lyophilized crystal, must be reconstituted with a 10 per cent invert sugar solution before it can be administered; also it is usually necessary to warm the solution to facilitate solubilizing the urea crystals. After reconstitution, urea represents a 30 per cent solution containing 5.8 milliosmols per ml, and is infused at a dosage of 1 to 1.5 gm per kilogram of body weight. Intravenous infusion time should be 45 to 60 minutes with mannitol or urea. Too rapid a rate of infusion of these hyperosmolar solutions may produce a sudden increase in the intravascular volume with resulting cardiac decompensation. Also, following infusion of these substances, a brisk diuresis develops and catheterization of the bladder may be necessary to prevent acute urinary retention in the unconscious patient.

The hyperosmolar solutions are most effective when the integrity of cerebral blood vessels has been maintained. Both urea and mannitol normally pass through these vessels into the cerebral tissue to some extent; after clearance of these substances by the kidneys, the resulting increased osmolality of the cerebral tissue draws water back into the brain, transiently increasing the intracranial pressure—the so-called rebound phenomenon. Risk of this is increased in extensive injury to cerebral blood vessels, when hyperosmolar solutions may pass more readily from the intravascular compartment into surrounding brain tissue.

The technique of assisted ventilation also can reduce the intracranial pressure transiently by producing cerebral vasoconstriction, thereby decreasing the size of the vascular compartment. Through this mechanism of action, brain perfusion is reduced, together with the intracranial pressure which could accentuate the injury to brain tissue by enhancing the cerebral ischemia and resulting tissue anoxia.

When the clinical situation dictates emergency treatment—and action cannot be delayed while the precise nature or extent of the intracranial pathology is delineated—it is justified to utilize such temporizing maneuvers, despite the theoretical limitations of each method, until additional studies can be performed to define surgically remediable lesions. Extracerebral and intracerebral hematomas can be evacuated with very gratifying results. Unfortunately, there is no generally accepted surgical treatment for extensive contusion or laceration of brain substance or for cerebral edema.

Other proposed adjuncts to treatment include the lowering of the body temperature to decrease the metabolic requirements of compromised cerebral tissue and the use of anticonvulsants. Hypothermia, to be truly effective in this regard, would require lowering of the body core temperature to 90 to 92°F, a level usually resulting in violent shivering and heightened metabolic activity which nullifies the advantage sought in the treatment. Drugs such as promethazine hydrochloride (Phenergan) or chlorpromazine (Thorazine) will eliminate the shivering reflex but will frequently depress the level of consciousness and further accentuate any hypotensive tendency. Furthermore, at these low body temperatures, one can expect increasing cardiac irritability with the possibility of a serious arrhythmia. We therefore strive simply to keep the patient afebrile.

Although anticonvulsants probably do not lessen the liability to post-traumatic epilepsy, we advocate their use in severe head injury in which cerebral contusion or laceration is suspected, because of the impression that such therapy minimizes the occurrence of seizures during the immediate post-injury period. Either diphenylhydantoin sodium (Dilantin) at a dosage of 5 mg per kilogram of body weight per day, or phenobarbital at 4 mg per kilogram per day, is an acceptable drug, although the former is less likely to obtund the patient.

PROGNOSIS

Children as a group demonstrate a remarkable capacity for recovery even when substantial neurological disturbances follow acute head injury. In general, the total duration of post-traumatic amnesia can be correlated directly with the degree of brain damage, and as Smith[14] has concluded, with the ultimate prognosis. The long-term effects of severe closed head injury and protracted coma have been summarized by Richardson.[15] He evaluated 10 children, comatose for 7 to 47 days following severe head injury, with post-traumatic amnesia ranging from 25 to 65 days. All were rehabilitated and returned to school in the community despite substantial residual neurological and psychological deficits. Persisting specific defects in rote memory were demonstrated in most of these children on formal psychometric testing. In a larger and less severely injured group, Dencker examined 117 head-injured children, removed on the average 10 years from the acute injury, and as a control their uninjured twins; he failed to demonstrate any difference in the psychometric scores, range of symptoms, electroencephalograms, or personality integration.[16] This study further substantiates the capacity of the young child to recover after significant closed craniocerebral injury.

This capacity for functional recovery must be remembered when evaluating any program of physical rehabilitation. Many sophisticated programs have been credited with the quality and quantity of recovery in the injured child, and as such, have unjustifiably increased the total financial expense incurred by parents. Yet there is no evidence that elaborate and time-consuming programs of physiotherapy offer any more than do simple passive and active range of motion exercises to minimize joint contractures and maintain muscle tone and strength.

The possibility of post-traumatic epilepsy is largely dependent on the site of injury. Certain areas of the brain, when damaged, give rise to epileptogenic foci more frequently than do others. The most vulnerable areas include the cortex of the medial temporal, posterior frontal, and anterior parietal lobes. In the given case the site of injury appears more important in the etiology of post-traumatic epilepsy than does an underlying genetic predisposition.[17] The incidence of post-traumatic epilepsy following closed head injury is probably less than 10 per cent. Patients with evidence of significant contusions or lacerations are especially prone to this complication. Those suffering from seizures at or shortly after injury are no more likely to develop post-traumatic epilepsy than are others who have sustained comparable lesions without fits during the immediate post-traumatic period.

Electroencephalography is of little help in anticipating which children ultimately will develop a seizure disorder. Though many EEG recordings are focally or diffusely disordered and may show epileptiform activity during the acute period, serial tracings usually show a gradual return towards a more normal pattern. Occasionally, an abnormal electroencephalogram with some epileptiform activity persists in a clinically asymptomatic patient; conversely, a large percentage of patients with post-traumatic epilepsy demonstrate a relatively normal EEG between seizures.

Chronic subdural effusions represent a major problem because of the lack of any uniformly effective treatment. Diagnostically, such a lesion may be suspected in a child whose head is increasing too rapidly in circumference, particularly if the contour is brachycephalic and transillumination shows a marked increase in the glow of light. The outcome in such cases appears to correlate primarily with the extent of damage sustained by the underlying cerebral substance during the acute head injury.[18] This realization, coupled with the knowledge that the efficacy of all forms of treatment remains unproved, encourages us to be conservative in our approach, and to attempt only to discourage disproportionate increases in head size by periodic paracentesis.

Enlarging skull fractures associated with leptomeningeal cysts or erosion of the skull occur in a small minority of children who have suffered acute head injury. Taveras and Ransohoff have suggested that rupture of the dura mater during the acute injury, with herniation of the arachnoid membrane into the fracture line, produces this condition.[19] Aided by the normal pulsations of the brain, this entrapped arachnoidal hernia gradually erodes the edge of the bone and may also compress the underlying cerebral cortex.

In conclusion, it should be pointed out that much of the management of the patient with acute head injury has been arrived at empirically, and many of the clinical regimens suggested, including the choice and dose of various therapeutic agents, are arbitrary. Ritualistic adherence to any particular program will only serve to perpetuate our state of ignorance and preclude further clarification of the problems which attend head injury. As is true of so many areas of medicine, clinical and basic research are sorely needed in relation to common problems associated with head injury.

REFERENCES

1. Mealey, J., Jr.: Pediatric Head Injuries. Springfield, Ill., Charles C Thomas, 1968, Chapter 1.
2. Denny-Brown, D., and Russell, W. R.: Experimental cerebral concussion. Brain, *64*:93, 1941.
3. Strich, S. J.: Shearing of nerve fibers as a cause of brain damage due to head injury. A pathological study of twenty cases. Lancet, *2*:443, 1961.
4. Dodge, P. R.: Tangential wounds of scalp and skull. *In* Neurological Surgery of

Trauma, edited by L. D. Heaton, J. B. Coates, Jr., and A. M. Meirowsky. Washington, D.C., U.S. Government Printing Office, 1965, pp. 143–159.

5. Friede, R. L.: Experimental acceleration concussion. Arch. Neurol., *4*:449, 1961.

6. Friede, R. L.: Specific cord damage at the atlas level as a pathogenic mechanism in cerebral concussion. J. Neuropath. Exp. Neurol., *29*:266, 1960.

7. Ward, A. A., Jr.: The physiology of concussion. In Head Injury, Conference Proceedings, edited by W. F. Caveness and A. E. Walker. Philadelphia, J. B. Lippincott, 1966, pp. 203–208.

8. Griffith, J. F., and Dodge, P. R.: Transient blindness following head injury in children. New Eng. J. Med., *278*:648, 1968.

9. Pickles, W.: Acute focal edema of the brain in children with head injuries. New Eng. J. Med., *240*:92, 1949.

10. Pant, S. S., Benton, J. W., and Dodge, P. R.: Unilateral pupillary dilatation during and immediately following seizures. Neurology, *16*:837, 1966.

11. Sparacio, R. R., Lin, T. H., and Cook, A. W.: Methylprednisolone sodium succinate in acute craniocerebral trauma. Surg. Gynec. Obst., *121*:513, 1965.

12. Long, D. M., Hartmann, J. F., and French, L. A.: The response of experimental cerebral edema to glucosteroid administration. J. Neurosurg., *24*:843, 1966.

13. McLaurin, R. L.: Some metabolic aspects of head injury. *In* Head Injury, Conference Proceedings, edited by W. F. Caveness and A. E. Walker. Philadelphia, J. B. Lippincott, 1966, pp. 142–157.

14. Smith, A.: Duration of impaired consciousness as an index of severity in closed head injuries. Dis. Nerv. Syst., *22*:69, 1961.

15. Richardson, F.: Some effects of severe head injury. A follow-up study of children and adolescents after protracted coma. Develop. Med. Child. Neurol., *5*:471, 1963.

16. Dencker, S. J.: Closed head injury in twins. Arch. Gen. Psychiat., *2*:569, 1960.

17. Marshall, C., and Walker, A. E.: The value of electroencephalography in the prognostication and prognosis of post-traumatic epilepsy. Epilepsia (Amster.), *2*:138, 1961.

18. Rabe, E. F., Flynn, R. E., and Dodge, P. R.: Subdural collections of fluid in infants and children. Neurology, *18*:559, 1968.

19. Taveras, J. M., and Ransohoff, J.: Leptomeningeal cysts of the brain following trauma with erosion of the skull: a study of 7 cases treated by surgery. J. Neurosurg., *10*:233, 1953.

6

Status Epilepticus

Sidney Carter, M.D., and Arnold P. Gold, M.D.

Status epilepticus is the clinical definition of a state in which the patient has a series of recurrent convulsions without recovering consciousness between episodes.[1] It can occur with any seizure type, but a true medical emergency usually exists only with the generalized or focal motor varieties of status epilepticus. This definition of status epilepticus clearly exclude epilepsia partialis continua, in which there is no alteration of the state of consciousness, and serial epilepsy, in which consciousness is regained between attacks.

Petit mal status epilepticus is characterized by a prolonged blurring of the state of consciousness lasting minutes to hours, during which there may be repetitive movements of the mouth and eyelids. The EEG shows continuous discharges of the characteristic 3 per second spike and wave variety. In some epileptic children status epilepticus may be manifested only by behavioral changes that mimic psychotic or retarded states.

Status epilepticus occurs in 5 to 10 per cent of children with epilepsy and may result in postepileptic paralysis or psychosis.[2] It requires immediate and continued medical attention, for, if uncontrolled, death or permanent neuronal damage could result. Death occurs in approxi-

---

From the Division of Pediatric Neurology, Department of Neurology, Columbia University, College of Physicians and Surgeons, New York, New York.

mately 15 per cent of patients and may either be related directly to status epilepticus or, as emphasized by Lombroso,[3] may result from the untoward effect of intravenous sedatives or hypnotic compounds on the already depressed medullary centers. The immature nervous system is particularly vulnerable to status epilepticus; in one recently reported study, slightly over 50 per cent of the children were 2 years of age or less.[4] Prompt management is mandatory, as both the neurologic residua from irreversible cerebral damage and mortality are higher in this young age group.

The true pathophysiology of status epilepticus is poorly understood. However, the condition is more common in children with symptomatic epilepsy of infectious, metabolic, vascular, or structural etiology than in those with the so-called idiopathic variety. Status epilepticus may be the initial manifestation of meningitis or encephalitis, hypertensive encephalopathy, uremia, or acute electrolyte disturbances such as hyponatremia. Rapid or sudden withdrawal of anticonvulsants and intercurrent infections are the common triggering mechanisms. Injudicious withdrawal of drugs, either prior to an electroencephalogram or after a seizure-free state of relatively short duration, and a sudden change in the anticonvulsant regimen, are frequent precipitating factors.

MANAGEMENT

Status epilepticus must be considered a life-threatening condition which requires immediate treatment. The four essential steps in management are: (1) suppression of convulsions as rapidly as possible, (2) general supportive measures, (3) initiation of daily maintenance therapy, and (4) concomitant investigation of the condition responsible for the status epilepticus.

Suppressive Therapy

Suppressive therapy is of primary importance and is an indication for the immediate use of intravenous anticonvulsants. Specific compounds must always be given in amounts large enough to arrest all seizure activity. Common errors include the administration of the drug by the intramuscular route and use of small aliquots with resultant toxicity and continued status. A variety of agents have been used in the treatment of grand mal and focal motor status epilepticus. These range from barbiturates, hydantoins, local anesthestic agents, and paraldehyde to hypertonic solutions of glucose and urea. Petit mal status epilepticus has been treated by trimethadione (Tridione) and inhalation of 10 to 20 per cent carbon dioxide. Traditionally, sodium phenobarbital (10 mg/kg) and paraldehyde in a 4 per cent solution have been the drugs of choice. Diazepam (Valium) has largely replaced both these agents and should now be employed as the initial anticonvulsant in the management of all types of status epilepticus.[5-11] It has the capacity to suppress seizure activity within minutes, and the untoward effects, respiratory depression and hypotension, are rare.

Generally, 0.3 mg/kg of diazepam, with a maximum dose of 10 mg, is both safe and effective when administered by slow intravenous injection over a period of 1 to 2 minutes. Diazepam is commercially dispensed in 10 mg quantities in 2 ml of buffered solution. Cessation of seizures may occur before the total anticipated dose is administered. If the first dose is ineffective, the same quantity should be readministered in a similar fashion after a period of 15 minutes. When diazepam is ineffective, sodium phenobarbital or 4 per cent paraldehyde, or both, should be given intravenously in sufficient quantities to control all seizure activity. Respiratory depression and hypotension may occur when parenteral paraldehyde or phenobarbital is administered in addition to Valium. Diazepam, as presently available in its injectible form, is a potent bilirubin-albumin encoupler. It is of interest that the diazepam itself is not responsible for this uncoupling of bilirubin but rather the benzoic acid, as found in the stabilizer preservative. This hyperbilirubinemic effect poses a risk above all others to the neonate in status epilepticus.[12] When parenteral suppressive measures fail, it may be necessary to use volatile anesthetics.

On occasion specific therapeutic measures are indicated. Hypertonic sodium chloride is essential in the management of hyponatremic convulsions, calcium solutions in hypocalcemic seizures, and hypertonic glucose in hypoglycemic states.

Supportive Therapy

On arrival at the hospital the child, often in coma with failing vital signs, requires a vigorous program of supportive therapy. Ideally, such children are best managed in a pediatric intensive care unit. General supportive measures include maintaining an adequate airway, administration of oxygen, and intravenous hydration. Close observation is essential, and impending respiratory failure is an indication for tracheostomy and the use of an artificial respirator. Antibiotics are not used prophylactically but are employed if specific infectious conditions are delineated.

Maintenance Therapy

Concomitant with the acute emergency therapy of status epilepticus, long-acting drugs, preferably diphenylhydantoin sodium (Dilantin), 5 mg/kg, should be initiated by the intramuscular route. Once the child is able to swallow, these long-acting compounds should be given orally in divided doses. Ethosuximide (Zarontin) is the drug of choice in the treatment of petit mal. Children 5 to 10 years of age usually require 250 mg two to four times a day.

Investigation of the Etiologic Factors

This phase of the management is initiated almost immediately in order to determine those conditions which require specific therapy other than anticonvulsants. Blood samples are drawn for determination of electrolytes, glucose, calcium, and blood urea nitrogen. Cerebrospinal fluid is examined for inflammatory disease. Toxic conditions, above all lead poisoning, should be ruled out by appropriate tests. The other less common causes of status epilepticus are usually investigated when seizure control has been attained.

Electroencephalography is not essential in the acute management of status epilepticus but may be helpful when petit mal status is suspected. Subsequent investigations are designed to delineate an etiologic factor responsible for the convulsive disorder and the associated status epilepticus. These include skull x-rays, electroencephalograms, echoventriculograms, brain scans, and, on rare occasions, contrast studies such as pneumoencephalograms and cerebral arteriograms.

References

1. Schmidt, R. P., and Wilder, B. J.: Epilepsy. Contemporary Neurology Series, Vol. 2. Philadelphia, F. A. Davis Company, 1968.
2. Hunter, R. A.: Status epilepticus — history, incidence and problems. Epilepsia, *1*:162, 1959.
3. Lombroso, C. T.: Treatment of status epilepticus with diazepam. Neurology, *16*:629, 1966.
4. Calderon-Gonzales, R., and Mireles-Gonzales, A.: Management of prolonged motor seizure activity in children. J.A.M.A., *204*:544, 1968.
5. Gordon, N. S.: Treatment of status epilepticus with diazepam. Develop. Med. Child Neurol., *8*:668, 1966.
6. Prensky, A. L., Raff, M. C., Moore, M. J., and Schwab, R. S.: Intravenous diazepam in the treatment of prolonged seizure activity. New Eng. J. Med., *276*:779, 1967.
7. Lalji, D., Hosking, C. S., and Sutherland, J. M.: Diazepam (Valium) in the control of status epilepticus. Med. J. Aust., *1*:542, 1967.
8. Bailey, D. W., and Fenichel, G. M.: Treatment of prolonged seizure activity with intravenous diazepam. J. Pediat., *73*:923, 1968.
9. Sawyer, G. T., Webster, D. D., and Schut, L. J.: Treatment of uncontrolled seizure activity with diazepam. J.A.M.A., *203*:913, 1968.
10. Brett, E. M.: Diazepam — the new wonder drug. Develop. Med. Child. Neurol., *12*:655, 1970.
11. Tutton, J. C.: Status epilepticus treatment with diazepam. N. Y. State J. Med., *70*: 2425, 1970.
12. Schiff, D., Chan, G., and Stern, L.: Fixed drug combinations and the displacement of bilirubin from albumin. Pediatrics, *48*:139, 1971.

7

Acute Bacterial Meningitis

Paul F. Wehrle, M.D., Allen W. Mathies, Jr., M.D., Ph.D. and John M. Leedom, M.D.

Although many of the serious and life-threatening infectious diseases of childhood have been controlled, no effective preventive approach is presently available for bacterial meningitis. Reduction of disability and death due to this important group of infections is dependent upon early clinical recognition of the disease, accurate and specific laboratory diagnosis, vigorous supportive and antimicrobial therapy, and subsequent attention to rehabilitative measures. Despite improvements in both antimicrobial and supportive treatment, meningitis remains one of the most serious of the infectious diseases and should be regarded as a true medical emergency.

The most common cause of bacterial meningitis is *Hemophilus influenzae*, type B. This organism, *Neisseria meningitidis*, and *Diplococcus pneumoniae* are responsible for an overwhelming proportion of cases of

From the Departments of Pediatrics and Medicine, University of Southern California School of Medicine, the Communicable Disease Service, Los Angeles County–University of Southern California Medical Center, and the Hastings Foundation Infectious Disease Laboratory. This work was supported in part by U.S. Army Medical Research and Development Command, Department of the Army, under research contract DA-49-193-MD-2874, under the sponsorship of the Commission on Acute Respiratory Diseases of the Armed Forces Epidemiological Board; Training Grant AI-00275 from The National Institutes of Health; and the Hastings Foundation Fund.

TABLE 1   ORGANISMS RECOVERED FROM PATIENTS WITH ACUTE BACTERIAL MENINGITIS OF KNOWN ETIOLOGY*

Age Group	H. influenzae	Meningo-cocci	Pneumo-cocci	E. coli	Klebsiella–Aerobacter	Strepto-cocci	Miscel-laneous	Total†
<2 mo	9	1	6	62	23	22	40	163
2–11 mo	266	67	63	3	.....	4	12	415
1–4 yr	359	126	49	3	2	6	3	548
5–14 yr	41	74	39	.....	.....	.....	6	160
15+ yr	19	160	205	12	4	17	25	442
TOTAL	694	428	362	80	29	49	86	1728

*Periods considered: July 1, 1963–December 31, 1970, for ages 2 months and over; 1961–1970 data for <2 months group. Study performed at Los Angeles County–University of Southern California Medical Center.

†Total does not include an additional 302 patients with purulent meningitis partially treated prior to admission from whom no organism was recovered.

purulent meningitis in patients older than 2 months of age. These three organisms are the "usual" causes of bacterial meningitis. Occasionally other bacteria, which might be called "unusual" organisms, are found in patients more than 2 months of age. However, clinical features detectable at the time of admission, such as lesions permitting direct communication with the dura, endocarditis, immunological defects or other underlying diseases, should alert the clinician to suspect "unusual" organisms. In the neonatal period *Escherichia coli,* other enteric bacteria, and other organisms are found which do not commonly cause meningitis in older patients. The relative frequency of various causes of acute bacterial meningitis by age is shown in Table 1.

CLINICAL RECOGNITION

The clinical symptoms and signs characteristically associated with meningeal irritation, such as nuchal rigidity and postive Kernig and Brudzinski signs, are frequently absent in young infants and in children with fulminant or overwhelming disease. In infants, a high-pitched cry, fretfulness or irritability, frowning, poor feeding, or vomiting, together with fullness of the fontanelle, may be the only signs leading the physician to suspect meningitis. The frequent absence of fever, definite meningeal signs, or definite bulging of the fontanelle presents a particular problem in clinical diagnosis during early infancy.

The clinical symptomatology is more consistent in older infants and children. Fever, headache, and vomiting, together with the customary signs of meningeal irritation, are often the presenting complaints. At times the presence of cranial bruits, a recently described clinical sign,[1] may be helpful in the diagnosis. Fulminant illness, accompanied by convulsions, coma, and shock, is seen with greatest frequency in meningococcal infections. These grave signs are also seen with other types of meningitis, but they are not characteristically associated with fulminant disease, as in meningococcal infections. Indeed, they are apt to supervene if recognition and proper therapy of the early stages of the infections are delayed.

An exanthem is seen in two thirds of children with meningococcal disease and is usually most evident on the lower extremities. Although the skin lesions are typically petechial when fully developed, an evanescent morbilliform rash may appear initially. Rarely, skin lesions resembling erythema nodosum have been observed. Purpuric lesions, ranging in size from a few millimeters to many centimeters in diameter, are seen in fulminant cases of the disease. Petechiae or purpura may appear during the course of the acute meningococcemia, before definite clinical invasion of the meninges has occurred. Bullous lesions are infrequent but do occur. They usually appear after at least 24 hours of illness and are most frequently found adjacent to the larger purpuric areas. It should be noted that petechial skin lesions and purulent meningitis are not diagnostic of meningococcal disease. Meningitis and petechial skin lesions sometimes accompany endocarditis (particularly prominent in the acute staphylococcal variety) and are less common concomitants of severe sepsis due to other organisms.

Joint involvement occurs in about 5 per cent of patients with meningococcal disease. A few patients, particularly those with fulminant disease, present with arthritis of multiple joints due to direct seeding of the synovia with organisms. More characteristic, and presenting a diagnostic and therapeutic dilemma to the uninformed, is arthritis with onset late in the first week of the illness. Pain and sterile effusion, usually involving a single large joint, is characteristic. Fever may persist or return. Neither type of meningococcal arthritis requires special treatment; both subside within 2 weeks, and late sequelae are unknown. Arthritis may occur as a septicemic complication in bacterial meningitis due to other organisms. These arthritides are quite different from those due to the meningococcal infections. They are purulent arthritides; there is active replication of bacteria in the joint space; and prompt drainage (open or closed) is necessary to prevent sequelae.

Presence of Underlying Disease

The evaluation of the patient must include a careful history with special emphasis on evidence of prior trauma, particularly skull fracture, other mechanical defects of the dura, localized infections, and immunological defects. Meningitides in patients with prior skull fractures and two or more attacks of purulent meningitis are most frequently pneumococcal in etiology, as are those associated with mastoiditis and sickle cell disease.[2] The presence of acute endocarditis, particularly with a petechial rash, suggests staphylococcal or streptococcal meningitis. Communicating dermal sinuses and prior neurosurgical procedures, particularly those involving insertion of a foreign body, seem particularly likely to be associated with staphylococcal meningitis, often due to coagulase-negative organisms. Infections in patients with ruptured meningomyeloceles, and those with immunological defects are likely to be due to "unusual" organisms, often those found in the enteric flora, or associated with the hospital environment.

Specific Diagnosis

Blood and cerebrospinal fluid (CSF) cultures should be obtained when the patient is first suspected of having meningitis and before antibiotic therapy has been initiated. Determination of the cell count, type of cells present, glucose and protein content of the CSF, plus gram stain of sedimented CSF, will indicate in most instances the type of infection present (Table 2). Exceptions to the findings listed in Table 2 may occur. Patients with acute meningococcemia may present to the physician prior to invasion of the central nervous system. In overwhelming pneumococcal infections of the newborn and older individuals with impaired resistance, organisms may be present without cellular response or a decrease in glucose.

The direct examination of CSF, using the gram-stain technique on sediment, is particularly important as it provides a presumptive-specific diagnosis in approximately two thirds of patients at the time of admission to the hospital. This examination should be completed, regardless of cell count, since bacteria may be present without cellular response. The use of fluorescent antibody techniques, while theoretically providing additional accuracy, does not significantly improve the frequency or accuracy of clinical diagnosis in laboratories with experienced person-

**TABLE 2   DIFFERENTIAL CHARACTERISTICS OF CEREBROSPINAL FLUID
IN MENINGITIS OF VARIOUS ETIOLOGIES**

CSF Findings	Type of Meningitis		
	Bacterial	AFB and Fungi	Viral
Total Cells	High: 500 to several thousand	Low: usually <500	Low: usually <500
Cell Type	Predominantly neutrophils	Predominantly mononuclear	Predominantly mononuclear
Glucose	Low	Low	Normal
Protein	Elevated	Elevated	Elevated
Organisms	Present*	Present*	Absent

*Present—usually detectable by microscopic examination of CSF sediments or by cultural techniques.

nel,[3] although it may permit a rapid specific diagnosis in individual instances. If *H. influenzae* is suspected after examination of the gram stain, a quellung reaction should be attempted by use of type-specific antiserum.

Gram-stained smears of scrapings from petechial lesions will frequently provide presumptive-specific bacteriologic diagnosis upon admission to the hospital.

SUPPORTIVE THERAPY

Blood pressure must be monitored frequently; if instability of the blood pressure is noted, an indwelling central venous catheter should be inserted. Rapid infusion of fluids (saline, albumin, dextran, or blood) will frequently restore an effective arterial circulation. If central venous pressure increases without concomitant improvement in arterial circulation, isoproterenol by intravenous drip may lead to restoration of the arterial blood pressure. Digitalis may be helpful in those patients not responding to this approach.

While pharmacologic doses of hydrocortisone or other glucocorticoids have been suggested (and data are available indicating their effect in the restoration of arterial circulation), satisfactory data indicating increased survival after their administration are not yet available. Low plasma cortisol levels have been observed in children with adrenal hemorrhage,[4] but clinical benefit from replacement therapy has not been established.

Attention to the maintenance of an adequate airway is essential. Tracheostomy or assisted ventilation or both are occasionally required.

Cerebral edema represents a serious problem and does not respond as well to urea or mannitol therapy as does edema following acute brain trauma. If either of these agents is used, full therapeutic doses are required, and relatively rapid infusion is suggested to insure maximum diuresis. Attention to electrolyte balance is particularly important in patients in whom extensive diuresis has been induced. Dexamethasone also appears to be of no definite value in reducing cerebral edema associated with infection.

Persistent fever may indicate continued sepsis, brain abscess formation, improper therapy, subdural effusion, lateral sinus thrombosis, sinusitis, mastoiditis, or localized tissue necrosis (particularly at the sites of large ecchymotic lesions in meningococcal disease). Persistent fever may also indicate nosocomial infections, such as urinary tract infections (in patients who have been catheterized during their acute illnesses), or pneumonia (most frequently after aspiration and in those patients requiring respiratory assistance). Drug fever, perhaps the most frequently overlooked cause of persistent fever, is readily suspected when fever returns after the fourth day. The patient does not appear toxic, lacks localizing signs, and none of the readily diagnosed causes noted here are found. The impression may be confirmed by discontinuing or changing therapy, with the prompt return of the temperature to normal levels.

Diffuse intravascular clotting has been described in meningococcal disease.[5-7] This phenomenon is associated with poor prognosis; and, while the clotting defect may be corrected by the use of heparin, there is a lack of convincing clinical evidence proving that such therapy is beneficial.

Obstruction to spinal fluid flow with resultant hydrocephalus occurs occasionally. While enzymes of various types (e.g., plasmin activators such as streptokinase) can produce lysis of fibrin clots, insufficient experimental data are available to justify their intrathecal use, even with grossly purulent CSF.

Hypothermia has also been suggested by some. Insufficient data are available indicating potential benefit to justify the real hazard of this procedure when used in an acutely ill child.

SPECIFIC ANTIMICROBIAL THERAPY

In the selection of specific therapy for an individual with meningitis, three patient categories should be considered: (1) infants less than 2 months of age, (2) "normal" individuals more than 2 months of age who have no underlying diseases, and (3) individuals more than 2 months of age who have underlying or concomitant diseases known to be associated with an increased frequency of "unusual" organisms. The antibiotic regimens suggested for the first two categories are depicted in Table 3. Ex-

TABLE 3 SUGGESTED THERAPY FOR MENINGITIS IN PATIENTS WITHOUT EVIDENT IMMUNOLOGICAL OR MECHANICAL DEFECT OR UNDERLYING DISEASE

Age of Patient	Initial Therapy (Until Organism Identified)	Definitive Therapy (After Organism Identified)
< 2 mo.	Ampicillin,* 75–150 mg/kg/day I.V. plus kanamycin sulfate, 15 mg/kg/day (or gentamicin sulfate, 5 mg/kg/day)	Dependent upon specific susceptibilities of organisms
2 mo. and older	Ampicillin 150 mg/kg/day I.V.	Meningococci – Penicillin G or ampicillin Pneumococci – Penicillin G or ampicillin *H. Influenzae* – Ampicillin Purulent unknown – Ampicillin

*Must be given intravenously. One-third of estimated daily dose by rapid I.V. infusion followed by 1/6 of daily dose by rapid I.V. infusion at 4 hour intervals. Dose is 75 mg/kg/day during the first week of life – 150 mg/kg/day thereafter.

ceptions to these recommendations and therapy for patients in the third category are discussed in the following paragraphs.

For infants less than 2 months of age, and for those patients more than 2 months old in whom there is reason to suspect the presence of "unusual" organisms, initial therapy must include one of the penicillins, usually ampicillin together with another drug, preferably kanamycin sulfate. (Methicillin should be substituted for ampicillin if staphylococcal disease is suspected.) Gentamicin has shown some promise as a replacement for kanamycin sulfate in these regimens,[8] but judgment as to its relative efficacy in comparison with kanamycin sulfate must be reserved at this time. Since serum levels of gentamicin sulfate do not appear to be as predictable as those of kanamycin sulfate, monitoring of levels may be necessary. After identification and specific antimicrobial susceptibility testing of an etiologic organism has been accomplished, the use of two drugs should be interrupted. Therapy should then be continued with the single least toxic drug demonstrated to be effective against the organism *in vitro.* Demonstrably bactericidal antimicrobials are to be preferred. Therapy should be continued for a minimum of 3 weeks in infants less than 2 months of age, despite earlier return of CSF to normal, because relapses requiring additional therapy are particularly frequent in this age group.

For a patient more than 2 months of age in whom studies at admission fail to identify a specific etiologic agent, ampicillin alone is the drug of choice. In the past a combination of penicillin and chloramphenicol has been recommended for such patients, but such therapy is outmoded. In a controlled study,[9] single drug ampicillin therapy was shown to be more effective, overall, than a combination of ampicillin and chloramphenicol in the three common kinds of bacterial meningitis. Indeed, analysis of the data from that same controlled study showed that, combining etiologic groups, antibiotic antagonism probably existed in the treatment group who received combination therapy with chloramphenicol plus ampicillin.[10]

For patients who have known meningococcal or pneumococcal disease, penicillin G remains the drug of choice because of relative cost and ease of administration, but ampicillin is an equivalent alternate.[11] For patients with proved *H. influenzae* meningitis, ampicillin is presently the drug of choice; chloramphenicol or tetracycline are acceptable alternates for patients unable to tolerate penicillin, despite the hematologic toxicity of chloramphenicol and the toxicities and difficulty in administration of tetracycline.[12] Inadequate response has been seen in patients with meningococcal disease who have received cephalothin therapy.

For patients in whom unusual organisms are suspected or identified, other drugs may be required. Selection of the appropriate antimicrobial agent, or agents, for initial therapy should be based upon the overall evaluation of the patient at the time of admission. Selection of final definitive therapy should be based upon demonstrated *in vitro* efficacy and knowledge of the relative toxicities of the available effective agents.

Due to the increase in recent years of sulfonamide-resistant group B meningococci,[13, 14] and, more recently, similarly resistant group C meningococci,[15] there is no reason to include sulfonamides in any antibiotic regimen used in bacterial meningitis, except for the very rare entity of central nervous system nocardiosis. There is no evidence that sulfonamides increase the efficacy of penicillin, ampicillin, chloramphenicol, or tetracycline therapy in the common kinds of meningitis, and there is ample evidence that drug fever or other manifestations of sulfonamide toxicity frequently complicate the clinical management of the disease.

Routine intrathecal administration of antibiotics is unnecessary unless polymyxin B or other antibiotics which have similarly poor diffusibility are indicated. With use of such antibiotics serum and CSF levels characteristically are insufficient to permit inactivation of the etiologic agents without intrathecal therapy. Pseudomonas meningitis is the main indication for such therapy. Polymyxin B sulfate, 2.0 to 2.5 mg/kg/24 hours is given intramuscularly in two or three divided doses. Adjunctive intrathecal therapy in a dosage of 0.5 to 1.0 mg per day is administered by barbotage until the CSF is sterilized. Then, the frequency of the intrathecal injections is decreased to every other day for the remainder of the course of therapy.

Monitoring Antimicrobial Therapy

A CSF specimen should be examined 24 hours following the initiation of therapy. The gram stain of the sediment at this point should not contain demonstrable microorganisms, and cultures should be negative, although the white cell count and protein level may be increased over those at admission. Such increases, considered alone, are not causes for alarm. The CSF glucose concentration should be greater than that observed initially, provided therapy is effective. (It should be noted that such rapid CSF responses may not occur in young infants with meningitis due to bacteria of enteric origin. Responses are often delayed — at times for several days.)

With the exception of early infancy, when therapy must be continued for a minimum of 3 weeks, treatment is continued until the patient has been afebrile for a minimum of 5 days. At that time, another repeat CSF is obtained, and, if the cell count is less than 30 cells, the glucose is normal, the protein is normal, or almost normal, and no microorganisms are seen, therapy may be discontinued. It is well to observe the patient for 2 additional days, as relapses, although very rare, do occur. If these criteria are not met, it is desirable to reevaluate the patient for signs of subdural effusion, brain abscess, sinusitis, mastoiditis, and other foci of infection which might be causing continued reseeding of the meninges. Relapses, although rare, are seen most frequently in young infants with meningitis due to enteric bacteria, and we have observed none in meningococcal disease, regardless of age.

Several recent isolated case reports have discussed "failure" or "relapse" of *H. influenzae* meningitis despite ampicillin therapy.[16-20] In one patient orbital cellulitis with positive blood cultures for *H. influenzae,* type B, occurred after therapy was stopped; there was no recurrence of meningitis.[16] In another, the initial treatment was probably inadequate as a consequence of oral administration of the drug.[17] A third patient had subdural effusions.[18] The remaining two reports are quite brief, and reasons for treatment failure are not obvious.[19, 20] It is important to emphasize that such "treatment failures" occur with other drugs. *H. influenzae* may persist or recur in the CSF despite therapy with chloramphenicol or tetracycline.[10-12] During a 22-month period when we were conducting controlled trials of ampicillin versus "conventional therapy," six instances of persistence or recurrence of *H. influenzae,* type B, after 24 hours of treatment were observed among 107 patients who received chloramphenicol, or penicillin G plus chloramphenicol.[10, 11] Among 66 patients who received ampicillin only, none had persistence or recurrence of *H. influenzae,* type B, in the CSF after 24 hours.[10, 11] It is also important to emphasize that routine disc susceptibility testing of *H. influenzae,* type B, against ampicillin may yield misleading results. In our experience with *H. influenzae,* type B, most strains reported as "resistant" by the disc technique have been susceptible when tested by tube dilution. Occasionally (less than 1 per cent), *H. influenzae* isolates have been found relatively resistant in tube dilution tests. The response to therapy has not correlated well with *in vitro* testing.

PROPHYLAXIS

Secondary cases of *H. influenzae* meningitis occasionally occur in young siblings of patients, but the low frequency of incidence does not justify attempts at prophylaxis. In contrast, the frequency and severity of co-primary and secondary cases among household associates of patients with meningococcal disease[13, 14] suggest that a good prophylactic drug might be useful. The current prevalence of sulfonamide-resistant meningococci limits the usefulness of sulfonamides, the only drugs shown to eradicate susceptible strains from the nasopharynx of carriers.[13, 14] Although rifampicin has shown some promise in terminating the nasopharyngeal carrier state, rapid emergence of resistant strains is likely to present problems in the future, and its role is uncertain at present.

Currently available antibiotics will not terminate the carrier state, and no regimen has been proved definitely effective in the prevention of secondary cases. However, if antibiotics are given to family contacts during the period of greatest risk of disease (24 to 48 hours after onset of the primary case),[13, 14] it is possible that they may abort bacteremia and prevent some cases. Consequently, either oral phenoxymethyl penicillin (250 to 500 mg 4 times a day) or erythromycin (40 mg/kg/day, up to a maximum dose of 2.0 gm) is recommended for 4 days. Because some meningococci remain susceptible to sulfonamides, some clinicians continue to use sulfadiazine (2 gm daily, 1 gm for those below 6 years) in two divided doses for each of the 4 days of prophylaxis.

There is no satisfactory evidence that hospital personnel caring for patients with meningococcal disease are at increased risk, but strict medical aseptic technique is recommended.

Vaccines are under development for Group A and C infections. Initial studies have shown promise in military recruits, but final appraisal awaits further study. No Group B vaccine has been developed as yet.

SURGICAL CONSIDERATIONS

Although relatively few subdural effusions require surgical intervention, it should be noted that about 10 per cent of infants and young children with acute purulent meningitis will develop clinically significant effusions. Daily removal of subdural fluid to a maximum of 20 ml from each side is recommended. If significant quantities of fluid continue to form after 2 weeks of daily removal despite continuation of antibiotic therapy, surgical intervention should be considered. However, surgery should be deferred until after at least 3 weeks of antimicrobial therapy with daily fluid removal. Antibiotics should be continued during surgery and for at least a week thereafter.

Brain abscesses, although virtually unknown with meningococcal disease and uncommon with *H. influenzae,* occur occasionally as concomitants of meningitis due to pneumococci or "unusual" organisms. Brain abscesses are especially common in the patient with acute or chronic mastoiditis. A brain scan or cerebral angiogram is indicated to localize the lesion. Surgical therapy is customarily delayed until convalescence, as in the case of acute mastoiditis, unless progressive localizing signs necessitate an emergency procedure.

Repeated episodes of pneumococcal meningitis suggest a skull fracture, usually communicating with the mastoid, middle ear, a frontal sinus, or the ethmoid sinus through the cribriform plate. If the dural defect tract can be located during convalescence, surgical repair is indicated.

Other surgical therapy includes skin grafts for patients with extensive loss of tissue following the development of large cutaneous infarctions of ecchymotic areas after acute meningococcal disease.

REHABILITATIVE MEASURES

Although some patients have readily demonstrable sequelae during convalescence after bacterial meningitis and other acute central nervous system infections, the necessity for proper rehabilitative measures is frequently overlooked. During convalescence, careful serial evaluations of motor, sensory, and intellectual functions should be made. These evaluations should be repeated approximately 2 months after discharge from the hospital. For infants and young children, in whom specific evaluations of central nervous system functions (particularly the sensory and intellectual) may be more difficult, the evaluations should be repeated at 3- or 4-month intervals for a year or more. It is important to note that proper recognition and attention to such defects as hearing loss, impairment of vision, and motor disability are important if optimal function is to be achieved, and if necessary skills are to be developed for the future.

CONCLUSIONS

The presently available, effective antimicrobial therapy has substantially decreased the frequency of disability due to meningitis and has been even more effective in reducing mortality. Optimum therapeutic results are dependent upon prompt clinical recognition of disease, the specific identification of the infectious agent, the prompt administration of bactericidal drugs by the intravenous route, and proper monitoring of the patient with acute illness. Indeed, rapid diagnosis, monitoring the patient for shock with prompt restoration of effective circulation, early detection of complications, and proper concern toward rehabilitative measures are features of therapy which may be as important as choosing the right antimicrobial agent.

References

1. Mace, J. W., Peters, E. R., and Mathies, A. W., Jr.: Cranial bruits in purulent meningitis in childhood. New Eng. J. Med., 278:1429, 1968.
2. Robinson, M. G., and Watson, R. J.: Pneumococcal meningitis in sickle cell disease. New Eng. J. Med., 274:1006, 1966.
3. Fox, H. A., Hagen, P. A., Turner, D. J., Glasgow, L. A., and Connor, J. D.: Immunofluorescence in the diagnosis of acute bacterial meningitis: a cooperative evaluation of the technique in a clinical laboratory setting. Pediatrics, 43:44, 1969.
4. Migeon, C. J., Kenny, F. M., Hung, W., and Voorhess, M. L.: Study of adrenal function in children with meningitis. Pediatrics, 40:163, 1967.
5. Abildgaard, C. F., Corrigan, J. J., Seeler, R. A., Simone, J. V., and Schulman, I.: Meningococcemia associated with intravascular coagulation. Pediatrics, 40:78, 1967.
6. McGehee, W. G., Rapaport, S. I., and Hjort, P. F.: Intravascular coagulation in fulminant meningococcemia. Ann. Int. Med., 67:250, 1967.
7. Hardman, J. M.: Fatal meningococcal infections: the changing pathologic picture in the '60's. Mil. Med., 133:951, 1968.
8. Leedom, J. M., Wehrle, P. F., Mathies, A. W., Ivler, D., and Warren, W. S.: Comments about the role of gentamicin in the treatment of meningitis in neonates. Adapted

from discussion presented at Gentamicin Conference, University of Illinois College of Medicine, Chicago, Illinois, October 31, 1968.

9. Wehrle, P. F., Mathies, A. W., Jr., Leedom, J. M., and Ivler, D.: Bacterial meningitis. Ann. N.Y. Acad. Sci., *145*:488, 1967.

10. Mathies, A. W., Jr., Leedom, J. M., Ivler, D., Wehrle, P. F., and Portnoy, B.: Antibiotic antagonism in bacterial meningitis. *In* Antimicrobial Agents and Chemotherapy — 1967. Proceedings, Seventh Interscience Conference on Antimicrobial Agents and Chemotherapy, Chicago, Illinois, October, 1967. Ann Arbor, Michigan, Amer. Soc. Microbiol., 1968, pp. 218–224.

11. Mathies, A. W., Jr., Leedom, J. M., Thrupp, L. D., Ivler, D., Portnoy, B., and Wehrle, P. F.: Experience with ampicillin in bacterial meningitis. *In* Antimicrobial Agents and Chemotherapy — 1965. Proceedings, Fifth Interscience Conference on Antimicrobial Agents and Chemotherapy and Fourth International Congress of Chemotherapy, Washington, D.C., October, 1965. Ann Arbor, Michigan, Amer. Soc. Microbiol., 1966, p. 610–617.

12. Lepper, M. H., and Spies, H. W.: Nontuberculous bacterial infections of the central nervous system. GP, *25*:83 (Feb.), 1962.

13. Leedom, J. M., Ivler, D., Mathies, A. W., Thrupp, L. D., Portnoy, B., and Wehrle, P. F.: Importance of sulfadiazine resistance in meningococcal disease in civilians. New Eng. J. Med., *273*:1395, 1965.

14. Leedom, J. M., Ivler, D., Mathies, A. W., Jr., Thrupp, L. D., Fremont, J. C., Wehrle, P. F., and Portnoy, B.: The problem of sulfadiazine-resistant meningococci. *In* Antimicrobial Agents and Chemotherapy — 1966. Proceedings, Sixth Interscience Conference on Antimicrobial Agents and Chemotherapy, Philadelphia, Pennsylvania, October, 1966. Ann Arbor, Michigan, Amer. Soc. Microbiol., 1967, pp. 281–292.

15. U. S. Public Health Service: Current trends, meningococcal infections — United States. Morbidity and Mortality Weekly Report. *18*:135, 1969.

16. Young, L. M., Haddow, J. E., and Klein, J. O.: Relapse following ampicillin treatment of acute *Hemophilus influenzae* meningitis. Pediatrics, *41*:516, 1968.

17. Cherry, J. D., and Sheenan, C. P.: Bacteriologic relapse in *Hemophilus influenzae* meningitis. New Eng. J. Med., *278*:1001, 1968.

18. Sanders, D. Y., and Garbee, H. W.: Failure of response to ampicillin in *Hemophilus influenzae* meningitis. Amer. J. Dis. Child., *117*:331, 1969.

19. Greene, H. L.: Failure of ampicillin in meningitis (Letter to the Editor). Lancet, *1*:861, 1968.

20. Hall, B. D.: Failure of ampicillin in meningitis (Letter to the Editor). Lancet, *1*:1033, 1968.

8

The Care of the Infant in Cardiac Failure

David Goldring, M.D., Antonio Hernandez, M.D.,
and Alexis F. Hartmann, Jr., M.D.

Cardiac failure in the infant is a medical emergency and the responsible physician must be able to make this diagnosis with confidence and institute immediate treatment if the patient is to be salvaged. The physician must, therefore, have an understanding of the generally accepted hypothesis of the pathogenesis and etiology of cardiac failure. He must also be able to recognize and appreciate the significance of the signs and symptoms. Finally, he must be well versed in the general and special aspects of treatment of this life-threatening cardiovascular derangement.

PATHOGENESIS OF CARDIAC FAILURE

The fundamental pathophysiologic mechanism underlying heart failure has been the subject of intensive research and can be treated only

From the Washington University School of Medicine: The Edward Mallinckrodt Department of Pediatrics, Division of Cardiology, and St. Louis Children's Hospital, Saint Louis, Missouri. Aided in part by the Arthur Fund, St. Louis Children's Hospital Heart Mother Fund, Scott Gentsch Memorial Fund, William T. Beauchamp Memorial Fund, John Clay Seier Fund, and the John Brewer Fund.

briefly here. The reader who wishes to review the subject in greater depth is referred to standard texts[1, 2] and other published studies which discuss special aspects of heart failure, such as myocardial energetics and biochemical derangements[3, 4, 5] and the roles of the sympathetic nervous system[6] and peripheral circulation[7] in this condition.

Any single definition of cardiac failure may be open to criticism because of the complex nature of this disorder and the controversial aspects of the subject. However, most cardiologists would agree that heart failure may be defined simply as the inability of the heart to pump blood commensurate with the body's needs. Cardiac failure may result from a primary abnormality of the heart muscle caused, for example, by inflammatory disease (rheumatic fever) or may be secondary to structural defect, such as a stenotic valve which produces a pressure overload, or volume overload, as in a left to right shunt (ventricular septal defect). When the right ventricle fails it cannot eject as much blood as it does under normal conditions. The output of that chamber is, therefore, diminished and its residual blood volume is increased. The end-diastolic pressure rises and there is a corresponding rise in the right atrial and venous pressure. In similar fashion, when the left ventricle fails there is an increase in the end-diastolic pressure of that chamber as well as in the left atrium and pulmonary veins. In most instances, right-sided failure results from and is associated with left-sided failure. In an effort to preserve cardiac output and accommodate the larger volume of residual blood, cardiac dilatation occurs, in accordance with the Frank-Starling concept which states that the contractile force of the heart muscle is a function of the length of the muscle fibers, or the more the heart is filled in diastole, the greater the force of the following contraction. This principle operates until the optimum degree of myocardial fiber length is reached. Thereafter, further dilatation stretches the fibers beyond the length for optimum function and the force of contraction declines.

The sympathetic nervous system has been shown to play a vital role in reflexly initiating compensatory mechanisms in heart failure. The increase in venous pressure mentioned above is an example of this, as is tachycardia, which helps preserve or increase cardiac output. Arteriolar vasoconstriction tends to preserve blood pressure in the face of a falling cardiac output.

In advanced heart failure the rate of blood flow to the kidneys and skin is reduced so that blood can be diverted to the heart, brain, and skeletal muscle, which have high metabolic requirements. The decrease in renal blood flow is thought to stimulate aldosterone secretion by way of the renin-angiotensin system[8, 9] which then causes renal retention of sodium and water. This, in turn, increases the circulating blood volume and thus helps to preserve cardiac output. Therefore, the elevations of pressures, the disturbances in blood flow, and the abnormal distribution of water and electrolytes which characterize heart failure may be looked upon as homeostatic mechanisms whereby the body attempts to preserve cardiac output. The clinician who can recognize the signs and symptoms which appear in the wake of these compensatory mechanisms will be able to diagnose heart failure.

Etiology of Cardiac Failure in Infancy

The experience at most pediatric cardiology centers has shown that about 20 per cent of infants and children with organic heart disease develop cardiac failure at some time. Ninety per cent of these children develop failure during the first year of life, and the majority have congenital cardiac malformations.[10] This presentation will, therefore, be focused on the recognition and treatment of heart failure during the first year of life.

The cardiac malformations most commonly complicated by heart failure in order of frequency, according to Keith,[10] are transposition of the great vessels, coarctation of the aorta, ventricular septal defect, aortic atresia, endocardial fibroelastosis, atrioventricularis communis, total anomalous pulmonary venous return, single ventricle, and patent ductus arteriosus. These defects account for more than 80 per cent of all cases of heart failure due to cardiovascular malformations. Ostium secundum atrial septal defects and tetralogy of Fallot, though relatively common defects, are seldom complicated by congestive failure. The reason for this is not entirely understood.

Characteristically, infants with congenital defects, such as aortic atresia or hypoplasia of the left ventricle and aortic arch, will usually develop cardiac failure in the first week of life. In contrast, the infant with a large interventricular septal defect may not develop heart failure until 1 to 6 months of age. A newborn infant with aortic atresia will be in difficulty soon after birth because of the mechanical obstruction to the outflow of blood from the left ventricle and the constriction of the ductus arteriosus in the first 24 to 48 hours. An infant with a large interventricular septal defect will not develop failure for the first 4 to 6 weeks because the pulmonary vascular resistance is sufficiently high, initially, to prevent excessive blood flow from the left to the right ventricle. However, as pulmonary vascular resistance normally falls with age as a result of dilation of the pulmonary arterioles, the left to right flow progressively increases. If the capacity of the pulmonary vasculature is exceeded, as well as that of the left atrium and left ventricle, cardiac failure will result. This mechanism of left ventricular failure which is seen in relation to the postnatal decrease in pulmonary vascular resistance applies to other congenital heart defects which involve a large communication between the ventricles or great vessels, i.e., atrioventricularis communis, patent ductus, and others.

Signs and Symptoms[11, 12, 13]

The common signs and symptoms in the infant with congestive heart failure (combined right and left ventricular failure) are tachypnea, tachycardia, cardiomegaly, hepatomegaly, pulmonary rales and rhonchi, feeding difficulties, growth failure, and cyanosis. Less common manifestations include peripheral edema, ascites, and gallop rhythm. Large, clinically demonstrable pleural and pericardial effusions have rarely been seen in our experience.

The purpose of the following discussion on the pathogenesis of the signs and symptoms is to develop a picture of the distinct clinical syndrome which the physician can recognize as cardiac failure.

Cardiomegaly. Since 90 per cent of infants who present in heart failure will have a congenital structural defect of the heart (either on the basis of pressure or volume overload), compensatory hypertrophy of the heart is to be expected as a result of the chronic stress imposed upon the heart muscle by the altered hemodynamics. If congestive heart failure is superimposed, there will be, in addition, compensatory dilatation in accordance with the Frank-Starling principle.

There are some types of congenital heart malformations which do not present with cardiomegaly by physical examination or roentgenography, such as total anomalous venous drainage below the diaphragm, cor triatriatum, and pulmonary venous atresia. In these conditions there is pulmonary venous obstruction which results in pulmonary arterial hypertension and right ventricular pressure overload but not volume overload; the left heart is usually hypoplastic. The clinical picture is that of congestive heart failure, cyanosis, marked right ventricular hypertrophy shown by electrocardiography but a normal overall heart size, and pulmonary vascular congestion detected by chest roentgenography.

Tachypnea and Dyspnea. Tachypnea during sleep, with rates that range from 50 to 100 per minute, is commonly seen in infants in failure. Dyspnea, especially while suckling the bottle, is also frequently observed.* Both tachypnea and dyspnea are primarily manifestations of left ventricular failure and are thought to be due to pulmonary congestion and increased pulmonary capillary pressure which result in pulmonary interstitial, alveolar, and bronchiolar edema. The viscoelastic properties of the lung are altered and this results in diminished compliance, with consequent restrained inspiration and expiration, i.e., shallow breathing. An increased respiratory stimulus, most probably neurogenic

---

*The paroxysmal dyspnea, tachypnea, and increased cyanosis ("blue spells," "syncopal episodes") occasionally seen in patients with tetralogy of Fallot, usually subside spontaneously or respond to oxygen administration and morphine sulfate. These spells are not a consequence of heart failure but are thought to result from a sudden transient increase in right to left flow or an increased demand of the tissues for oxygen, as with fever, excitement, or exercise.

(exaggerated Herring-Breuer reflex),[14] and occasionally hypoxema increase ventilation by increasing the rate. Pulmonary rales will be heard when the failure is severe. Very often there is a superimposed *pulmonary infection* which usually precipitates congestive heart failure. Under these circumstances, the rales may be a result of the infection or failure, or both. In the face of elevated left ventricular end-diastolic pressure, left atrial and pulmonary venous pressure, pulmonary edema may be seen and the chest will be filled with rales and rhonchi, although bloody, frothy sputum is not commonly seen.

Hepatomegaly. The elevation in the atrial, central, and peripheral venous pressure has been attributed to heightened venous tone, probably induced by reflex stimulation of the sympathetic nervous system and secretion of norepinephrine.[6, 7] In infants, the evidence of increased venous pressure is not as obvious as in adults. Distention of the external jugular vein is rarely observed in infants because of their short necks and the marked compliance or vascular distensibility of the liver. *Hepatomegaly* is, therefore, regularly seen in infants with heart failure, although liver tenderness, so frequently observed in adults and older children, is not commonly seen.

Tachycardia. This is almost always present in cardiac failure. The rate may be as high as 200 per minute. This is a major compensatory response which initially helps preserve or increase cardiac output. The pathogenesis of this response is thought to be the following: In congestive failure there is a rise in pressure in the right atrium and great veins. This sets in motion the Bainbridge reflex[15] by which vagal effect is diminished and the heart rate increases. Another mechanism proposes that the increased level of circulating catecholamines commonly observed in heart failure is responsible for this tachycardia. The compensatory effect of the tachycardia is limited by the shortening of diastole and consequent reduction in coronary and ventricular filling as the rate increases.

Edema. In infants edema is not readily apparent. The first indication may be a sudden weight gain (200 to 300 gm) in 24 hours. Upon close inspection there may be puffiness on the dorsum of the hands or feet and around the eyes. The pathogenesis of peripheral edema is incompletely understood but is thought to result from the increased venous and, therefore, capillary hydrostatic pressure, as well as sodium-water retention. (See earlier discussion of *Pathogenesis of Cardiac Failure.*)

Feeding Difficulties. Feeding difficulties with resultant growth failure are commonly seen in infants with heart failure. The tachypnea, dyspnea, and cough, especially if there is a superimposed lower respiratory infection, will make it difficult for the infant to suck, and the calorie and fluid intake will fall below the daily requirement. Growth failure will therefore result.

Gallop Rhythm. The presence of an *accentuated* third heart sound should make one suspect heart failure in an infant. This is a protodiastolic sound which appears 0.10 second after the second sound and it has been attributed to the sudden distention of the ventricles during the rapid filling phase of diastole. This same mechanism is believed to produce the third heart sound normally heard in most infants, though sometimes very faintly.

Cyanosis. Varying degrees of cyanosis may be seen in infants who present in severe congestive heart failure. One or a combination of the following three mechanisms may be responsible. The first type is seen in congenital heart disease with a right to left shunt. The second type is central cyanosis which is caused by inadequate oxygenation of the blood in the lungs on account of congestion, infection, or both. The third type is caused by an excessive extraction of oxygen from the capillary blood in the tissues. This last type is observed especially in severe congestive failure when the circulation time is prolonged beyond the normal range of 6 to 12 seconds for the infant or young child.[1]

Diseases Confused with Heart Failure

There are a number of disease states which may be confused with congestive heart failure. For example, the respiratory distress syndrome, severe acute bronchiolitis, pneumonia, tracheoesophageal fistula, diaphragmatic hernia, hypoglycemia, renal disease, sepsis, central nervous system disorders (trauma, hemorrhage, infection), and neonatal polycythemia. Indeed, in some cases it may be difficult to rule out primary cardiac disease without resorting to cardiac catheterization and angiocardiography. In most instances, however, the correct diagnosis can be made after a careful history, physical examination (presence of a murmur), demonstration of single or biventricular enlargement by the electrocardiogram, and the finding of cardiomegaly and pulmonary congestion by chest roentgenography.

TREATMENT[1, 2, 11, 12]

Cardiac failure in infants has a very serious prognosis and the reported mortality rate ranges from 50 to 85 per cent, because a significant number of the deaths occur in babies born with inoperable cardiac malformations. Although the mortality rate is high, the spectrum of congenital cardiac malformations which are amenable to either palliative or corrective surgical therapy is ever increasing. An aggressive and enthusiastic approach to medical treatment is therefore vital if a baby is to be salvaged by surgical therapy. Since most infants in cardiac failure have congenital structural malformations of the heart, the initial medical therapy should be aimed at expeditious stabilization of the hemodynamic state so that the sick infant can be studied by cardiac catheterization and angiocardiography as soon as possible. A definitive anatomic diagnosis can thus be made and the plan for therapy outlined, be it immediate surgical intervention or continued medical treatment. At times, cardiac catheterization and angiocardiography may have to be done upon an emergency basis. For example, a baby with complete transposition of the great vessels will need, in most instances, a balloon septostomy at time of catheterization for sheer survival.[16]

The salvage rate of critically ill infants in cardiac failure will be improved if the diagnostic studies are done at a medical center which has the necessary equipment and trained medical personnel. If a physician's practice is some distance from a medical center, he can initiate treatment at his office which will improve the probability of survival of the patient. If the doctor suspects congestive heart failure, the patient should be given one half the digitalizing dose of digoxin (see following section on *Digoxin* for dosage schedule) parenterally and placed in oxygen and sent to the hospital. If the patient is restless, a dose of morphine sulfate (see later discussion of *morphine sulfate* for dosage schedule) should be given, and if he suspects bacterial infection, antibiotic therapy is strongly recommended (see later discussion on *antibiotics*).

Monitoring

At the hospital, the infant should be admitted to a well-equipped and well-staffed *intensive care unit* where he can be monitored; i.e., *daily weights, recorded intake* and *output*. The vital signs should be carefully monitored with regard to his *respiratory rate, electrocardiographic changes*, and *blood pressure*. (We have used the Doppler ultrasound method which measures the systolic and diastolic pressures. This method is uniquely suited for the infant under six months of age.)[17] In addition, the *blood gases* (PaO_2, $PaCO_2$) as well as the serum pH should be followed at regular intervals, and periodic determinations of the *serum electrolytes* are vital guides to rational fluid therapy. All of these data should be kept on a daily chart at the bedside.

Digoxin

Although the mechanism of action of digitalis is still imperfectly understood, there is universal agreement that it is the most valuable drug in the treatment of cardiac failure because digitalis increases the force of contraction of the failing myocardium, thereby increasing cardiac output. The most popular glycoside of digitalis for pediatric use has been digoxin. Numerous dosage regimens have been proposed, depending upon the age of the patient, and different dosage schedules have been proposed for oral and parenteral routes. There is questionable basis for both practices. Digoxin is absorbed equally well when given orally or parenterally, and there is questionable evidence that premature and newborn infants are more sensitive to the drug than older children.[18] We prefer to start with a digitalizing dosage of 0.03 mg per kg of body weight. One half the dose is given immediately and one fourth in 6 hours and the other fourth again in 6 hours. A maintenance dose of 10 per cent of the total digitalizing dosage is then given every 12 hours. We prefer to give the drug parenterally to a critically ill infant because of the probability of vomiting. If the initial dose is found to be inadequate, the amount of glycoside may be increased to as much as 0.1 mg/kg as a total digitalizing dose. It should be emphasized that each patient has to be managed individually and the treatment of each patient should be carried out as a biologic titration. One is not as apt, therefore, to encounter digoxin intoxication with this regimen.*

Since infants rarely vomit with digoxin intoxication, one has to rely upon electrocardiographic monitoring for evidence of overdosage. This is not a sensitive method for detecting digoxin intoxication, but the appearance of a significant prolongation of the AV conduction time (0.04 second or greater) when compared with the predigitalization electrocardiogram and the appearance of premature ventricular contractions should be looked for as signs of intoxication.

Diuretics

Essentially all diuretic agents function by suppressing the resorption of sodium by the kidney, with subsequent decrease in the edema. The mercurial diuretic, meralluride, has largely been replaced by ethacrynic acid. The dose of ethacrynic acid is 1 mg/kg of body weight for intravenous use and this may be repeated in 12 hours, if necessary. One may expect a response in 15 minutes to an hour. This drug may also be given orally (3 mg/kg/day).

The administration of *oxygen* (oxygen concentration in incubator, 30 to 40 per cent) to the infant is of benefit, especially if there is superimposed bacterial infection or atelectasis. In addition, the relative humidity in the incubator should be 40 to 50 per cent. The *temperature* inside the incubator should be adjusted so that the infant's rectal temperature is maintained at 37° C. A hot humid environment should be avoided because an infant in congestive heart failure cannot initiate the compensatory mechanisms, such as an increase in cardiac output, increase in dermal blood flow, and increase in perspiration, which a normal infant calls into play for thermal regulation.[19] The *posture* of the patient should be adjusted so that his head and chest are on an incline of 10 to 30

---

*Higher doses of digoxin have been recommended[1, 11, 12] but we feel the regimen recommended in this discussion provides the greatest factor of safety to the patient.

degrees. In the recumbent position the shift of blood to the thorax from the lower extremities and splanchnic viscera increases the degree of pulmonary congestion which is already present as a result of congestive heart failure. This undesirable effect is lessened by the semi-sitting position. Also, by elevation of the head and chest the work of breathing will be reduced because the compression on the diaphragm by the abdominal viscera will be decreased.

Feeding and Metabolism

Critically ill infants should be supported by parenteral fluids. Small feedings or gavage may provoke vomiting and aspiration. A fluid containing 10 per cent glucose (on rare occasions an infant in heart failure may be hypoglycemic), with sodium, 1 to 4 mEq/kg/24 hours, and potassium, 0 to 3 mEq/kg/24 hours, depending upon the serum electrolytes, may be used. The total fluid administered in 24 hours should be 50 to 100 ml/kg. If the baby has rales and obvious edema, the lower figure should be used. When the baby has improved, small oral feedings may be started. A low salt formula, such as Similac PM 60/40 (Ross Laboratories), may be used for several days, but infants tolerate the conventional formulas quite well without aggravation of the edema.

Respiratory and metabolic acidosis may be seen in infants with heart failure. There are alveolar and bronchiolar transudates which compromise gas exchange at the alveolar level and are reflected in a low PaO_2 and elevated $PaCO_2$. In extremely severe heart failure the hypoxemia encourages anaerobic metabolism with a consequent increase in the production of lactic acid. Under these circumstances, cautious treatment with sodium bicarbonate is indicated. One may calculate, in the conventional manner, the amount of bicarbonate needed to correct the metabolic acidosis. For example: Desired bicarbonate level (20 to 25 mEq/L) minus the patient's actual bicarbonate level $\times$ 0.6 $\times$ kg body weight is equal to mEq of bicarbonate to be given. We usually give one fourth to one half of this amount during a 6 to 8 hour period to reduce the possibility of untoward reactions such as hypernatremia, water retention, and alkalosis, because the initially high serum lactic acid content may be quickly metabolized with reduction in the metabolic acidosis if the heart function improves after digitalization. Thus the full dose of bicarbonate initially determined may not be needed.

Additional Therapeutic Measures

Morphine sulfate is a valuable drug in the treatment of heart failure, especially for the extremely restless infant, as well as the patient who presents either with impending or overt pulmonary edema. The benefit of the drug in pulmonary edema is its effect upon the peripheral circulation. The capacity of the total vascular bed is increased, thereby encouraging venous pooling and thereby decreasing venous return.[20] The recommended dose is 0.5 to 1 mg per 5 kg of body weight. This dose may be repeated in 3 to 4 hours.

Antibiotics are usually indicated in patients with acute heart failure because of the high incidence of superimposed pulmonary infection. After appropriate cultures are obtained, initial broad coverage should be instituted. For infants (birth to 3 months) ampicillin, 100 to 200 mg/kg per 24 hours, and kanamycin sulfate, 10 to 15 mg/kg per 24 hours, should be given intramuscularly. For infants (3 to 12 months), ampicillin, 100 to 200 mg/kg per 24 hours and methicillin, 100 mg/kg per 24 hours, should be given intramuscularly.[21] The ampicillin may be given intravenously if the situation dictates this. If a specific infecting organism is isolated, the appropriate antibiotic drug can then be substituted.

Anemia (Hgb <7 gm per 100 ml), if present, should be corrected so that there is an optimum hemogloblin level for oxygen transport. A packed red blood cell solution should be given cautiously and slowly (5 mg/kg) so that the hemoglobin is raised to 10 grams per 100 ml or higher. This should be administered after the baby has had the benefit of the treatment outlined previously.

Emergency measures are sometimes indicated for the infant who presents with heart failure in a moribund state. Because one can presume that the baby has severe metabolic acidosis, a rapid intravenous or, in desperate circumstances, intracardiac infusion of *sodium bicarbonate* (2 to 5 mEq/kg) may be given. An *Isuprel* drip is also indicated (0.2 μg/kg/min) and should be given preferably by an infusion pump while the heart rate and blood pressure are continuously monitored. This drug is especially useful in bradycardia and has an added advantage because of its positive inotropic effect. Upon occasion, a mechanical ventilator will be necessary if the patient cannot maintain adequate gas exchange, as is commonly seen in the immediate postoperative period after cardiac surgery. Since most of these infants in congestive failure are weak and have superimposed pulmonary infection with increased or changing lung compliance, a volume limited ventilator is the instrument of choice.[22] *Rotating tourniquets* are worth a try to three extremities. The cuffs should occlude the venous but not the arterial flow. The tourniquet blood pressure cuffs should be removed every 10 minutes. In cases with extreme bradycardia or cardiac arrest, the physician has to resort to *external cardiac massage* and *assisted respiration* with an endotracheal tube.

SUMMARY

Heart failure may be defined simply as the inability of the heart to pump blood commensurate with the body's needs. Although it is possible for the right or left ventricle to fail separately, it is much more common for infants to present with failure of both chambers. When a ventricle fails, the end-diastolic pressure in that chamber rises and the pressure in the atrium and central and peripheral veins is increased. There is a decrease in blood flow to the kidney and this decrease is thought to be responsible for the renal retention of sodium and water which, in turn, increases blood volume. Thus, the elevations in pressure, the disturbances in blood flow, and abnormal distribution of water and electrolytes are homeostatic mechanisms which help preserve cardiac output. Because of these compensatory mechanisms, signs and symptoms develop which the clinician recognizes as heart failure.

Infants under one year of age account for 90 per cent of pediatric patients who develop congestive heart failure, and the majority of these have congenital heart disease.

Although the mortality rate in infants with congestive heart failure is high (50 to 85 per cent), the spectrum of congenital cardiac malformations which are amenable to corrective surgery is ever increasing. The physician must, therefore, be able to make the diagnosis of heart failure with confidence and institute immediate therapy. The patient, ideally, should be transferred to a medical center and admitted to a well-equipped and well-staffed intensive care unit where 24 hour monitoring is available and therapy can be initiated.

Since most of the infants will have congenital structural malformation of the heart as the basis for their failure, the treatment should be aimed at expeditious stabilization of the hemodynamic state so that the patient can then be evaluated by cardiac catheterization and angiocardiography as soon as possible. A definitive anatomic diagnosis can thus be made and the plan for therapy decided, whether it be immediate surgical intervention or continued medical treatment.

The approach just outlined will continually improve the salvage rate of infants in congestive heart failure.

References

1. Keith, J. D., Rowe, R. D., and Vlad, P.: Heart Disease in Infancy and Childhood. New York, Macmillan, 1967.
2. Friedberg, C. K.: Diseases of the Heart. Philadelphia, W. B. Saunders Company, 1966.
3. Braunwald, E., Ross, J., and Sonnenblick, E. H.: Mechanism of Contraction of the Normal and Failing Heart. Boston, Little, Brown, 1967.
4. Spann, J. F., Jr., Mason, D. T., and Zelis, R. F.: Recent advances in the understanding of congestive heart failure (I). Mod. Conc. Cardiovasc. Dis., 39:73, 1970.
5. Spann, J. F., Jr., Mason, D. T., and Zelis, R. F.: Recent advances in the understanding of congestive heart failure (II). Mod. Conc. Cardiovasc. Dis., 39:79, 1970.
6. Braunwald, E.: The sympathetic nervous system in heart failure. Hosp. Prac., 31:31, 1970.
7. Mason, D. T.: Control of the peripheral circulation in health and disease. Mod. Conc. Cardiovasc. Dis., 36:25, 1967.
8. Haber, E.: The renin-angiotensin system in curable hypertension. Mod. Conc. Cardiovasc. Dis., 38:7, 1969.

 9. Romero, J. C., and Hoobler, S. W.: The renin-angiotensin system in clinical medicine. Amer. Heart J., *80*:701, 1969.
10. Keith, J. D.: Congestive heart failure. Pediatrics, *18*:491, 1956.
11. Lees, M. H.: Heart failure in the newborn infant. J. Pediat., *75*:139, 1969.
12. Nadas, A. S., and Hauck, A. J.: Pediatric aspects of congestive heart failure. Circulation, *21*:242, 1960.
13. Braunwald, E.: Physiology of congestive heart failure. Ann. Int. Med., *64*:904, 1966.
14. Marshall, R., and Widdecombe, J. G.: The activity of the pulmonary stretch receptors during congestion of the lung. Quart. J. Exp. Physiol., *43*:320, 1958.
15. Bainbridge, F. A.: The influence of venous filling upon the rate of the heart. J. Physiol., *50*:65, 1915.
16. Rashkind, W. J., and Miller, W. W.: Creation of an atrial septal defect without thoracotomy. J.A.M.A., *196*:991, 1966.
17. Hernandez, A., Hartmann, A. F., and Goldring, D.: Measurement of blood pressure by Doppler ultrasonic technique. Pediatrics, *48*:788, 1971.
18. Hernandez, A., Burton, R. M., Pagtakhan, R. D., and Goldring, D.: Pharmacodynamics of ^{3}H-digoxin in infants. Pediatrics, *44*:418, 1969.
19. Burch, G. E., and Giles, T. D.: The burden of a hot humid environment on the heart. Mod. Conc. Cardiovasc. Dis., *39*:115, 1970.
20. Vasko, J. S., Henney, R. P., Oldham, H. N., Brawley, R. K., and Morrow, A. G.: Mechanism of action of morphine in the treatment of experimental pulmonary edema. Amer. J. Cardiol., *18*:876, 1966.
21. Feigin, R. D.: Personal communication, 1971.
22. Smith, R. M.: The critically ill child: respiratory arrest and its sequelae. Pediatrics, *46*:108, 1970.

9

Acute Hepatic Failure

Charles Trey, M.B., Ch.B., M.D.

The clinical syndrome of acute liver failure is the manifestation of severe hepatic dysfunction or massive hepatic necrosis. The child usually presents with a history suggestive of viral infection. There may have been exposure to hepatitis, blood products, or presumed hepatotoxins. Progressive jaundice is usual, except in the liver failure of Reye's syndrome; other symptoms include fetor hepaticus, decrease in liver size, and asterixis ("liver flap"). Mental confusion or coma may develop as the disease progresses. The biochemical abnormalities usually include elevated serum bilirubin and glutamic oxaloacetic transaminase (G.O.T.). Increased serum alpha amino-nitrogen and blood ammonia, and a prolonged prothrombin time, unaffected by parenteral vitamin K administration, are useful indications of increasing severity of the disease. Hypoglycemia can occur in severe liver failure and is common in Reye's syndrome. Serum albumin decreases as the failure

From the Thorndike Memorial Laboratory, Harvard Medical Unit, Boston City Hospital, the Children's Hospital Medical Center, and the Harvard Medical School, Boston, Massachusetts.

progresses. The patient's course may fluctuate, and improvement or recovery is possible at almost any stage.[1-3]

While the underlying cause may not be immediately apparent, diagnosis is usually not difficult if other varieties of coma, such as those from metabolic or intracranial causes, are excluded. In encephalopathy and fatty degeneration of the liver and viscera (Reye's syndrome), the child is not jaundiced and the diagnosis may be confused with other forms of toxic encephalitis.[4-7] Reye's syndrome must thus be suspected in nonicteric children in coma with high levels of serum G.O.T. and other enzymes, increased blood ammonia, and prolonged prothrombin time. These laboratory measurements should be performed at frequent intervals in the child in whom the diagnosis is suspected, as the abnormalities may not at first be evident but can become manifest during the course of illness.

Histological examination of the liver in acute hepatic failure shows severe hepatocellular necrosis. In Reye's syndrome and in tetracycline-associated liver disease, the hepatocytes are diffusely infiltrated by small fat droplets without displacement of the nucleus, and only a few cells are necrosed. Liver biopsy, if the child's coagulation studies are normal, is useful in differentiating these two conditions and also in detecting granuloma, lymphoma, and other systemic diseases which can manifest with acute hepatic failure. Usually the hepatic failure is part of the systemic involvement.[8]

In children who have been presumed to have normal liver function prior to liver failure, infectious hepatitis can only be suspected, as there are no definitive tests to differentiate between this and other causes. The demonstration of Australia antigen may prove useful in this respect, as it often is present with viral hepatitis.[9, 10] Table 1 shows the presumed causes and outcome in our own experience with 24 children up to 14 years of age, and in the Fulminant Hepatic Failure Surveillance Study

TABLE 1 PRESUMED CAUSES AND OUTCOME OF FULMINANT HEPATIC FAILURE IN CHILDREN

| | Author's Experience | | Fulminant Hepatic Failure Surveillance Study | |
Cause	Number of Cases	Number Surviving	Number of Cases	Number Surviving
Infectious hepatitis	12	6	26	16
Serum hepatitis	2	2	5	2
Halothane	1	1	2	2
Drugs	2	2	0	0
Reye's syndrome	6	3	7	4
Others	1	1	2	2
TOTAL	24	15	42	26

(FHFSS).[1] Patients who did not progress to severe hepatic coma (unresponsiveness, except in a reflex manner, to painful stimuli) had a much better chance of survival. Of 318 FHFSS patients of all ages in hepatic failure with hepatic coma, 42 (13 per cent) were children up to 14 years. Twenty-six of these 42 children survived; 38 of the 42 were in severe hepatic coma, and 13 of these survived. Four children who had infectious hepatitis did not progress to that state; of these, three survived and one died of septicemia and subacute hepatic necrosis. The overall experience is similar to that with our own 24 patients (Table 1), 11 of whom are also included in the Surveillance Study. The others were seen either before the initiation of that study or since the third report to members of FHFSS.

PREVENTION

Prevention of acute liver failure may be possible; early recognition can improve the prognosis. Prophylaxis, by the early administration of gamma globulin to children who have been in contact with patients with infectious hepatitis, may prevent or attenuate that infection.[11] The dangers of drug abuse should be stressed, as this forms the second commonest cause of fulminant hepatic failure in the age group over 14. In two of our patients, prolonged intravenous administration of tetracycline may have led to fulminant hepatic failure.[12, 13] Generalized allergic reaction and hepatic disease have been reported with para-aminosalicylate.[14] In such patients the discontinuance of the medications in the early stages of reaction may prevent hepatic failure.

The clinical entity of halothane-associated hepatic disease should be considered in a child who develops unexplained fever and jaundice after repeated exposure to this anesthetic agent. These events are sometimes confused with the diagnosis of postoperative infection or cholestatic jaundice and can thus lead to further surgery. No test detects the occasional child at risk from this complication of the use of halothane. Thus, unexplained and unexpected fever following surgery should be a relative contraindication to further use of halothane, and postoperative jaundice should be an absolute contraindication.[1, 15]

On occasions, patients with chronic liver disease can present in hepatic coma. This is usually precipitated by infections, gastrointestinal bleeding, or electrolyte imbalance which might have been preventable. The child has signs of chronic liver disease, such as spider angioma, palmar erythema, or portal hypertension. As in the investigation of comatose patients with fulminant hepatic failure, other causes of coma must be excluded. The principles of therapy are similar in both groups.

TREATMENT

General Principles

The purposes of treatment are to alleviate the systemic effects of hepatic failure and to promote liver cell regeneration. Our knowledge of the latter is so limited that therapy is aimed essentially at supporting the patient in the hope that sufficient hepatic regeneration to sustain life will occur. The rationale of treatment is based on clinical observations and experimental studies. In regard to the central nervous system, the response of the child in hepatic coma will depend on the severity of the liver disease and the presence of complications. In the mild form agitation and confusion are noted, while in the severe stage the child may be unresponsive to painful stimuli and in decorticate or decerebrate posture.[16] Mental confusion and restlessness are not indications for sedation, but rather they are warnings that the patient may lapse into severe hepatic or hypoglycemic coma, which will be discussed later. Sedatives metabolized in the liver, such as morphine or paraldehyde,[17] are contraindicated. If sedation is necessary, drugs excreted in the kidneys, such as long-acting barbiturates or meperidine, should be chosen.

In patients or animals with liver disease and portal-systemic shunts, high protein diets or ammonia salts can precipitate or aggravate hepatic coma. The mechanism of these effects is not clear. The practical application of these observations to children with liver failure is that protein intake or degradation in the intestinal tract should be reduced. Protein is either eliminated entirely from the diet during the acute disease or markedly restricted; protein degradation by intestinal bacteria is decreased by altering the intestinal flora with antibiotics (such as neomycin), and its products are removed by frequent enemas. The early detection or prevention of gastrointestinal bleeding, should it develop, is important, as the added protein in the gastrointestinal tract can aggravate the coma, while the shock from volume depletion can endanger the life of the patient.

Hypoglycemia can be a manifestation of severe liver dysfunction and is frequently seen in Reye's syndrome. Blood sugar should be frequently estimated and an adequate blood glucose concentration should be maintained. We have encountered hypoglycemia despite the administration of intravenous glucose, in cases in which the quantity administered has been inadequate.[18] Frequent bedside estimation of blood glucose by "Dextrostix"* as well as laboratory determination can aid in detecting this complication.

---

*Ames Company, Elkhart, Indiana

Ascites is seen in both acute and chronic liver disease. While peritoneal fluid should be aspirated for diagnostic tests and cultures, the only indications for removal of larger volumes are respiratory embarrassment or esophageal variceal bleeding in the presence of tense ascites. In patients with chronic liver disease, injudicious use of diuretics and inadequate replacement of lost potassium can result in severe depletion. Electrolyte imbalance, especially hypokalemia, can aggravate or precipitate hepatic coma. Supplementary potassium (as potassium chloride) may need to be given intravenously or orally.

The effects of hepatic failure on the kidney are apparently unrelated to organic lesions.[19] The characteristically low urinary sodium (e.g., 5 mEq/L) and the high urinary potassium (e.g., 35 mEq/L) do not suggest renal tubular malfunction or acute tubular failure. The 24-hour urinary potassium is useful in calculating the minimum potassium requirement. The serum creatinine level rises, and oliguria occurs in the late stages. Treatment is aimed at maintaining normal serum electrolyte concentrations, intravascular volume, and colloid osmotic pressure. The intravascular volume can be roughly estimated by the central venous pressure (CVP); if the CVP is low, colloid is given as salt-poor human albumin or plasma. The liver cannot adequately maintain the serum albumin.

The child in severe liver failure is prone to infection, the site and organism of which may be difficult to detect. The temperature may not be elevated; in severe illness it may actually be lower than normal. If intravascular coagulation (as manifested by thrombocytopenia and low fibrinogen) occurs, it is usually due to septicemia rather than liver disease *per se*. Sputum, urine, blood, and cerebrospinal fluid cultures, as well as chest roentgenograms, may be necessary to detect the site and extent of infection. If there is indication of infection, an appropriate antibiotic should be given. If the child cannot cope with his oral secretions or has respiratory distress, a cuffed endotracheal tube will be required. Loss of swallowing reflex usually precedes respiratory depression.

Steroids are frequently used in patients with acute hepatic failure, but it is difficult to judge their value.[20, 21] Contraindications to their use are infection and gastrointestinal hemorrhage, which is commonly due to superficial gastritis and usually responds to fresh blood replacement and intravenous pituitrin, although it occasionally requires surgery.

The results of the approach described here have been good in the child with chronic liver disease and superimposed strain on the decreased liver metabolism. As these patients improve, protein is slowly reintroduced in the diet and oral antibiotics reduced. The initial addition of protein is only 10 gm or less daily. If the child does not become very drowsy or confused, low salt milk (8 ounces of whole milk contains 9.1 gm protein) is then tried as an addition and, if tolerated, that quantity of protein is included in the diet. In this way the response to increased protein intake can be assessed. The hypoalbuminemia which usually occurs during the course of acute liver failure may need to be combated by intravenous administration of salt-poor albumin, especially if the serum albumin is under 2 gm per 100 ml. As a diuretic when ascites and peripheral edema cause discomfort, spiranolactone (Aldactone) should be tried, but many patients usually require the concomitant use of benzothiadiazides such as chlorothiazide. If these latter are used, they should be supplemented with potassium chloride.

Specific Procedures

Fulminant hepatic failure has a high mortality.[1] Procedures such as hemodialysis, peritoneal dialysis, and blood and plasma exchange transfusions have therefore been advocated to eliminate or dilute the unknown metabolites and thus reduce the degree of encephalopathy and other systemic effects of severe disease.[22-28]

Exchange transfusion with whole blood and plasmapheresis and return of packed cells and platelets with fresh plasma have been the most common procedures used. These can be performed in most medical centers. The indications are severe hepatic coma without response to treatment after about 24 hours, or rapid deterioration with respiratory distress. Because the child is usually in a high cardiac output state and sensitive to volume depletion, the blood pressure, CVP, and blood volume should be stable before the procedure is begun. About 150 per cent of the calculated blood volume is exchanged by administration and withdrawal of blood simultaneously into and from two vessels, with the patient's vital signs monitored. The procedure is repeated about every 24 hours if the patient does not improve. Fresh blood must be used in order to replace platelets. If heparinized blood is used, clotting time is estimated following the replacement and protamine sulphate is administered to maintain a normal clotting time.

Although such transfusions are often used, their therapeutic value is difficult to gauge. In our experience over 60 per cent of children so transfused awoke sufficiently to talk, but many of these children subsequently died of complications or relapsed into coma. The survival of about 40 per cent may be related to the ability of the liver to regenerate. We have demonstrated improvement in cardiac output and prothrombin time after exchange transfusion. In the third report of the Fulminant Hepatic Failure Surveillance Study,[1] 33 of 38 children with deep hepatic coma had exchange transfusion and of these 33, 30 died; the five children who were not so treated all died. We have seen one patient with Reye's syndrome who was in coma for one day survive without replacement, and there are other reports of such patients. In experiments on rhesus monkeys, repeated exchange transfusions have been shown to reverse hepatic coma and significantly prolong life.[28] While exchange transfusions are recommended for liver failure in humans, more experience is necessary to define their value.

Once facilities and blood are available for transfusions, it is difficult to discontinue such supportive therapy in the child who does not respond. Continual improvement in prothrombin time is a most useful sign, whereas the lowering of serum G.O.T., of other enzymes, and of blood ammonia does not necessarily indicate good prognosis. The electroencephalogram is useful only in terminal events, in which flat voltage may be a sign of permanent brain damage. Complications such as renal failure, respiratory failure, and sepsis (which can occur at any stage) need not be indications for stopping such a program of therapy. There have been reports of survival despite all of them.[29, 30] On the other hand, hepatic coma is but one manifestation of liver failure, and patients who have recovered from coma can succumb to any of the other complications mentioned.

Treatment by human cross circulation has been used in adult patients, but ethical considerations and the risk of transmitting the disease to the normal volunteer add special difficulties. Cross circulation with a baboon has been reported,[31] but it is still in experimental stages. Repeated cross circulation between two normal baboons usually results in severe reactions.[32] Pig or bovine livers have been used in extracorporeal perfusions in the treatment of hepatic failure. There are reports of improvement in consciousness while the patient is connected to the human donor or animal liver, but long-term cures are few. These procedures need to be performed in specially equipped centers. In patients who have not responded to usual conservative treatment and in whom liver failure is fulminant, such procedures may be indicated. The overall results are difficult to assess, as are also those of any of these procedures performed on adult patients whose chronic liver disease tends to have a highly variable course.

SUMMARY

The aim of treatment in liver failure in children is to maintain the child until the liver function is improved. (See accompanying chart for outline of suggested regimen.) Possible causes of coma other than liver failure must be investigated; hypoglycemia, infection, electrolyte imbalance, or gastrointestinal hemorrhage must be prevented if possible or promptly recognized and treated if they occur. Dietary protein is restricted and alimentary protein breakdown by bacteria is decreased by oral antibiotics and purgatives. Glucocorticosteroids may be administered. If the deeply comatose child does not improve or deteriorates rapidly, procedures such as exchange blood transfusions should be used. All aspects of therapy may be required in the child recovering from the acute phase or in the child with chronic liver failure. The mortality rate is high, and prevention or early detection of this syndrome is important.

REGIMEN FOR TREATMENT OF HEPATIC FAILURE

Acute Phase
Diet
Stop protein.
Add glucose and carbohydrate.
Administer parenterally vitamins K, B complex, folic acid, and ascorbic acid.
Antibiotics
Oral, and poorly absorbed (e.g., neomycin, 1 to 4 gm daily).
Combat infection if present.
Purgation and Enema
Use if indicated.
To Prevent Precipitating or Aggravating Factors
1. Protein restriction.
2. Treat gastrointestinal bleeding.
3. Fluid and electrolyte correction.
4. Avoid diuretics — except spiranolactone.
5. Avoid paracentesis.
6. Maintain adequate blood glucose.
7. Sedation, if necessary by drugs excreted by the kidney.

Ascites
Diagnostic tap
Spiranolactone (Aldactone 25 mg, t.i.d.)
Salt-poor albumin
Further Procedures (possibly indicated in rapid deterioration or severe hepatic coma not responding to other treatment)
1. Exchange blood or plasma transfusion (one and one-half to two times blood volume).
2. Cross circulation with human or primate donors.
3. Perfusion with *ex vivo* liver.
4. Liver transplantation.

References

1. Trey, C., Lipworth, L., Chalmers, T. C., Davidson, C. S., Gottlieb, L. S., Popper, H., and Saunders, S. J.: Fulminant hepatic failure. Presumable contribution of halothane. New Eng. J. Med., *279*:789, 1968.
2. Trey, C., Burns, D. G., and Saunders, S. J.: Treatment of hepatic coma by exchange blood transfusion. New Eng. J. Med., *274*:473, 1966.
3. Ritt, D. J., Whelan, G., Werner, D. J., Eiglerbrodt, E. H., Schenker, S., and Combes, B.: Acute hepatic necrosis with stupor or coma: An analysis of thirty-one patients. Medicine, *48*:151, 1969.
4. Reye, R. D. K., Morgan, G., and Baral, J.: Encephalopathy and fatty degeneration of the viscera. A disease entity in childhood. Lancet, *2*:749, 1963.
5. Bradford, W. D., and Latham, W. C.: Acute encephalopathy and fatty hepatomegaly. Amer. J. Dis. Child., *114*:152, 1967.
6. Randolph, M., and Gelfman, N. A.: Acute encephalopathy in children associated with acute hepatocellular dysfunction. Reye's syndrome revisited. Amer. J. Dis. Child., *116*:303, 1968.
7. Huttenlocher, P. R., Schwartz, A. D., and Klatskin, G.: Reye's syndrome. Ammonia intoxication as a possible factor in the encephalopathy. Pediatrics, *43*:443, 1969.
8. Sherlock, S.: Diseases of the Liver and Biliary System, 4th Edition. Philadelphia, F. A. Davis Co., 1968, p. 518.
9. London, W. T., Sutnick, A. I., and Blumberg, B. S.: Australia antigen and auto viral hepatitis. Ann. Int. Med., *70*:55, 1969.
10. Prince, A. M.: Relation of Australia and SH antigens. Lancet, *2*:462, 1968.
11. Pollock, T. M., and Reid, D.: Assessment of British gammaglobulin in preventing

infectious hepatitis. A report to the Director of the Public Health Laboratory Service. Brit. Med. J., 2:451, 1968.

12. Lepper, M. H., Wolfe, C. K., Zimmerman, H. G., Caldwell, E. R., Spies, W. H., and Dowling, H. F.: Effects of large doses of aureomycin on human liver. Arch. Int. Med., 88:271, 1951.

13. Schultz, J. C., Adamson, J. S., Workman, W. W., and Horman, T. D.: Fatal liver disease after intravenous administration of tetracycline in high dosage. New Eng. J. Med., 269:999, 1963.

14. Lederman, R. J., Davis, F. B., and Davis, P. J.: Exchange transfusion as treatment of acute hepatic failure due to anti-tuberculous drugs. Ann. Int. Med., 68:830, 1968.

15. Trey, C., Lipworth, L., and Davidson, C. S.: The clinical syndrome of halothane hepatitis. Anesth. Analg., 48:1033, 1969.

16. Plum, F., and Posner, J. B.: The Diagnosis of Stupor and Coma. Philadelphia, F. A. Davis Co., 1966, p. 138.

17. Hayward, J. N., and Boshell, B. R.: Paraldehyde intoxication with metabolic acidosis. Report of 2 cases, experimental data and critical review of the literature. Amer. J. Med., 26:965, 1967.

18. Sampson, R. I., Trey, C., Timme, A. H., and Saunders, S. J.: Fulminant hepatitis with recurrent hypoglycemia and hemorrhage. Gastroenterology, 53:291, 1967.

19. Summerskill, W. H.: Hepatic failure and the kidney. Gastroenterology, 51:92, 1965.

20. Katz, R., Velasco, M., Klinger, J., and Alessandri, H.: Corticosteroids in treatment of acute hepatic coma. Gastroenterology, 42:258, 1962.

21. Schiff, L.: Use of steroids in liver disease. Medicine, 45:565, 1966.

22. Neinhuis, L. I., Mulmed, E. I., and Kelley, J.: Hepatic coma, treatment emphasizing merit of peritoneal dialysis. Amer. J. Surg., 106:980, 1963.

23. Krebs, R., and Flynn, M.: Treatment of hepatic coma with exchange transfusion and peritoneal dialysis. J.A.M.A., 199:430, 1967.

24. Lee, C., and Tink, A.: Exchange transfusion in hepatic coma; report of a case. Med. J. Australia, 1:40, 1958.

25. Berger, R. L., and Stohlman, F., Jr.: Evaluation of blood exchange in treatment of hepatic coma. Amer. J. Surg., 112:412, 1966.

26. Burnell, J. M., Thomas, E. D., Ansell, J. S., Cross, H. E., Dillard, D. H., Epstein, R. B., Eschbach, J. W., Jr., Hogan, R., Hutchings, R. H., Motulsky, A., Ormsby, J. W., Poffenbarger, P., Scribner, B. H., and Volwiler, W.: Observations on cross circulation in man. Amer. J. Med., 38:832, 1965.

27. Burnell, J. M., Dawbon, J. K., Epstein, R. B., Gutman, R. H., Leinbach, G. E., Thomas, E. D., and Volwiler, W.: Acute hepatic coma treated by cross circulation of exchange transfusion. New Eng. J. Med., 276:935, 1967.

28. Trey, C., Garcia, F. G., King, N. W., Lowenstein, L. M., and Davidson, C. S.: Massive liver necrosis in the monkey. The effects of exchange blood transfusion of fulminant liver failure. J. Lab. Clin. Med., 73:784, 1969.

29. Thompson, E. N., Cowdery, J., and Martin, J.: Hepatic coma with renal failure, treated by repeated exchange transfusions. Arch. Dis. Child., 43:368, 1968.

30. Trey, C., and Davidson, C. S.: The management of fulminant hepatic failure. Progress in Liver Diseases, Vol. III. H. Popper and F. Schaffner, editors. New York, Grune and Stratton, 1970, pp. 282–298.

31. Bosman, S. C. W., Lerblanche, J., Saunders, S. J., and Harrison, G. G.: Cross circulation between man and baboon. Lancet, 2:583, 1968.

32. Starb, R., Buckner, C. D., Epstein, R. B., Graham, T., and Thomas, E. D.: Clinical and hematologic effects of cross circulation in baboons. Transfusion, 9:23, 1969.

10

Acute Renal Failure

Robert S. Dobrin, M.D.,
C. Duane Larsen, M.D., and
Malcolm A. Holliday, M.D.

The syndrome of acute renal failure in children evolves from many causes. The prognosis of a particular episode may be modified by the particular process causing the impairment in function and by the speed with which the condition is detected and treated. Over 140 children have been admitted to the University of California Pediatric Service during the past 8 years in whom this diagnosis was made. The survival rate during both the acute and the long-term treatment has steadily improved. In this 8-year interval, there have been three developments which have influenced this improvement. Physicians have become more alert to the causes and early signs of acute renal failure; pediatric nephrology has developed as a subspecialty in medical school hospitals so that experienced teams of physicians, nurses, and technicians have become experts in managing the care of patients with extended (> 1 week) renal failure; dialysis and transplantation have become available as treatment for irreversible renal failure.

From the Department of Pediatrics, University of California, San Francisco, and San Francisco General Hospital, San Francisco, California. Supported by Training Grant HD 00182 from the National Institute of Child Health and Human Development.

The authors are indebted to Dr. Carolyn Piel, Dr. Donald Potter, house staff, fellows, and nurses on the renal service at the University of California, San Francisco, and San Francisco General Hospital. We gratefully acknowledge their assistance in the medical management of these patients.

This article deals primarily with the recognition of the causes and their therapy, the identification and treatment of manifestations, and the management of the patient who is handicapped by lacking excretory capacity.

CAUSES OF ACUTE RENAL FAILURE AND THEIR TREATMENT

The causes of acute renal failure include acute reversible impairment in function, acute parenchymal disease that is irreversible, and chronic parenchymal disease, often undetected, in which the signs of failure develop suddenly. In acute reversible disease, a good result depends only on successful management of the acute phase.[1] In both acute irreversible disease and chronic destructive disease, ultimate recovery depends upon the availability of dialysis and transplantation. Our 140 cases were nearly evenly divided among those three categories.

The basis for the diagnosis of acute renal failure may be oliguria, chemical uremia (elevated blood urea nitrogen [BUN] or creatinine), or an obvious nephrotoxic state, as in myoglobinuria.[2] Children with chronic renal disease and acute renal failure may not have oliguria.[3]

The causes may also be divided into prerenal, renal, and postrenal.

Prerenal

In prerenal cases, hypotension and hypovolemia lead to poor renal perfusion.[4] The causes are:

(a) Blood loss or aortic or renal vessel injury following trauma or surgical operations. The condition has occurred in newborn infants following cardiac surgery where aortic clamping was used. Renal vessel thrombosis is an extreme example.

(b) Dehydration or contraction of extracellular fluid volume (ECFV). This occurs mostly where malnutrition and diarrheal dehydration are prevalent.[5]

(c) Pooling of interstitial fluid into a local area of injury. Burns are the most important example.[6] Postoperatively, there may be pooling of ECFV into an operative site. Peritonitis and other exudative processes may cause hypovolemia. A clysis containing too little sodium chloride, e.g., 5 per cent glucose and water, may produce dislocation of ECFV. (For treatment, see p. 116.)

Renal

These conditions comprise by far the largest number of cases of acute renal failure. In this group there is damage to glomeruli or tubules so that renal function is directly impaired. The process may be sudden or it may have proceeded slowly, but suddenly reaches a stage of clinical uremia. The injury may be an extension of prerenal hypoperfusion in which ischemia led to necrosis. The various causes include:

(a) Intravascular coagulation (acute): the hemolytic uremic syndrome;[7, 8] septic shock[9] (particularly in an asplenic patient, including those who have had a kidney transplant); and severe hemorrhagic shock.

Heparin is used in the belief that it will lessen the thrombosis and the progressing injury to the kidney.[7]

(b) Glomerulonephropathies (acute): these are presumed to be immunological disorders in a number of instances, e.g., acute post-streptococcal glomerulonephritis,[10] lupus nephritis, and "rapidly progressive" glomerulonephritis. Acute and chronic rejection of a donor kidney is another example.[11]

Steroids, azothiaprine, cyclophosphamide, and heparin all have been used in acute severe glomerulonephritis. Their effectiveness in preventing renal failure is uncertain.

(c) Neoplastic diseases (acute): leukemia, lymphoma, and other tumors may directly infiltrate the kidney and cause damage. They may be associated with hyperuricemia or xanthinuria and cause damage.[12, 13] Allopurinol, to reduce uric acid formation, and alkali treatment, to facilitate urine excretion of uric acid, may be required, If oliguria already is present, dialysis to lower uric acid concentration in plasma is indicated.

(d) Renal necrosis (acute): acute tubular necrosis follows prolonged shock and renal ischemia (see p. 114), certain nephrotoxins (chloroform, heavy metals, organic insecticides, and so forth), and hemoglobinuria and myoglobinuria. Cortical necrosis, which may result from severe ischemia, is irreversible. Medullary necrosis, usually associated with diabetes mellitus, is rare and poorly understood.

Acute tubular necrosis can be averted by early treatment of shock (see p. 116). Inducing a mannitol diuresis in a patient with hemoglobinuria or myoglobinuria will lessen the toxic effect of these pigments.

(e) Pyelonephritis: Acute pyelonephritis rarely causes renal failure. Chronic recurrent pyelonephritis either as a primary disorder or complicating any structural disease can lead to progressive loss of function. Successful control of chronic infection may be associated with some restoration of renal function.

(f) Structural anomalies: These include either familial, e.g., certain forms of cystic and hypoplastic kidneys, oligomeganephronie, medullary cystic disease, or sporadic, e.g., dysplastic kidneys and anomalies of the lower genitourinary tract.

(g) Chronic familial nephritides: These include a number of syndromes, some associated with deafness, anomalies of the eye, retinitis, and platelet defects. Characteristically, hematuria is an early finding. Renal insufficiency is most prone to develop in the second decade. No treatment is effective. Cystinosis is a familial metabolic disorder with multiple system involvement and early onset of tubular dysfunction. Uremia usually develops by 10 years of age. Treating the consequences of tubular dysfunction—e.g., rickets, polyuria, and acidosis—will prolong life until glomerular failure results in uremia.

(h) Chronic glomerulonephritis of any form in which there is progressive loss of function: This may be recognized or silent—usually recognized in children. "Steroid-resistant" nephrosis, anaphylactoid purpura, and other entities are included. The relation of these to "immunological disorders" is not clear. Steroids, or immunosuppressive therapy, once there is renal failure, are ineffective.

Postrenal

Postrenal obstruction includes congenital anomalies, ureteral stricture, tumor, inflammation, hematoma, and lithiasis. There may be acute oliguria, but more often there is an undetermined period of infection and/or chronic obstruction made apparent by the development of uremia. Where obstruction is acute, the earlier it is recognized and treated, the greater will be the return in function.

TREATMENT OF MANIFESTATIONS OF RENAL FAILURE

Failure of kidney function leads to a variety of disorders which become fatal unless they are controlled. A patient who develops renal failure is most likely to have developed some of these manifestations prior to hospitalization. This section enumerates the most important of these manifestations and describes methods for their treatment.

Contraction of Extracellular Fluid Volume (ECFV)

Probably the most urgent task is to recognize and restore any deficit in plasma and interstitial fluid volume. Treatment is the infusion of an expander of ECFV, i.e., a solution containing 115 to 154 mEq/L sodium and 70 to 154 mEq/L chloride chosen from those listed in Table 1 and given at a rate of 20 ml/kg every 15 to 60 minutes until skin turgor is normal. In dehydration, the total fluid administration required to achieve this is between 60 and 120 ml/kg body weight. In trauma, particularly with burns, a total of up to 200 ml/kg[6] may be needed. Plasma and other colloid solutions are not indicated under

TABLE 1   I.V. SOLUTIONS FOR EXPANDING ECFV

Solution	mEq/L	
	Na	Cl
0.9% saline ("isotonic")	154	154
Ringer's lactate solution	130	109
0.5 L of 0.45% saline + 50 ml		
7.5% NaHCO$_3$	152	72
1.0 L of 0.45% saline + 50 ml		
7.5% NaHCO$_3$	116	73

these conditions unless hypoproteinemia already exists, as in nephrosis and shock, ileitis, malnutrition, and dehydration. If colloids, e.g., plasma-like solutions, are given as in burns, their amount should not exceed 20 ml/kg in the first 24 hours.

Once ECFV is expanded and if urine formation is scant, or there is hemo- or myoglobinuria, 0.5 gm/kg of mannitol (2.5 ml/kg of a 20 per cent solution) can be given. This should generate 6 to 10 ml/kg of urine in 1 to 3 hours. If it does not do so, it is *not* appropriate to give additional mannitol and it is assumed that acute necrosis has developed. If there is urine formation but continued hemo- or myoglobinuria, 5 per cent mannitol in 0.2 per cent saline can be given in an amount equal to urine flow for a period of 2 to 8 hours, or until urine is free of pigment. Five per cent mannitol in 0.2 per cent saline is approximately equal to the composition of urine during mannitol diuresis, so that if volume infused is made equal to volume excreted for 2 to 8 hours, significant imbalance is unlikely. However, careful monitoring of sodium concentration in serum (Na$_S$) and weight, in addition to urine flow, are important. Bladder catheterization for this period is desirable.

Hyperkalemia

Hyperkalemia may cause heart block, bradycardia, fibrillation, and death. Patients with suspected hyperkalemia should have an electrocardiogram (ECG) promptly, and blood obtained for determination of serum concentration of potassium (K$_s$). If arrhythmias are noted or the ECG has abnormalities typical of hyperkalemia (prolonged QRS complexes, depressed ST segment, high T wave, or heart block), treatment should be instituted immediately. If K$_s$ > 7.0 the same urgency exists.

The priorities of treatment are:

(1) Intravenous injection of 0.5 ml/kg 10 per cent calcium gluconate over 2 to 4 minutes; the effect is very transient. ECG monitoring, during this infusion, is desirable. A second dose may be used but is not likely to be effective.

(2) Injection of 2.5 mEq/kg (approximately 3 ml/kg) of 7.5 per cent $NaHCO_3$ to increase pH_s, lower K_s, and counteract arrhythmia. This effect also is very rapid but transient; repetition is not recommended.

(3) Injection of 1 ml/kg 50 per cent glucose to increase blood sugar to approximately 250 mg/100 ml which will lower K_s to some extent. Then, infusion of 30 per cent glucose solution at a rate commensurate with insensible water loss may begin (see p. 121). Effect may be noted within 1 to 2 hours.

(4) After monitoring blood sugar, in the face of persistent hyperkalemia, one may give a single dose of insulin (1 unit/kg I.V.) so long as the hypertonic glucose infusion continues.

(5) If K_s is above 5.5 mEq/L and below 7.0 mEq/L, and the ECG is normal, neither calcium nor alkali need be given. Instead, 1 gm/kg of sodium polystyrene sulfonate (Kayexalate—a sodium-potassium exchange resin) may be given orally or by retention enema. If these measures have not restored K_s to below 6.0 mEq/L in 2 to 3 hours, they may be repeated and dialysis planned for the treatment of "intractable hyperkalemia."

Sodium polystyrene sulfonate may also be used concurrently with Measures 1 to 4, and may be used at any subsequent point in management to treat hyperkalemia.

Hypertonic glucose and water should be used initially, as described below (see p. 121), regardless of K_s. This will assist in retarding a subsequent rise of K_s.

(6) Peritoneal dialysis or hemodialysis should be undertaken when K_s remains above 6.5 in spite of the above treatment (see p. 122).

Seizures and Coma

Convulsions may be an initial presentation for acute renal failure. They may occur secondary to: (1) hyponatremia, (2) hypocalcemia, usually associated with hyperphosphatemia, (3) hypertension, and (4) the "uremic state."

In general, the treatment of seizures encompasses three important principles: (1) maintaining cerebral oxygenation and blood flow, i.e., assuring an adequate airway and circulation; (2) diagnosing and treating the underlying cause, e.g., hypertension; and (3) using anticonvulsant drugs.

Hyponatremia (Na_s <130 mEq/L) may be treated immediately by giving 3 per cent saline (12 ml/kg will increase Na_s by 10 mEq/L). If hypertension coexists, this treatment will be hazardous. The condition can be treated by dialysis, although the response is slow. If Na_s is <120 mEq/L, 3 per cent saline is recommended coincident with arranging for dialysis; 1 ml/kg 50 per cent glucose (0.5 gm/kg glucose) will have a transient effect to correct the hypo-osmotic state secondary to hyponatremia. Mannitol (0.5 gm/kg) will have a more prolonged effect if there is anuria.

Hypocalcemia is regularly associated with uremia. Its contribution to convulsions is always difficult to assess. Intravenously administered calcium gluconate may reduce seizures. Where serum phosphorus concentration is elevated above 8 to 10 mg/100 ml, dialysis and phosphate binding antacids are needed, in that order.

When convulsions coexist with hypertension, treatment of the hypertension clearly receives a high priority (see following section).

The relation between "chemical uremia," convulsions, and/or coma is very poorly understood. However, when a patient has a BUN >100 mg/100 ml and has neurological symptoms,[14] dialysis often is associated with relief of convulsions and improvement in sensorium. It is important to avoid lowering urea concentration too rapidly when hemodialysis is used. A reduction of BUN no greater than 30 mg/100 ml each hour usually will avoid the brain swelling ("disequilibrium syndrome")[15] noted when BUN is lowered more abruptly.

Anticonvulsants, such as barbiturates, are needed for immediate control. Diazepam (Valium) and/or diphenylhydantoin sodium (Dilantin) are also recommended. Our practice has been to give paraldehyde by rectum in conjunction with either giving phenobarbital intramuscularly, or diazepam intravenously.

Hypertension

The commonest reason for hypertension is ECFV overload. Blood pressure (BP) is most effectively controlled by reducing this overexpansion. Hypertension also arises from poor renal perfusion and increased secretion of renin in a closed overexpanded system. Other renal factors, i.e., postaglandins, may contribute.[16]

When ECFV is overexpanded the best treatment for its removal is peritoneal or hemodialysis (see p. 122).

Hypotensive drugs are also used in lowering blood pressure. Intravenous hydralazine (Apresoline) 0.3 to 0.5 mg/kg up to 15 to 20 mg per dose, given at 20-minute intervals, if necessary, for no more than three doses, is usually effective. If not, alpha-methyldopa (Aldomet) given intravenously over 5 to 10 minutes (6 to 20 mg/kg) may be effective. This dose may be repeated at 6-hour intervals. The drug can be given for long-term effect orally in a dose of 6 to 25 mg/kg repeated at 6 to 8-hour intervals. Hydralazine can be given for an acute rise of BP when chronic alpha-methyldopa therapy is being maintained.

Prevention of hypertension also is important. This is achieved in part by the absolute restriction of sodium chloride intake. Nothing should be given that will expand blood volume unless it is contracted to begin with. Children with renal failure have a very restricted vascular compliance so that blood volume expansion of a minor degree may precipitate severe hypertension and convulsions. Consequently, transfusions should be given only by an exchange technique (see section on *Anemia*, following), unless there is acute blood loss or shock.

Cardiac Failure and Pulmonary Edema

Cardiac failure (including pulmonary edema) like hypertension, is usually due to ECFV overload and its treatment is removal of extracellular fluid. What determines why one patient is hypertensive and another has heart failure is not clear. They may coexist. Uremia may, to a varying degree, affect the myocardium, and changes in electrolyte composition may also affect myocardial efficiency. The degree of ECFV overload often is obscured by a concomitant degree of cachexia. Persistence in its removal, until clear signs of ECFV depletion develop, may be necessary. Plasma volume determinations are useful.

Digitalis is the most difficult drug to use in uremia, and usually it is not needed. Changes that occur in K_s, in particular, modify the effect of digitalis considerably. The priming and maintenance doses must be kept smaller than usual, but adequate digitalization is always uncertain.

Peritoneal dialysis is effective in removing edema fluid (4 to 7 per cent glucose, rather than $1\frac{1}{2}$ per cent glucose, is used in the dialysate). Complications include hypernatremia and hyperosmolarity, when cycling is too rapid. Ultrafiltration during hemodialysis may be more effective, although small children may experience shock during the process of ultrafiltration.

Anemia

Anemia almost always coexists with renal failure. If there is bleeding, direct replacement is appropriate. Otherwise, blood transfused to correct anemia should be accompanied by withdrawal of an equal volume of the patient's blood so that his total vascular volume does not increase. An exchange of 10 ml/kg of packed red cells (hemoglobin — 25 gm/100 ml) for 10 ml/kg of the patient's blood (hemoglobin — 5 gm/ 100 ml) should increase hemoglobin by 2.5 gm/100 ml.

Acidosis

Acidosis develops in acute renal failure because excretion of endogenous acid is insufficient. Acid production is lessened by glucose administration (see p. 121). Acute acidosis is most effectively treated by dialysis. Adequate dialysis and intake control usually will prevent significant acidosis from recurring.

Uremia

Uremia as a clinical entity refers to those symptoms of stupor, anorexia, excess bleeding, and other indeterminate symptoms which cannot be related to any of the other specific manifestations but which improve with dialysis.[17] The relation of BUN to these findings is variable. However, there is a general impression that dialysis is indicated when symptoms as described are present and the BUN exceeds 80 to 100 mg/100 ml.

MANAGEMENT OF THE PATIENT LACKING EXCRETORY FUNCTION

This entails the control of intake, knowing there is no means for the excretion of any excess, but that minimal requirements must be met. Patients who are anuric also have a lower resistance to infection.

(a) Fluid and electrolyte intake: Water intake is limited to meet extrarenal water loss, i.e., insensible water loss less water of oxidation. This equals 20 to 30 ml per 100 kcal per day,* and is usually given as 30 per cent glucose. If there is urine excretion, it may represent loss of edema fluid and need not be replaced. If partial or total replacement of urine loss is considered appropriate, this should be done independent of the prescribed 30 per cent glucose and water noted above. The sodium concentration in the replacement fluid should be equal to the sodium concentration observed in the excreted urine. Generally, no potassium is given. As noted earlier, no sodium chloride is given except to replace renal or extrarenal losses which are associated with undesired contraction of ECFV.

(b) Nutrition: In the acute phase of management, it is impossible to meet all nutritional needs. Giving 30 per cent glucose as described above provides from 25 to 35 per cent of the calories needed and is effective in reducing endogenous protein catabolism. This solution, containing 1 U heparin/ml, can be given into a peripheral vein, a Scribner shunt if one is in place, or a catheter inserted in the manner recommended by Dudrick, et al.,[18] and should be delivered by an intravenous pump. We have used 70 per cent glucose solution to provide 50 to 80 per cent of the total calories. We have not used and do not recommend

---

*Calculation of calorie expenditure is done as follows: 1 to 10 kg: 100 kcal/kg/day. 12 to 20 kg: 1,000 kcal + 100 kcal for each 2 kg > 10 (e.g., 12 kg = 1,100 kcal/day; 20 kg = 1,500 kcal/day). 25 kg and up: 1,600 kcal + 100 kcal for each 5 kg > 25 (e.g., 30 kg = 1,700 kcal/day; 45 kg = 2,000 kcal/day; 70 kg = 2,500 kcal/day).

using amino acid solutions intravenously in the acute phase of renal failure. Even in chronic renal failure, should total intravenous feeding be indicated, the most stringent monitoring of plasma composition is necessary, and indeed additional nutritional studies are needed before the hazards or the value of total parenteral feeding in renal failure can be assessed. When hypertonic glucose is given, blood sugar must be monitored to avoid hyperglycemia and hyperosmolarity.

(c) Calcium and phosphorus: Hypocalcemia and hyperphosphatemia, when not treated by dialysis, may be partially controlled by giving oral $CaCO_3$ (Titralac), 1 to 4 gm/day, and phosphate binding gels (Amphojel), 10 to 120 ml/day.

(d) Control of infection: As patients survive the acute phase of renal failure they are particularly susceptible to infection.[19, 20] Careful technique in using intravenous catheters is very critical. Careful observation for early infection is important. Antibiotics should be used only to treat identified infections, and in specially modified doses, because of the uremia. Recent reviews describe the modifications appropriate to this condition.[21, 22]

(e) Peritoneal and hemodialysis: Dialysis has been cited throughout as one means of treating several of the manifestations of acute renal failure. Until very recently, peritoneal dialysis was used in nearly all instances of acute renal failure. As experience with hemodialysis has accumulated in children with chronic renal failure,[23] hemodialysis has been used in preference to peritoneal dialysis in acute failure.

In either case experienced personnel who are used to working with children greatly improve the results and lower the incidence of complications.

Children with acute renal failure often are debilitated. As they recover enough to eat, more frequent dialysis will permit more food intake with less uremia or salt retention. At this point the distinction between acute renal failure and chronic renal failure is best bridged by the term "extended renal failure," with treatment as described in other reports.[23, 24]

References

1. Merrill, J. P.: Acute renal failure. J.A.M.A., *24*:289, 1970.
2. Holliday, M. A.: Acute renal failure. Pediatrics, *35*:478, 1965.
3. Vertel, R., and Kochel, J. P.: Non-oliguric acute renal failure. J.A.M.A., *200*:598, 1967.
4. Hollenberg, N. K., Adams, D. F., Oken, D. E., Abrams, H. L., and Merrill, J. P.: Acute renal failure due to nephrotoxins: Renal hemodynamic and angiographic studies in man. New Eng. J. Med., *282*:1329, 1970.
5. Gordillo, G.: Acute renal failure. Proceedings of the Third International Congress on Nephrology, 1966, p. 20; Personal communication.
6. Moyer, C. A., Margraf, H. W., and Monafo, W. W.: Burn shock and extravascular sodium deficiency—Treatment with Ringer's solution with lactate. Arch. Surg., *90*:799, 1965.

7. Gianantonio, C. A., Vitacco, M., Mendilaharzu, F., and Gallo, G.: The hemolytic uremic syndrome. J. Pediat., *72*:757, 1968.
8. Piel, C. F., and Phibbs, R. H.: The hemolytic uremic syndrome. Pediat. Clin. N. Amer., *13*:295, 1966.
9. McCracken, G. H., and Dickerman, J. D.: Septicemia and disseminated intravascular coagulation: Occurrence in 4 asplenic children. Amer. J. Dis. Child., *118*:431, 1969.
10. Michael, A. F., Drummond, K. N., Good, R. A., and Vernier, R. L.: Acute poststreptococcal glomerulonephritis: Immune deposit disease. J. Clin. Invest., *45*:237, 1966.
11. Coman, R. W., Braun, W. E., Busch, G. J., Dammin, T. J., and Merrill, J. P.: Coagulation studies in the hyperacute and other forms of renal allograft rejection. New Eng. J. Med., *281*:686, 1969.
12. Gutman, A. B.: Uric acid nephrolithiasis. Amer. J. Med., *45*:756, 1968.
13. Band, P. R., Silverberg, D. S., Henderson, J. F., Ulan, R. A., Wensel, R. H., Banerjee, T. K., and Little, A. S.: Xanthine nephropathy in a patient with lymphosarcoma treated with Allopurinol. New Eng. J. Med., *283*:354, 1970.
14. Tyler, H. R.: Neurologic disorders in renal failure. Amer. J. Med., *44*:734, 1968.
15. Maher, J. F., and Schreiner, G. E.: Hazards and complications of dialysis. New Eng. J. Med., *273*:370, 1965.
16. Muehrcke, R. C., Mandal, A. K., and Volini, F. I.: A pathophysiological review of the renal medullary interstitial cells and their relationship to hypertension. Circ. Res. (Suppl. I) *27*:109, 1970.
17. Schreiner, G. E., and Maher, J. F.: Uremia: Biochemistry, Pathogenesis and Treatment. Springfield, Illinois: Charles C Thomas, 1961.
18. Dudrick, S. J., Wilmore, D. W., Vars, H. M., and Rhoads, J. R.: Long-term total parenteral nutrition with growth, development, and positive nitrogen balance. Surgery, *64*:134, 1968.
19. Montgomerie, J. Z., Kalmanson, G. M., and Guze, L. B.: Renal failure and infection. Medicine, *47*:1, 1968.
20. Lawrence, H. S.: Uremia, nature's immunosuppressive device. Ann. Intern. Med., *62*:166, 1965.
21. Kunin, C. M.: A guide to use of antibiotics in patients with renal disease. Ann. Intern. Med., *67*:151, 1967.
22. Bulger, R. J., and Petersdorf, R. G.: Antimicrobial therapy in patients with renal insufficiency. Postgrad. Med., *47*:160, 1970.
23. Potter, D., Larsen, D., Leumann, E., Perin, D., Simmons, J., Piel, C. F., and Holliday, M. A.: Treatment of chronic uremia in childhood. II. Hemodialysis. Pediatrics, *46*:678, 1970.
24. Holliday, M. A., Potter, D. E., and Dobrin, R. S.: Treatment of renal failure in children. Pediat. Clin. N. Amer., *18*:613, 1971.

11

Respiratory Arrest and Its Sequelae

Robert M. Smith, M.D.

The term respiratory arrest is at once an admission of inaccuracy and confusion, since it can only stand for the chaos of a bad accident or, worse, the unhappy occasion when a patient has been allowed to slip through the measurable stages of respiratory failure because of neglect, poor judgment, or inadequate therapy.

Unfortunately, we do find ourselves confronted by children in respiratory arrest all too frequently. Regardless of the cause, salvage of many of them depends not only upon management of the emergency itself, about which there has been considerable discussion, but also upon management of the sequelae, an area which deserves more attention. Actually, the two phases are markedly different: the emergency period demands instant action, rapid thinking, and efficient organization, while the recovery period requires more sophisticated evaluation and grueling observation and sometimes ends in painful decision.

From the Department of Anesthesia, Children's Hospital Medical Center and Harvard Medical School, Boston, Massachusetts.

124

MANAGEMENT OF EMERGENCY PHASE

The two principal factors in emergency care of children in respiratory arrest are: (1) the preparation for such incidents, and (2) an organized response to the emergency when it occurs.

Preparation

Suitable Treatment Areas. Well-equipped hospitals should have apparatus for resuscitation in emergency rooms for accidents and outpatient care and in intensive care units for long-term respiratory therapy.[1] Also, the hospitals should have portable resuscitation kits on all nursing divisions.[2]

Equipment. In each of the aforementioned areas, suction apparatus, oxygen, airways, laryngoscopes, endotracheal tubes, self-inflating breathing bags, masks, syringes, needles, and suitable drugs (Table 1) are stocked, easily available, and ready for use. Mechanical ventilators are seldom necessary for emergency use, but they might be available in intensive care units where more extensive monitoring and diagnostic equipment should be maintained. Since tracheostomy is rarely performed as a primary measure, this equipment may be stored in operating theatres.

Personnel. Most important and most difficult to establish is an around-the-clock coverage by suitably equipped personnel. A properly prepared individual should have the diagnostic competence of a pediatrician and an internist, the technical skills of an anesthesiologist and a surgeon, and the organizational ability of a gang boss. Because of the

TABLE 1   DRUGS FOR CARDIORESPIRATORY EMERGENCIES[2]

Agent	Concentration	Dosage	
		Under 10 lb	Over 10 lb
Epinephrine	1/1,000 (0.1%)	0.2 ml	0.25 ml/25 lb
Calcium gluconate	100 mg/ml (10%)	1 ml	1 ml/15 lb
Glucose	500 mg/ml (50%)	1 ml	1 ml/15 lb
Sodium bicarbonate	3.75 gm/50 ml (44.6 mEq/50 ml)	3–4 ml	1 ml/3 lb
Tris (hydroxymethyl) aminomethane (THAM)	200 mg/ml (1.5 M)	3–4 ml	1 ml/3 lb
Isoproterenol (Isuprel)	1/5,000	0.2 ml	0.1 ml/15 lb

rarity of such a combination in any one person, it is customary to rely upon teams and hope that the cumulative talents of the team will be sufficient to meet the situation.

Of the preceding requirements, diagnostic acuity usually is the most important. Though treatment must be immediate, each step should be determined by previous accurate diagnosis. That which is life-saving in one situation (e.g., strong positive pressure respiration in respiratory distress syndrome)[3] may be fatal in another outwardly similar situation (diaphragmatic hernia).[4]

The importance of early diagnosis in these emergencies cannot be overemphasized. Although the possible causes of respiratory arrest are innumerable, several clinical situations are basically different. The differential diagnosis can be considerably narrowed, depending upon

TABLE 2   HOSPITAL LOCATIONS OF COMMON CAUSES OF RESPIRATORY DISTRESS

Delivery Room and Newborn Nursery

Prematurity[5]
Central nervous system lesions[6]
  developmental pathology
  birth injuries
  drug overdosage
Hyperbilirubinemia
Sepsis
Respiratory lesions
  airway obstruction
  respiratory distress syndrome[7]
  diaphragmatic hernia
  spontaneous pneumothorax[8]
Cardiovascular lesions[9]
  truncus arteriosus
  transposition of the great vessels

Emergency Room

Trauma
  head, chest or abdominal injury
  drowning[10]
  foreign body in airway[11]
Respiratory infection
  epiglottitis,[12, 13]
  tracheobronchitis[14]
  status asthmaticus[15]
  pneumonia
Central nervous system disease
  encephalitis[16]
  epilepsy[17]
  tumor
  cardiovascular disease

whether the respiratory arrest is encountered in (1) the delivery room or newborn nursery, (2) the out-patient emergency room, (3) the post-operative room or surgical ward, or (4) the medical ward. In the operating room respiration is usually under the control of the anesthesiologist and respiratory arrest seldom constitutes an emergency. Table 2 suggests a few of the more common causes of respiratory arrest in each of the situations mentioned. The physicians involved should have these in mind and should have a practical knowledge of their diagnosis and early treatment. While sorting out the proper diagnosis and organizing emergency care, one must bear in mind three important precepts: (1) Don't harm the patient by using wrong methods. (2) Don't waste time with useless diagnostic or therapeutic procedures. (3) Don't initiate a costly effort to prolong dying when the situation is irreversible.

TABLE 2   **HOSPITAL LOCATIONS OF COMMON CAUSES OF RESPIRATORY DISTRESS — Continued**

Surgical Ward and Recovery Room

General surgery
  shock, hypovolemia, hypothermia
  aspiration of blood and vomitus[2]
  pneumothorax
  atelectasis, pneumonia
Cardiac surgery
  hemothorax
  pulmonary hypertension[18]
  cardiac failure[19]
  arrhythmia
Neurosurgery
  increased intracranial pressure
  coma[17]
Ear, nose, and throat surgery
  postoperative hemorrhage[20]
  tracheostomy obstruction or displacement[21]

Medical Ward

Respiratory
  pneumonia
  cystic fibrosis
  status asthmaticus[15]
Central nervous system
  encephalitis
  Guillain-Barré disease
  epilepsy[17]
  tetanus
Cardiac
  cardiac failure, arrhythmia
  digitalis poisoning
Hepatorenal failure[22]
Metabolic
  hypoglycemia[23]
  endocrine disorders

Therapeutic Action Pattern in Response to Respiratory Arrest

The physician's response to respiratory arrest is multiphasic and includes simultaneously scanning the scene, calling for assistance and information, and starting therapy. As previously stated, there is no standard routine to be followed. Ventilation and circulation must be restored and maintained. To accomplish this, the following basic approach is suggested which must be altered to suit each situation:

Begin with brisk, 5-second external cardiac massage.[24] (*Note*: cardiac massage in infants is most effective when both hands are used, thumbs at mid-sternum. To avoid rupture of liver or stomach, it is better to stand above the patient, as shown in Figures 1 and 2.) The anoxic patient's last act often is regurgitation. Initial mouth-to-mouth resuscitation can fill the trachea with vomitus.

Clear the mouth and pharynx of obstructing material with finger or suction.[25] Seconds taken here are not wasted.

Ventilate gently with mouth-to-mouth or bag and mask method. Neonates require only small 20 cc puffs. Watch for chest expansion and listen for bilateral chest sounds. Rule out diaphragmatic hernia before increasing pressure in newborn infants. Add oxygen to the system.

Intubate the trachea. This is delayed until initial oxygenation has occurred, as it often takes longer than direct methods. For intubation, elevate the head (sniffing position) (Fig. 3), but don't hyperextend the

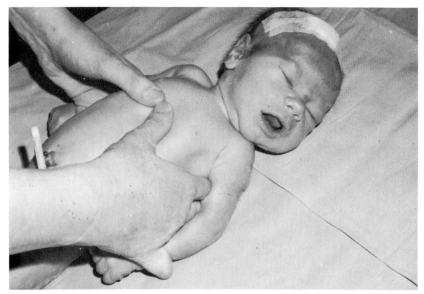

Figure 1. Closed cardiac massage. Thumbs press at mid-sternum, but hands may compress stomach or liver.

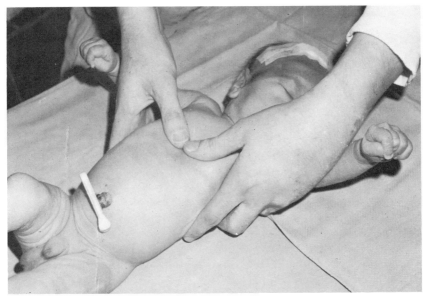

Figure 2. Closed cardiac massage applied from above child's head to avoid compression of abdomen.

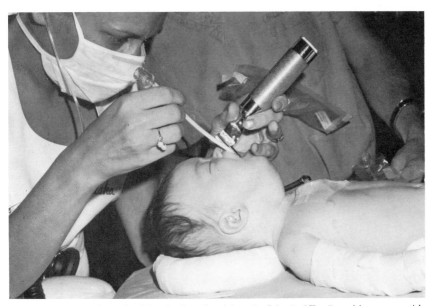

Figure 3. Endotracheal intubation; head is raised in "sniffing" position to provide best exposure of glottis.

head and neck over side of bed; check tube position by chest expansion and stethoscope.

Ventilate with self-inflating bag or anesthesia apparatus. Anesthesia apparatus is better for severe hypoxia; 40 per cent oxygen may be the maximum attained when oxygen is added to self-inflating bag. In case of gastric distention, express gas manually or pass nasogastric tube.

Continue cardiac massage until spontaneous pulse is easily palpable. Rate of massage is 180 per minute for neonates, 100 per minute for adults. Adequacy is shown by palpable pulsation and regular pupils. Do not interrupt massage for ventilation, which may be interposed between every fourth cardiac compression. Remember that overinflation causes pneumothorax. Take early chest films.

Use narcotic antagonist if indicated. Levallorphan (Lorfan), 0.02 mg/kg of body weight, or nalorphine (Nalline), 0.01 mg/kg.[26] Other respiratory stimulants (epinephrine and calcium gluconate by direct intracardiac injection) are indicated if heart action is not promptly restored; hypertonic glucose, isoproterenol, and buffering agents can be added by the intravenous route.

Assistants are immediately directed to aid in cardiac massage, start infusion, check breath sounds, attach electrocardiogram, and check initial diagnosis, early and recent history, operative and postoperative course, last oral intake, medication, sensitivity, hyperactivity, seizure, respiratory problems, fever, weakness, and other relevant data. Chest x-ray is taken, and blood is drawn for cross matching, culture, cell counts, hematocrit, glucose level, electrolytes, pO_2, pH, and pCO_2. The umbilical artery is cannulated in neonates, and the radial artery may be cannulated in older children. A thermistor is attached for continuous temperature recording, and a warming lamp and blankets are used to preserve body temperature in infants.[27] Lumbar puncture, pupillary and fundus examination, and other neurological procedures are in order for nervous system lesions. The bladder is catheterized for a urinary specimen.

To reduce the dangers caused by confusion and overenthusiastic helpers, it is highly advisable to post one intelligent observer at an early stage as coordinator and recorder, to list each drug and procedure, and to assist in overall organization. After 30 minutes of resuscitative efforts, the chaos that otherwise results makes further therapy grossly inaccurate.

MANAGEMENT OF SEQUELAE

Although treatment of later stages of respiratory arrest is less frantic and allows time to sort out and evaluate some of the problems, many of the answers are extremely elusive.

Management of these children varies considerably, depending upon whether they are among those who recover promptly, those in whom recovery is delayed, or those in whom recovery does not occur.

Group 1: Prompt Recovery Following Respiratory Arrest

A child who chokes on a peach stone or who is submerged underwater for 1 or 2 minutes may develop respiratory arrest and then, after a few minutes of effective treatment, start to breathe spontaneously, move, gag, cough, open his eyes, awaken, and regain full mental and physical control.

Recovery is actually 100 per cent in many of these children, and no subsequent therapy will be indicated; however, some precautions are always advisable, and serious errors may occur. As soon as a patient begins to breathe spontaneously after a period of apnea, there is a tendency to withdraw assistance and let him do it all by himself. This is a grave error, for there is usually an appreciable period when spontaneous respiration is present but inadequate, and marked hypoxic damage and respiratory acidosis may result. Respiration must be assisted until the patient is exchanging actively and adequately.

If the child has had endotracheal intubation, extubation should be preceded by careful clearing of pharynx, mouth, and nose of any foreign material that could be aspirated.

Following any use of positive pressure ventilation and cardiac massage, it is advisable to rule out by chest x-ray pneumothorax or rib cage fracture. Even when children appear to recover promptly, it should be noted that any period of hypoxia may be followed by hyperexcitability, fever, visual disturbance, memory loss, incoordination, seizures, renal shutdown, and other complications. Immediately following any hypoxic episode, a child should be kept under continuous observation for 3 or 4 hours and released only when the parents have been adequately alerted. The child should return for reexamination within 2 weeks.

Group 2: Delayed Recovery Following Respiratory Arrest

Days or weeks of supportive therapy may be required during recovery from severe hypoxic damage caused by the respiratory arrest, or from a prolonged underlying process, such as Guillain-Barré disease or encephalitis.

When acute hypoxia has caused tissue damage, all efforts are centered upon supportive care and reduction of oxygen requirements by control of muscular activity and body temperatures. If there is a specific disease process in addition, definitive antibiotics, medication, and other measures are added.

The problems of prolonged support are chiefly related to ventilation. Although this aspect has been discussed widely,[7, 28-34] several points are controversial and remain unsettled. On two points there is general agreement. The first is the importance of moving all patients who require prolonged respiratory care to an area especially designed and equipped for this purpose. Equipment will include resuscitation apparatus, ventilators, and monitoring devices, plus laboratory facilities for 24-hour blood gas analysis. The second feature is the necessity of staffing this area, or unit, with physicians, nurses, and technicians who will render top-level care on a continuous basis.

Type of Airway. Use of nasal or oral endotracheal tube or tracheostomy will be necessary, but each method carries disadvantages and serious complications.[3, 21, 35-37] Endotracheal intubation has greater advantages in infants and for short-term use. Nasal intubation is more difficult but more easily tolerated. Endotracheal tubes may cause tissue irritation unless especially made and implant-tested (tubes should be marked IT and Z79).[38] The tapered tube is undesirable for long-term use, since the shoulder puts additional pressure on the vocal cords. Many believe that all intubated patients should have tracheostomy after 3 or 4 days, but this is open to discussion.

Indication for Mechanical Ventilation. A mechanical ventilator will be necessary if the patient cannot maintain adequate gas exchange. Determination of adequate exchange is not always easy. If the child remains apneic after the arrest, the answer is obvious. When respiration is present, but weak or obstructed, the decision must be guided by some standards, such as those suggested by Downes and Wood[39] and others.[31, 40]

The type of ventilator chosen depends upon the size of the patient and the type of lesion.[31, 41] When muscular weakness is the chief problem and lungs are normal, a pressure-limited ventilator may suffice; but, when there is pulmonary disease and increased or changing lung compliance, volume-limited devices will provide more dependable ventilation.[42] It is essential to be able to control the oxygen concentration when dealing with small infants. Since pressure-limited ventilators entrain oxygen[43] and the concentration varies with rate of flow, these are less desirable for premature infants. Ventilators still leave much to be desired; they have many mechanical weaknesses and inadequate alarm systems. Most have short periods of satisfactory performance, and all require continuous and immediate attendance by alert personnel.

Starting Patient on Ventilator. Use of a mechanical ventilator should not be initiated when the patient's condition is obviously irreversible (seldom an easy decision), for once thus committed, it is much more difficult to discontinue this form of treatment. When ventilator care is indicated, the ventilator must be adjusted to provide proper respiratory rate, tidal volume, pressure, inspiratory-expiratory ratio, oxygen concentration, and humidification, and the choice must be made between assisting or controlling ventilation. Initial settings are calculated from physiologic data such as the Radford nomogram,[44, 45] with practical modifications,[46] and subsequently altered as indicated by blood gas determination. Rapid correction of acid-base alteration may be dangerous.[47] It may be preferable in dealing with a patient in severe respiratory acidosis to start ventilator treatment and refrain from use of buffering agents until the initial response to improved ventilation can be evaluated. Measured resistance to expiration may also be indicated.[47a]

If patients are hyperactive, or fail to breathe with the ventilator, their activity may be controlled by morphine or d-tubocurarine in small repeated intravenous or intramuscular doses (0.1 mg/kg and 0.3 mg/kg, respectively).

Strict sterile precautions must be employed when suction is used with endotracheal or tracheostomy tubes, since infection is commonplace and dangerous. Good humidification[48] is an essential factor in ventilating devices, not only for physiologic and anti-inflammatory effects but also because it prevents secretions from drying and occluding endotracheal tubes. With adequate humidification, endotracheal tubes may be left in place indefinitely without fear of such occlusion. Antibiotics should be used if sufficient indications are present.

Problems of Continuing Ventilator Care. Once ventilatory support has been initiated, many clinical signs are lost, and numerous parameters must be followed to maintain a correct physiologic course. It is extremely helpful to start a large, time-flow chart that can be posted on the wall, with interim recordings of important vital functions, including temperature, pulse rate, blood pressure, respiratory rate, minute volume, maximum inspiratory pressure, dead space/tidal volume ratio, inspired oxygen concentration, oxygen flow in liters, arterial pH, pO_2, pCO_2, electrolytes, hematocrit, white blood count, urinary specific gravity, volume, osmolality, fluid in and out volumes, and medications. Demonstrations of these values will give all personnel an easy and rapid summary of the patient's progress and greatly facilitate management.

Space in this article allows a minimum of suggestions on ventilatory management. Of special importance are avoidance of (1) rapid change in acid-base balance, and (2) the belief that respiratory alkalosis is a safer

TABLE 3   INDICATIONS FOR USE OF MECHANICAL VENTILATOR

Signs and Symptoms	Arterial pH and Blood Gases
Apnea	pH less than 7.25
Retraction or crowing with rising pulse	pO_2 less than 50 mm Hg
Fatigue or hyperexcitability	pCO_2 65 mm Hg or over
Restlessness	
Cyanosis, coma	

state than respiratory acidosis.[49] Actually, it is preferable to hold the patient in a slight respiratory acidosis with arterial pH near 7.25 and pCO_2 40 to 45 mm Hg.

An error frequently made is to allow the hemoglobin to fall to levels that reduce oxygen-carrying power of the blood. In critical conditions a transfusion will make it possible to avoid use of dangerously high oxygen concentrations.

Vigorous supportive care should include moving and turning the child, intermittent positive pressure respiration, suctioning of airway with the aid of irrigating saline as indicated, and addition of aerosols for bronchodilation. Manual compression and thumping of the rib cage is also helpful. X-rays are taken at frequent intervals. General supportive measures include feeding through nasogastric tube, or preferably a gastrostomy, plus intravenous therapy. The jugular "life line"[50] has proved invaluable in infant support. Urethral catheterization is often indicated as well. Monitoring of electrocardiogram, temperature, and arterial pressure is helpful if available, with temperature control by water-circulating mattresses plus use of parenteral chlorpromazine when temperature is elevated.

Termination of Ventilator Care. This is another problem, since patients must relearn breathing and often have serious psychologic problems as a result of prolonged dependence on mechanical support. Standards for termination are as rigid as for initiation and include mental clarity, normal nutrition and blood gases, temperature, chest x-ray, and Vd/Vt ratio less than 0.5. It is essential to attempt weaning only when expert personnel are available (preferably on weekdays before 3:00 *p.m.*).

If the child's respiration has been controlled, as with an Engstrom ventilator, it is usually necessary to allow a period of spontaneous respiration with a ventilator that can assist respiration (Bird, Bennett, and others). Removal of the tracheostomy or endotracheal tube is a similarly critical step in recovery, because of the possibility of the occurrence of granuloma, subglottic membrane, or subsequent scarring.

Complications of Long-Term Ventilator Care. The variety and severity of complications encountered during and following ventilator therapy make it reasonable to attempt to get the child "off" the ventilator as soon as possible. While trouble may arise from mechanics of the ventilator performance and from leakage, kinking, plugging, or displacement of endotracheal tubes or tracheostomy,[51] pneumothorax and tracheostomy wound sepsis are the most frequent major problems to be avoided.[52] Tracheal ulcerations appear to result from inadequate circulation in which the pressure of the cuffs of endotracheal tubes and tracheostomy tubes plus hypotension of critically ill patients play a combined role. Newly available ventilators that inflate the cuff with each breath seem advantageous, while granuloma and scarring probably may be reduced by avoiding motion, poor fit, and contamination during ventilator care.

Pathological changes in brain and lung that have been ascribed to ventilators are more confusing than these local disturbances. Thus, a marked softening of brain tissue found at postmortem examination after prolonged ventilatory support has been pointed at as one of the evils of mechanical respirators. Probably factors underlying this so-called "ventilator brain" are cerebral vasoconstriction due to prolonged hyperventilation,[53] plus the fact that many patients have been supported so long after clinical death that the brain has undergone early decomposition.

Pulmonary lesions associated with oxygen and ventilator therapy remain a major problem; they are varied in nature and involve considerable morbidity and mortality. The mechanism of their production is not clear and prevention has been unsuccessful. The high concentration of oxygen by itself is undoubtedly one factor,[54, 55] and increased ventilatory pressure probably has additional damaging effects; both agents act in proportion to degree and duration of their use.[56] The response of lungs includes hyperemia, atelectasis, and consolidation of the pulmonary tissue; the initial defect probably is damage and swelling of the endothelial lining of pulmonary capillaries.[57] A vicious cycle is thus begun, in which the reduced oxygen uptake makes continued oxygen administration necessary. The process leads to complete consolidation of the lungs and an anoxic death.[58, 59]

Because of the dangers involved, the general beliefs are that, when possible, inspiratory pressure should be less than 40 mm Hg, pO_2 less than 125 mm Hg, and inspired oxygen concentration less than 40 per cent.

Group III: The Child Who Cannot Recover

This group offers the unhappy problem of the decision to terminate support. In the emergency phase, in case of obvious brain trauma, rigor mortis, agonal stages of irreversible disease, or with the patient who has had repeated cardiac arrests without hope of recovery, the decision may be obvious. Ventilatory support should not be initiated in these patients. Those whose outcome was at first uncertain and who fail to recover have been the source of much professional and ethical concern. Diagnosis of irreversible brain damage is still difficult and, if made, must be followed by the more harrowing decision of what to do next. At present it has been stated that a patient whose depressed responses are not under the effect of temperature change or drugs, whose pupils remain fully dilated and unreacting, and who remains unresponsive to all stimuli and repeatedly shows a flat electroencephalogram may be considered to have irreversible brain damage.[60, 61]

Even this definition often leaves enough doubt in one's mind to prolong support several days after the diagnosis has been made. By this time, withdrawal of circulatory vasopressor stimulation often is sufficient to terminate cardiac action, and the discontinuation of ventilation is a rational and obvious procedure.

References

1. Hamilton, W. K.: Workshop on intensive care units. Anesthesiology, 25:192, 1964.
2. Smith, R. M.: Anesthesia for Infants and Children, ed. 3. St. Louis, C. V. Mosby Company, 1968.
3. Reid, D. H. S., and Tunstall, M. D.: Treatment of respiratory distress syndrome of newborn with nasotracheal intubation and intermittent positive pressure respiration. Lancet, 1:1196, 1965.
4. McNamara, J. J., Eraklis, A. J., and Gross, R. E.: Congenital posterolateral diaphragmatic hernia in the newborn. J. Thorac. Cardiov. Surg., 55:55, 1968.
5. Abramson, H.: Resuscitation of the Newborn Infant. St. Louis, C. V. Mosby Company, 1960.
6. Matson, D. D.: Neurosurgery of Infancy and Childhood, ed. 2. Springfield, Illinois, Charles C Thomas Company, 1969.
7. Adamson, T. M.: Mechanical ventilation in newborn infants with respiratory failure. Lancet, 2:227, 1968.
8. James, O. C., and Marx, G. F.: Spontaneous bilateral pneumothorax in a newborn infant. Anesthesiology, 28:629, 1967.
9. Cassels, D. E., ed.: The Heart and Circulation in the Newborn Infant. New York, Grune and Stratton, Inc., 1966.
10. Modell, J. H., Davis, J. H., Giammona, S. T., Moya, F., and Mann, J. F.: Blood gas and electrolyte changes in human near-drowning victims. J.A.M.A., 203, 337, 1968.
11. Robinson, C. L., and Mushin, W. W.: Inhaled foreign bodies. Brit. Med. J., 2:324, 1956.
12. Berenberg, W., and Kevy, S.: Acute epiglottitis in childhood: A serious emergency readily recognized at the bedside. New Eng. J. Med., 258:870, 1958.
13. Raj, P., Larard, D. G., and Diba, Y. T.: Acute epiglottitis in children. A respiratory emergency. Brit. J. Anaesth., 41:619, 1969.
14. Proctor, D. F., and Safar, P.: Management of airway obstruction in respiratory therapy. In Safar, P. ed.: Respiratory Therapy. Philadelphia, F. A. Davis Company, 1965.
15. Downes, J. J., Wood, D. W., Striker, T. W., and Pittman, J. C.: Arterial blood gas and acid base disorders in infants and children with status asthmaticus. Pediatrics, 42:238, 1968.
16. Plum F., and Posner, J. F.: Diagnosis of Stupor and Coma. Philadelphia, F. A. Davis Company, 1966.
17. Hunter, R. A.: Status epilepticus: History, incidence, and problems. Epilepsia, 1:162, 1959.
18. Dammann, J. F., Jr., Thung, N., Christlieb, I. J., Littlefield, J. B., and Muller, W. H., Jr.: The management of the severely ill patient after open heart surgery. J. Thorac. Cardiov. Surg., 45:80, 1963.
19. Brown, K., Johnston, A. E., and Conn, A. W.: Respiratory insufficiency and its treatment following paediatric cardiovascular surgery. Canad. Anaesth. Soc. J., 36:244, 1964.
20. Davies, D. D.: Reanesthetizing cases of tonsillectomy and adenoidectomy because of persistent postoperative hemorrhage. Brit. J. Anaesth., 36:244, 1964.
21. Kuner, J., and Goldman, A.: Prolonged nasotracheal intubation in adults versus tracheostomy. Dis. Chest, 51:270, 1967.
22. Locke, S., Merrill, J. P., and Tyler, H. R.: Neurologic complications of acute uremia. Arch. Intern. Med., 108:519, 1961.
23. Hazeltine, F. G.: Hypoglycemia and erythroblastosis. Pediatrics, 39:696, 1967.
24. Kouwenhoven, W. B., Jude, J. R., and Knickerbocker, G. G.: Closed-chest cardiac massage. J.A.M.A., 173:1064, 1960.
25. Safar, P.: Recognition and management of airway obstruction. J.A.M.A., 208:1008, 1969.
26. Shirkey, H.: Pediatric Therapy, ed. 3. St. Louis, C. V. Mosby Company, 1968.
27. Smith, R. M.: Temperature monitoring and regulation. Pediat. Clin. N. Amer., 16:643, 1969.

28. Bendixen, H. H., Egbert, L., Hedley-Whyte, J., Laver, M. D., and Pontoppidan, H.: Respiratory Care. St. Louis, C. V. Mosby Company, 1965.
29. Safar, P., ed.: Clinical Anesthesia: Respiratory Therapy. Philadelphia, F. A. Davis Company, 1965.
30. Crocker, D.: Principles and Practices of Inhalation Therapy. Chicago, Year Book Medical Publishers, Inc., 1970.
31. Moore, F. D., Lyons, J. H., Jr., Pierce, E. C., Jr., Morgan, A. P., Jr., Drinker, P. A., MacArthur, J. D., and Dammin, G. J.: Post-traumatic Pulmonary Insufficiency. Philadelphia, W. B. Saunders Company, 1969.
32. Thomas, D. V., and Fletcher, G.: Prolonged respirator use in newborn pulmonary insufficiency. J.A.M.A., *193*:183, 1965.
33. McCaughey, T. J., Kuwabara, S., and Fund, H.: Respiratory distress syndrome of the newborn: A critique of current management of the ventilation-oxygenation problem. Canad. Anaesth. Soc. J., *13*:476, 1966.
34. Ahlgren, E. W., and Stephen, C. R.: Experience in the management of hyaline membrane disease with a new mechanical ventilator. Anesthesiology, *28*:237, 1967.
35. MacDonald, I. H., and Stocks, J. G.: Prolonged nasotracheal intubation: A review of its development in a paediatric hospital. Brit. J. Anaesth., *37*:161, 1965.
36. Allen, T. H., and Steven, I. M.: Prolonged endotracheal intubation in infants and children. Brit. J. Anaesth. ,*37*:566, 1967.
37. Striker, S. T., Stool, S., and Downes, J. J.: Prolonged nasotracheal intubation in infants and children. Arch. Otolaryng., *85*:210, 1967.
38. Stetson, J. B.: Apparatus for anaesthetics for children. Endotracheal tube irritation paper. Fourth World Congress of Anesthesiologists, London, September 9–13, 1968.
39. Downes, J. J., and Wood, D. W.: Mechanical ventilation in the management of status asthmaticus in children. *In* Eckenhoff, J. E., ed.: Science and Practice in Anesthesia. Philadelphia, J. B. Lippincott Company, 1965.
40. Fairley, H. B.: Respiratory insufficiency. Int. Anesth. Clin., *1*:351, 1963.
41. Fairley, H. B.: The selection of a mechanical ventilator. Canad. Anaesth. Soc. J., *6*:219, 1959.
42. Mapleson, W. W.: The effect of changes of lung characteristics on the functioning of automatic ventilators. Anaesthesia, *17*:300, 1962.
43. Lewisohn, G. F., Channin, E. A., and Tyler, J. M.: Oxygen concentration in pressure cycled ventilators. J.A.M.A., *211*:961, 1970.
44. Radford, E. D., Jr.: Ventilated standards for use in artificial respiration. J. Applied Physiol., *7*:451, 1957.
45. Brown, S. A., and Drinker, P. A.: Nomograms for gas mixtures in respiratory therapy. Anesthesiology, *29*:830, 1968.
46. Robbins, L., Crocker, D., and Smith, R. M.: Tidal volume losses of volume-limited ventilators. Anesth. Analg., *46*:428, 1967.
47. Roth, D. A., Rengachary, S. S., Andrew, N. W., Mark, V. H., and Norman, J. C.: Alteration of the blood-brain by hyperventilation. Surg. Forum, *17*:410, 1966.
47a. Gregory, G. A., Kitterman, J. A., Phibbs, R. H., Tooley, W. H., and Hamilton, W. K.: Treatment of idiopathic respiratory distress syndrome with continuous positive airway pressure. New Eng. J. Med., *284*:1333, 1971.
48. Bosomworth, P. P., and Spencer, F. C.: Prolonged mechanical ventilation: I. Factors affecting delivered oxygen concentration and relative humidity. Amer. Surg., *31*:377, 1965.
49. Rotheram, E. B., Jr., Safar, P., and Robin, E. D.: CNS disorder during mechanical ventilation in chronic pulmonary disease. J.A.M.A., *189*:993, 1964.
50. Filler, R. M., Eraklis, A. J., Rubin, V. G., Das, J. B.: Long-term total parenteral nutrition in infants. New Eng. J. Med., *281*:589, 1969.
51. Londholm, C. E.: Prolonged endotracheal intubation. Acta Anaesth. Scand. (Suppl.) *33*:1969.
52. Goldberg, J. D.: Mediastinal emphysema and pneumothorax following tracheostomy for croup. Amer. J. Surg., *56*:448, 1942.
53. Sokologg, L.: The effects of carbon dioxide on the cerebral circulation. Anesthesiology, *21*:664, 1960.
54. Morgan, A. P.: The pulmonary toxicity of oxygen. Anesthesiology, *29*:570, 1968.
55. Nash, G., Blennerhassett, J. B., and Pontoppidan, H.: Pulmonary lesions associated with oxygen therapy and artificial ventilation. New Eng. J. Med., *276*:368, 1967.

56. Welch, B. E., Morgan, T. E., Jr., and Clamann, H. G.: Time-concentration effects in relation to oxygen toxicity in man. Fed. Proc., 22:1053, 1963.
57. Kistler, G. S., Caldwell, P. R. B., and Weibel, E. R.: Development of fine structural damage to alveolar and capillary lining cells in oxygen-poisoned rat lungs. J. Cell Biol., 32:605, 1967.
58. Tilney, N. L., and Hester, W. J.: Physiologic and histologic changes in the lungs of patients dying after prolonged cardiopulmonary bypass: An inquiry into the nature of post-perfusion lung. Ann. Surg., 166:759, 1967.
59. Veith, F. J., Hagstrom, J. W. C., Parossian, A., Nehlsen, S. L., and Wilson, J. W.: Pulmonary microcirculatory response to shock, transfusion, and pump-oxygenator procedures: A unified mechanism underlying pulmonary damage. Surgery, 64:95, 1968.
60. A definition of irreversible coma: Report of the ad hoc committee of the Harvard Medical School to examine the definition of brain death. J.A.M.A., 205:337, 1968.
61. Silverman, D., Saunders, M. G., Schwab, R. S., and Masland, R. L.: Cerebral death and the electroencephalogram. J.A.M.A., 209:1505, 1969.

ADDENDUM

Lawrence Finberg, M.D.

The use of $NaHCO_3$ therapy intravenously has sufficient hazards to warrant amplification of the preceding discussion, especially in view of current practices in the management of hypoventilation in hyaline membrane disease and in severe asthma.

The known hazards of $NaHCO_3$ therapy reside in two general areas, osmolar and pH disturbances. The first problem has been discussed in detail elsewhere and is avoidable by using isotonic solutions, administering them relatively slowly and by using a reasonable total dosage of under 6 mEq/kg/day in a neonate. The importance of the metabolic fate of $NaHCO_3$ during hypoventilation represents another frequently ignored hazard.* Upon intravenous injection, some of the bicarbonate combines with hydrogen ions to form carbonic acid which rapidly dissociates into carbon dioxide and water. In an organism with adequate ventilatory reserve (an open system) the carbon dioxide produced in this reaction can be rapidly excreted in the expired air, in effect reducing the body acid content so that bicarbonate may act as an effective buffer and diminish the hydrogen ion concentration (raise pH).

In a closed system, as is the case with apnea or marked hypoventilation, in which the CO_2 produced will not be readily excreted, bicarbonate would be a very poor buffer. In addition, since carbon dioxide diffuses rapidly across cell membranes while HCO_3^- diffuses relatively slowly, this could lead to a severe and precipitous drop in intracellular and cerebrospinal pH. This last hazard may be prevented by the provision of adequate ventilation when using sodium bicarbonate. Conversely, $NaHCO_3$ should not be given if ventilation is absent or minimal. For example, an asthmatic patient with a high and rising P_{CO_2} needs ventilation *first* and then appropriate bicarbonate therapy.

---

*Ostrea, E. M., and Odell, G. B.: Influence of bicarbonate administration on blood pH in a "closed system": Clinical implications. J. Pediat., 80:671, 1972.

12

Management of Tracheostomy

Dean Crocker, M.D.

The indications for and methods of performing a tracheostomy in children are many and varied. There is still controversy as to the size, types, and placement of the tube; the type of incision; the relative indications for tracheostomy in infants and older children; the use of prolonged endotracheal intubation in preference to tracheostomy; and even the type of instruments used to perform the tracheostomy. However, problems discussed here are mainly the proper care of the child with a tracheostomy tube, including those associated with its removal.

Whatever the disease state from which the child suffers, certain basic principles must be kept in mind during all tracheostomy care. These relate to: (1) inspired gas mixtures, (2) humidification in inspired gas, (3) suctioning of secretions, (4) positive pressure breathing, (5) chest physiotherapy, (6) weaning of a patient from tracheostomy, (7) home care of tracheostomy by parent, and (8) complications of tracheostomy. Let us now examine these factors in detail.

From the Departments of Anesthesia and Respiratory Therapy, Children's Hospital Medical Center, Boston, Massachusetts.

INSPIRED GAS MIXTURES

Gas mixtures most commonly administered via tracheostomy are of oxygen and air, in percentage that will maintain arterial oxygen tension (PaO_2) at near normal. Sometimes this will require 100 per cent oxygen. or sometimes 100 per cent air, which is, of course, 20 per cent oxygen. Whatever the mixture, the PaO_2 should never exceed 250 mm Hg; ideally, it should never approach this figure.

Immediately following tracheostomy, arterial blood gases should be measured with the patient breathing room air, provided that his clinical condition will tolerate this minimal oxygen percentage. If by clinical judgment additional oxygen is required, the inspired percentage should be carefully measured at the time blood is drawn for gas determination. The most common means of administering gas to a tracheostomy is via a "Briggs" adaptor, which is a "T" shaped connector (Fig. 1). Measuring the exact oxygen percentage delivered through such a tube is difficult because this varies with the child's respiration, and each measurement requires repeated sampling of gas. It is better to calculate the percentage of oxygen by comparing liter flow from the oxygen source with minute volume of respiration, in hospitals where this can be measured.

HUMIDIFICATION OF THE INSPIRED GAS MIXTURES

Dry gas of any composition should never be administered to a tracheostomized patient. When a tracheostomy is performed and the upper airway system (particularly the nose) is thus bypassed, the body's normal means of warming, filtering, and humidifying the inspired air are lost. The filtration effect of the extensive and moist nasal surfaces, upon which particles can settle out, can hardly be artificially replaced. Warming and humidification may be imitated, but their interrelation complicates the process.[1, 2] Nevertheless, the trachea and lungs must be supplied, if possible, with warm air of proper relative humidity.

Some definitions are necessary here since, unfortunately, many physicians fail to distinguish relative from absolute humidity, the water

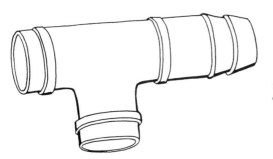

Figure 1. Briggs adaptor, for gas administration to tracheostomy.

vapor content of air, in grams per cubic centimeter. Relative humidity expresses the ratio of the actual pressure of the water vapor in the air at a given temperature to the maximum or saturated vapor pressure possible at that temperature. Absolute humidity may remain constant, while relative humidity changes as air is warmed or cooled. Dew point is the temperature to which a gas must be cooled for moisture to condense or precipitate.

In the nose and nasopharynx, air is simultaneously warmed and moistened to a physiological relative humidity. Bypass of these areas by tracheostomy not only reduces the warmth and moisture but also removes their control, with resultant irritation of the mucous membranes of the tracheobronchial tree and predisposition to infection.[3]

Ideally, inspired gas should be warmed to near body temperature and saturated with water vapor. This can be accomplished by heating water to a vapor above body temperature at a fixed distance back on the inspiratory gas tubing. The cooling effect of the air surrounding the tubing causes a fall in temperature of the vapor to body temperature at the tracheostomy, where the temperature must nevertheless be measured in order to prevent too high an inspired gas temperature. Although water will condense in the inspiratory gas tubing as the gas stream is cooled and the vapor reaches the dew point, it is, fortunately, impossible by the administration of gas saturated to the body temperature dew point to administer too much water (i.e., too high a relative humidity) to a patient. Such a saturation should always be maintained.

However, a very different situation exists when particulate water suspended in the gas stream is administered via a tracheostomy tube. Apparatus generating liquid particles in a gas stream usually employs agitation of the liquid by a Venturi device or a spinning disc. More recently, by use of ultrahigh frequency sound, a water content supplying as much as 6 ml per minute has been nebulized into inspiratory gas mixtures; particularly in intubated infants, water intoxication rapidly occurred. Continuous ultrasonic nebulization should never be used in infants, nor, probably, in older children. It is possible to supply the entire daily water requirements of an infant or child from one of these units, but it has been found that, in children with tracheostomies and with thick or purulent bronchorrhea, the intermittent use of particulate water to provide a lavage of the tracheostomy tube is useful. The toxic properties of dry gases, particularly oxygen, have been demonstrated both experimentally and clinically.[4]

SUCTIONING OF SECRETIONS

For a procedure seemingly so easy and effortless, an infinite variety of problems occur during and after suctioning. An obvious one is the danger of infection, for it has been conclusively shown that suctioning of the airway has the immediate potential of carrying bacteria into the trachea and bronchi. Sterile technique has become of paramount importance.[5]

The use of a catheter of proper diameter relative to the lumen of the trachesotomy tube, always necessary to prevent the rapid aspiration of oxygen from the airway system with subsequent hypoxia, is especially important in infants and children. The ratio of catheter size to tube lumen is 1:3, but, as a further precaution, particularly in children with lowered pO_2, it is recommended that assisted ventilation be performed with a suitable bag and adaptor for 3 to 5 minutes prior to the suctioning episodes.

In patients with complicating hypoxia, such as those suffering from primary cardiac disease, vagal stimulation may occur with severe slowing or arrest of the heart.[6] Vagal effects are particularly active in children and, whenever problems are anticipated, suctioning should be carried out by the physician. Preoxygenation and the use of the appropriate dosage of atropine may obviate these vagal effects.

Catheters should have a "T" or side-arm opening to ambient air, and the suction should not be applied until the catheter, properly inserted into the tracheostomy tube, is being withdrawn. If the catheter does not have a side-arm opening and is closed off by kinking as it is passed down the tracheostomy, vacuum will continue to rise to maximum proximal to the catheter. When the suction is then initiated, a very high vacuum pressure will draw mucosa in at the catheter tip, performing an unintentional biopsy. Problems with bleeding and infection result. The side-arm hole should be of adequate size to allow complete air flow, thus creating no negative pressure during the time the catheter is inserted.

There is a further hazard in patients who have tracheostomy tubes with inflated cuffs. Secretions accumulate above the cuff of the tube and, upon deflation, immediately descend into the lungs, with attendant risks of atelectasis and pneumonia. To prevent this problem, the cuff of the tube should be deflated and positive pressure should be applied to the airway via the tracheostomy tube. This causes the secretions to be ejected over the vocal cords where they may be swallowed or suctioned from the oropharynx.

The standard procedures and routines listed below and on page 144 should be available and familiar to anyone entrusted with suctioning and care of tracheostomy tubes.

Procedure for Tracheostomy Tube Care

Care should be taken in nursing involving a patient with a tracheostomy tube in place. Tubes are easily dislodged, leaving the patient without an airway. All nursing procedures (bath, skin care, positioning, and so forth) should be done with attention to the prevention of airway obstruction from aspiration of fluid, powder, tissue paper, and so forth, or by positioning, bed linen, patient's hands, and toys. Frequent and repeated explanations to the patient about his tube, its purpose, and the procedures being done are essential. The fact that most patients with tubes in place are inarticulate necessitates all the more reassurance and, if age and condition permit, an alternate means of communication.

The nurse should be aware of the size and type of tube the patient is using. The cuff, if in use, should be released as ordered by the physician. An extra, sterile tube of the same size and type as the one in place should be available. Extra parts and the obturator of the tracheostomy tube should be wrapped, labeled, and kept near the patient. A sterile, wrapped, and labeled Kelly clamp also should be available for emergency maintenance of the tracheostomy stoma in case of tube displacement.

It is important to remember that tracheostomy suctioning is a sterile procedure; therefore, a sterile catheter and gloves are imperative. However, during the course of the procedure, it will be necessary to contaminate one hand. Indications for and frequency of suctioning are specified in the Doctors' Order Book. Prolonged suctioning, suctioning with too large a catheter, or failure to allow the patient time to ventilate between suction attempts can lead to hypoxia, predisposing the patient to cardiac arrest. The heart rate should be monitored during the suctioning procedure.

At the first sign of any respiratory distress, interrupt suctioning and provide humidified oxygen. The left main stem bronchus may be entered by positioning the head to the right, and vice versa. When the patient also requires oral or nasopharyngeal suctioning, separate clean equipment should be used.

POSITIVE PRESSURE BREATHING

Although a number of available texts deal with this facet,[7, 8] a few basic comments relative to the use of intermittent positive pressure breathing (IPPB) devices with tracheostomy are presented here. Interconnections of standard size, usually with 15 mm tapered male and female connectors, should be employed to allow adaptation of IPPB machines, ventilators, anesthesia equipment, and resuscitative, self-inflating bags to the tracheostomy. There must be no traction or pressure from the positive pressure breathing device which might cause deviation or pressure on the tracheostomy tube. A number of swivel-type devices are available for tube and machine connection, but all of them introduce some "mechanical dead space," which may add greatly to the carbon dioxide retention of small patients.

In children, inflatable cuffs should be avoided when possible. It is better to rely upon the multiplicity of sizes of tracheostomy tubes and fit the proper size to the trachea. Nevertheless, a cuff may be required in conjunction with a positive pressure device where the peak inspiratory pressure is high and a leak develops around the tube. A cuff may also be required to prevent aspiration of foreign material down the trachea in diseases where the swallowing mechanism is lost.

Patients who have tracheostomies attached to positive pressure breathing devices should have frequent x-ray examinations of the chest to ensure proper location of the tip of the tube. Repeated connection and disconnection from the ventilator for suctioning, instillation, or weaning may push the tracheostomy tube in until it enters either the left or right main stem bronchus. Because of the large shunt developed in the nonventilated lung, blood gases will usually reflect this accident, as will lack of breath sounds over this area and progressive atelectasis. The peak inspiratory pressure of the ventilator will show a sudden rise, for example, from 20 cm of water to 30 cm. If this happens, the tube should be pulled back slightly after deflation of the cuff (if present), and the patient should be given periodic deep breaths and suctioned.

Steps in Procedure

1. Check suction unit and humidified oxygen for working order.
2. Be sure all necessary equipment is close at hand during the procedure.
3. Explain the procedure to the patient if his age and condition allow.
4. Wash hands.
5. Open gloves, catheter, and bottle of normal saline, making sure all are sterile.
6. Don gloves and remove catheter from wrapper, protecting tip while enfolding catheter in palm of sterile-gloved hand.
7. Attach suction unit tubing to the end of the catheter with gloved hand to be contaminated.
8. Moisten catheter with sterile, normal saline.
9. Turn patient's head to one side, using contaminated hand (Fig. 2).
10. With suction off, introduce catheter into tracheostomy tube until patient coughs.
11. On inspiration following cough, advance catheter to main stem bronchus and apply suction.
12. With a continuous twisting motion, remove catheter from tube while applying intermittent suction.
13. Rinse catheter with sterile, normal saline.

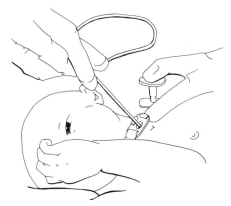

Figure 2. Suction of baby with tracheostomy. Patient's head is turned to the right for insertion of the catheter into left main bronchus. Suction is being performed while the catheter is removed. (From Young, J., and Crocker, D.: Principles and Practice of Inhalation Therapy, p. 137, 1970. Reprinted by permission of Year Book Medical Publishers, Inc.).

14. Allow patient several breaths of humidified oxygen to aid his ventilation and to rest him between suction attempts.

15. Repeat only as necessary to clear airway.

16. Turn the patient's head to the opposite side and repeat the procedure.

17. Remove gloves and detach catheter, discarding both.

18. Check if twill tape or adhesive tape is too loose or tight.

19. Check tissue area around the tube for cleanliness, irritation, and broken skin. (a) Clean area carefully when necessary with a cotton applicator moistened with warm tap water. (b) Dry area carefully with a dry sponge.

20. Change tracheostomy sponge when necessary.

21. Assess patient for comfort and report any respiratory distress.

As has already been discussed, humidification of the ventilatory systems should be as close to 100 per cent relative humidity as possible. If the ventilator system is of the mechanical-electrical type, all connections should be via grounded plugs, and circuits should be checked periodically for integrity of grounding. With a break in the grounding system, it is possible to build up an electrical charge on the patient via the wet tubing and the tracheostomy tube; such a charge becomes particularly dangerous when associated with electrical devices (e.g., cardiac or respiratory monitors or pacemakers) because electrocution can occur.

Another problem associated with ventilatory devices centers around the water which collects in the tubing. There must be some form of trap to hold this water, and it should be drained frequently. Tubes with water in them should never be raised above the tracheostomy, as even a relatively small collection of water may drown the patient.

The respirator may be a potent source of infection and should be sterile when the patient is placed on this machine. Despite all attempts to prevent it, any ventilator will become contaminated within a period of time. Work carried out by Kundsin and Walter[9] shows that the ventilator will be infected within 24 to 48 hours, and it should be changed at or before this time. An attempt should be made to keep the water within the humidifier sterile by using acetic acid or silver nitrate solutions.[10]

CHEST PHYSIOTHERAPY

A regular regimen of assisted coughing and postural drainage should be instituted for any child with a tracheostomy. An effective cough is the most important protection against respiratory complications; without it, sputum retention may lead to atelectasis, infection, and respiratory failure. The patient may drown in his secretions. Even the most critically ill patient should have the benefit of positional changes from side to back to side; and, for those who will tolerate it, both head-up and head-down positions should be used as well. A pillow placed in either flank will aid in the head-down position. Clapping and cupping by an experienced therapist while these positional changes are instituted aids in raising secretions. Infants and small children may often be positioned on the therapist's knees, and chest physiotherapy may thus be carried out (Fig. 3). A combination of chest physiotherapy, suctioning, and intermittent hyperinflation produces best results. Gentle hyperinflation following removal of secretions will often reinflate areas of atelectasis, particularly in the newborn infant.

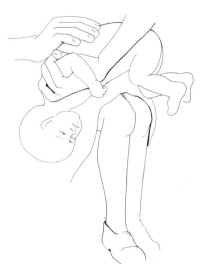

Figure 3. Clapping percussion with infant positioned across therapist's knees. This requires care but can be performed in tracheostomized child.

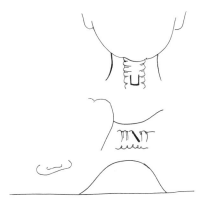

Figure 4. U-shaped incision, with ball-valving following tube removal. In some instances the incision may be inverted U, with similar risk.

WEANING PATIENTS FROM TRACHEOSTOMIES

Plans to remove a tracheostomy require that the patient's disease be well under control, with no acute pulmonary infection present. Coughing mechanisms must be intact and the patency of the upper airway ensured.

Infants tracheostomized for a prolonged period of time may present the special difficulty of insufficient air flow through the upper airway, perhaps, as suggested by Gross, because lack of air movement through the larynx results in retardation of local development.[11] But, patency of the airway at or below the tracheostomy site is more difficult to ensure. Obstruction by either tracheomalacia or fibrotic stenosis, well described by Cooper and Grillo,[12] occurs only when a cuffed tracheostomy tube has been used. Geffin and Pontoppidan have suggested the use of prestretched inflatable cuffs to reduce this type of tracheal damage.[13] Murphy and co-workers have described stenosis following the use of H-type incision for the tracheostomy insertion.[14] If ball-valving of the tracheostomy cartilage (by in-drawing of the flap of a U-type incision, Figure 4) occurs, the accident usually follows immediately after removal of the tracheostomy. Therefore, one should be prepared to replace the tube rapidly.

Without clear and published proof of effectiveness, many physicians use steroids in the hope of reducing edema surrounding the tracheal lumen. Large doses of dexamethasone (Decadron) are often prescribed for 24 hours following removal of the tube.

Among the numerous types of tracheostomy tubes commercially available (Fig. 5), some physicians recommend the use of progressively smaller sizes of unfenestrated tubes on successive days until the tube is removed. They point to the possible complications of ingrown tracheal mucosa into the fenestrated portion of the tube. If a fenestrated tube is used, tracheal plugs of increasing size may be inserted into the tube with

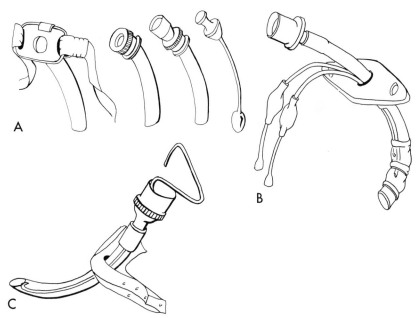

Figure 5.   Types of tracheostomy tubes in common use. *A*, Metal four-part special tracheostomy tube consisting of (*left to right*) fenestrated outer cannula, regular inner cannula special 15-mm adaptor inner cannula, and obturator. *B*, Double-cuffed tracheostomy tube of red rubber for alternation of cuffs. *C*, Lightweight, clear, inert Silon tracheostomy tube.

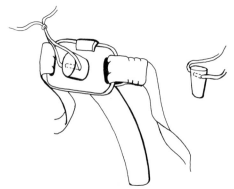

Figure 6.   Fenestrated tracheostomy tube, showing plug. The type illustrated here is a complete plug.

the inner cannula removed (Fig. 6), and a progressively greater percentage of the tidal volume may thus be diverted through the fenestration and less through the lumen of the tube. When the patient will tolerate complete plugging of the tube for 24 hours, it is removed.

Home Care of the Tracheostomized Child

Sending a child home with a tracheostomy is a most dangerous procedure. We have seen many deaths occur from acute plugging, inadvertent removal of the tube, or blockage of the lumen from external influences. Therefore, the decision to discharge such a patient must be made only after the physician is sure the circumstances warrant it. Before the child is sent home, he should be well adapted to the tube, and the parents should have been meticulously instructed by the nursing staff in its care. Practicing of suctioning techniques, cleaning, and, ideally, replacement of the tube should be performed under the controlled situation of the hospital.

Written instructions to the parents to take home with the child should be carefully explained and studied. An example of these instructions is outlined on page 150.

COMPLICATIONS OF TRACHEOSTOMY

Many of the specified complications of tracheostomies have already been discussed in previous sections. The two complications which cause the most difficulties during the first two weeks following tracheostomy are mechanical problems and infections.

Mechanical problems, probably the most common cause of acute airway obstruction in tracheostomized children, should be prevented by strict attention to their common causes. The child must be positioned well at all times; he should never be allowed to sleep in the prone position, and his coverings must be carefully placed. In infants, it is wise to provide a restraint to prevent pulling at the tracheostomy. A respirator should never be connected to a tracheostomy tube unless a nurse is in constant attendance.

Probably all tracheostomies develop infection at some time. The most pressing resultant problem is to prevent pulmonary involvement, especially if there are areas of atelectasis within the lung. Routine cultures and drug sensitivities are advisable during the period immediately following tracheostomy; and if positive, treatment with the appropriate antibiotic should be begun. The patient will eventually develop an immunity and symbiotic relationship with common bacteria. It is important that every attempt be made to introduce no pathogens to the tracheostomy.

HOME CARE PROGRAM FOR SUCTIONING AND CARE OF TRACHEOSTOMY TUBES

Equipment

1. Suction pump
2. Y piece
3. Catheters (French rubber)
4. 3 × 3 Telfa pad
5. Four 2 × 4 Pyrex dishes with covers
6. 3 × 3 unsterile plain gauze sponges without cotton filling
7. Hydrogen peroxide, 3 per cent solution
8. Zephiran Chloride, 1:750 solution
9. Bacitracin ointment
10. Paper bag
11. Pipe cleaners
12. 2-quart covered glass jar or bottle containing boiled water
13. Metal tongs soaking in alcohol

Preparation

1. Place four boiled Pyrex dishes with covers on small tray.
2. Label each dish: (a) hydrogen peroxide, (b) water—inner tube, (c) water—flushing catheter, (d) Zephiran Chloride for soaking catheter between uses.
3. Have pipe cleaners, jar of boiled water, Telfa pads, paper bag, suction pump, and Y piece by tray.
4. Boil equipment once a day: (a) boil dishes and 2-quart bottle for 10 minutes; (b) remove containers with metal tongs; (c) fill respective containers with boiled water.
5. Change peroxide and boiled water before each use.

Procedure for Suctioning

1. Check suction pump for working condition.
2. Wash hands thoroughly.
3. Remove inner tube and place in hydrogen peroxide.
4. Remove catheter from dish labeled Zephiran Chloride—catheter marked 3 inches from tip.
5. Attach catheter to Y piece.
6. Insert catheter to marked area.
7. Apply suction and remove with a rotating motion.
8. Rinse catheter with boiled water.
9. If necessary, repeat suctioning after child has rested a minute.

Cleaning Inner Tube

1. Clean inner tube in hydrogen peroxide with pipe cleaners.
2. Rinse inner tube in container of boiled water labeled: water—inner tube.
3. Replace inner tube and lock in place.
4. Inner tube should be cleaned at least every 4 hours during the day and suctioned as necessary between cleanings.

Care of Skin Around Tracheostomy Tube

1. Cleanse area around tracheostomy tube with 3 × 3 gauze sponge moistened with Zephiran Chloride.
2. Apply small amount of Bacitracin ointment to area.
3. Apply cut Telfa pad under outer tube.

References

1. Bang, B. G., and Bang, F. B.: Effect of water deprivation on mucous flow. Proc. Soc. Exp. Biol. Med., *106*:46, 1961.
2. Hilding, A. C.: Four physiological defenses of the upper part of the respiratory tract: ciliary action, exchanges mucin, regeneration and adaptability. Ann. Intern. Med., *6*:227, 1932.
3. Roche, H.: Air conditioning in relation to public health and to diseases of the respiratory tract. J. Roy. Inst. Public Health, *1*:473, 1938.
4. Lambertsen, C. J., Kough, R. H., Cooper, D. Y., Emmel, G. L., Loeschcke, H. H., and Schmidt, C. F.: Oxygen toxicity. Effects in man of oxygen inhalation at 1 and 3.5 atmospheres upon blood gas transport, cerebral circulation, and cerebral metabolism. J. Appl. Physiol., *5*:471, 1953.
5. Smith, H.: The virulence enhancing action of mucins: A survey of human mucins and mucosal extracts for virulence enhancing activity. J. Infect. Dis., *88*:207, 1951.
6. Fineberg, C., Cohn, H. E., and Gibbon, J. H.: Cardiac arrest during nasotracheal aspiration. J.A.M.A., *174*:410, 1960.
7. Mushin, W. W., Rendell-Baker, L., Thompson, P. W., and Mapleson, W. W.: Automatic Ventilation of the Lungs, ed. 2. Philadelphia, F. A. Davis Company, 1969.
8. Young, J. A., and Crocker, D.: Principles and Practice of Inhalation Therapy. Chicago, Year Book Medical Publishers, Inc., 1970.
9. Kundsin, R. A., and Walter, C. W.: Asepsis for inhalation therapy. Anesthesiology, *23*:507, 1962.
10. Reinarz, J. A., Pierce, A. K., Mays, B. B., and Sanford, J. P.: Potential role of inhalation therapy equipment in nosocomial pulmonary infection. J. Clin. Invest., *44*:381, 1965.
11. Gross, R. E.: Personal communication, 1971.
12. Cooper, J. D., and Grillo, H. G.: The evolution of tracheal injury due to ventilatory assistance through cuffed tubes. A pathological study. Ann. Surg., *169*:334, 1969.
13. Geffin, B., and Pontoppidan, H.: Reduction of tracheal damage by the prestretching of inflatable cuffs. Anesthesiology, *31*:462, 1969.
14. Murphy, D. A., MacLean, L. D., and Dobell, A. R. C.: Tracheal stenosis as a complication of tracheostomy. Ann. Thor. Surg., *2*:44, 1966.

13

The Respiratory Distress Syndrome of the Newborn

George W. Brumley, M.D.

Adaptation from intra-uterine to extra-uterine life is a dramatic and complex event in which the lung undergoes transition from a fluid-filled dormant organ receiving about 10% of fetal cardiac output[1] to an air-filled dynamic organ receiving almost all the cardiac output and responsible for oxygenation, carbon dioxide excretion, and indirectly acid-base stability.

When this transition is imperfect the result is either apnea or, more commonly, labored rapid breathing. The latter indicates a wide range of diagnostic possibilities to be considered for the proper choice of therapy. If congenital anomalies of the respiratory system, asphyxia, pneumonia, pneumothorax, aspiration (stomach contents, amnionic fluid, meconium, or blood), delayed resorption of alveolar fluid, and congestive heart failure are ruled out as diagnoses, there remains generalized atelectasis, due to incomplete expansion of the lung at birth, to surfactant depletion,[2] or to both. Such labored or distressed breathing with pulmonary

From the Department of Pediatrics, Division of Perinatal Medicine, Duke University Medical Center, Durham, North Carolina.

atelectasis persisting beyond the immediate newborn period, laboratory evidence of hypoxia, carbon dioxide retention, and metabolic acidosis represents the clinical entity once known as the idiopathic respiratory distress syndrome, and now by the last three words, or their initials, RDS. This is the clinical counterpart of the disease characterized by pathologists as hyaline membrane disease (HMD). Labored breathing from other causes will not be referred to as RDS in this presentation. Respiratory failure will be used to indicate pulmonary functional inadequacy of any etiology resulting in the accumulation of carbon dioxide ($Pco_2 > 65$ mm Hg).

Numerous unproven therapeutic regimens[3] have been proposed for RDS and have confused the physician and often placed the marginally involved infant at greater risk. Current information suggests that such hazards at least can be surmounted and that survivors may not only have normal lungs but may be comparable to their siblings in intelligence.[4, 5, 6] To achieve this outcome, management must be individualized. The following diagnostic and therapeutic approach is not curative, but attempts to rule out causes of distressed breathing other than RDS and provides compensation and stabilization until spontaneous recovery is possible.

DIAGNOSIS

History and Physical Examination

Almost all infants who go on to have RDS are born before 38 weeks gestation and most will require resuscitation at birth and have Apgar scores below 7 at 1 and 5 minutes. Their abnormal respirations persist after 20 minutes of age.[7] The maternal history is likely to include anemia, antepartum uterine bleeding, and delivery by Cesarean section before the onset of labor.[8] Observed in the nursery, the neonate with RDS is noted to have tachypnea and an apparent increase in the work of breathing characterized by retractions, nasal flaring, sternal rocking, decreased ventilation on auscultation, and grunting. The infant is also often obtunded, cyanotic in room air, and shows evidence of temperature instability, poor peripheral circulation, and edema. Frequently these signs worsen over the first 12 to 24 hours of life.

Laboratory Assessment

The infant who persists with distressed breathing after a satisfactory airway and normal body temperature are established requires blood analysis for oxygen and acid-base status. Blood samples for micro pH and blood gas assessment may first be obtained from the warmed finger, heel, or ear lobe. If these values are abnormal, i.e., pH < 7.20 and arterial CO_2 tension (P_aCO_2) > 60 mm Hg in a distressed infant, we catheterize the umbilical artery under sterile conditions with an Argyle 1980 catheter inserted (the distance from ear lobe to umbilicus) into the thoracic aorta. Subsequently the catheter's position is determined by chest x-ray; the proper placement is indicated by visualizing the ascending tip of the catheter in the center of the heart shadow on AP view. Like others reporting a relatively low incidence of major complications associated with umbilical arterial catheterization,[9] we believe performance of the procedure may be safer for the infant than its omission.

Blood samples may also be obtained through the umbilical vein with the catheter tip placed in the inferior vena cava as checked by x-ray, though the venous catheter is less satisfactory for oxygenation studies. If these umbilical sources cannot be used, serial radial or temporal artery sampling is feasible; capillary samples may be quite satisfactory for acid-base evaluation, though poor peripheral perfusion of many RDS babies invalidates the latter source for reliable oxygen sampling. We do not use the femoral artery for blood sampling because of the inherent dangers of this approach.

A moderate degree of asphyxia from compromise in placental blood flow during the last stages of labor may normally produce a pH of 7.20 with respiratory acidosis and P_aCO_2 as great as 60 mm Hg. This falls rapidly with the onset of breathing and the pH approaches normal within a few hours. Unless intra-uterine hypoxia is prolonged, the infant at birth has a normal serum bicarbonate level of approximately 21 mEq/L. A bicarbonate level below 17 mEq/L is indicative of a significant reduction if buffering capacity and will result in an acidotic pH unless adequate respiratory compensation occurs. After the first 12 hours, carbon dioxide retention in excess of 45 mm Hg in arterial or arterialized capillary blood is considered abnormal though no therapeutic measures are necessary unless significant acidosis results (pH < 7.30).[10] Oxygen tension in arterial blood should reach 65 mm Hg by 1 hour of age.[11]

As pulmonary atelectasis worsens and ventilation-perfusion imbalance increases, retention of carbon dioxide results in a persistent respiratory acidosis and respiratory failure (P_aCO_2 > 65 mm Hg). Larger degrees of atelectasis appear to be responsible for increasing right-left shunts through the parenchyma of the lung,[12] the clinically apparent cyanosis resulting from this admixture correlates well with the low arterial oxygen tension (P_aO_2) found in the presence of added inspired oxygen. Neonatal arterial oxygen levels below 30 mm Hg probably do not provide for adequate tissue oxygenation so that significant amounts of lactic acid are produced from anerobic glycolysis. The consumption of bicarbonate in buffering this added non-volatile acid produces a metabolic acidosis and compounds the respiratory acidosis already present. The acidosis may be further complicated by the inability of the neonatal kidney to excrete acid and effectively compensate the respiratory acidosis.[13]

Radiographic Examination

A chest x-ray should be obtained in all infants with respiratory distress and respiratory failure, provided the infant can tolerate the stress of the procedure. Irreducible risks of manipulation, hypothermia, and the disruption of oxygen and endotracheal tubes are acceptable, even in the most marginal infant, if a tension pneumothorax, diaphragmatic hernia, or misplaced endotracheal tube is suspected. In such instances, if portable x-ray equipment is not available, the physician should accompany the infant to the x-ray department and be prepared to minimize trauma and resuscitate his patient.

The radiographic differential diagnosis of respiratory distress of Capitano and Kirkpatrick[14] (Table 1) warrants a few added comments. In the immediate neonatal period, the appearance of amnionic fluid aspiration may not differ significantly from that of delayed resorption of alveolar fluid. Both show patchy to diffuse water densities scattered throughout all lung fields, but delayed resorption of alveolar fluid may be further characterized by increased vascular streaking, probably due to lymphatic engorgement of the perivascular spaces as the alveolar fluid is removed from the lung by the lymphatics.[15] Aspiration of meconium usually has been heralded by meconium in the posterior pharynx at birth and substantiated by the findings of perihilar streaking on x-ray.

TABLE 1   RADIOGRAPHIC DIFFERENTIAL DIAGNOSIS OF
RESPIRATORY DISTRESS IN THE NEWBORN INFANT*

Primary Pulmonary	*Nonpulmonary*
Abnormalities associated with a shift of the mediastinum	
Cystic adenomatoid malformation	Diaphragmatic hernia or eventration
Agenesis	Hydrothorax
Atelectasis	Pneumothorax
Congenital lobar emphysema	Tumor
Abnormalities not associated with shift of the mediastinum	
Fetal aspiration syndrome	Abnormal thoracic cage
Hemorrhage	Airway obstruction
Hyaline membrane syndrome	Cardiovascular abnormalities
Pneumonia	
Pulmonary dysmaturity	
Transient tachypnea of the newborn	

*From Capitano, M. A., and Kirkpatrick, J. A., Jr.: Roentgen examination in the evaluation of the newborn infant with respiratory distress. J. Pediat., 75:896, 1969.

The hallmark of RDS, diffuse atelectasis, appears as "ground-glass" opacification of peripheral lung fields upon which is superimposed an air brochogram.

The stronger infant with respiratory failure, however, may have an unimpressive x-ray at variance with the biochemical evidence of carbon dioxide retention. The better fixation of the thorax (in the larger infant) appears to permit the development of sufficient transpulmonary pressure to expand the atelectatic lung so that the radiographic evidence of atelectasis may be lacking at maximal inspiration. These findings need not negate other more basic evidences of respiratory failure in RDS.

Other conditions likely to produce parenchymal x-ray findings are pneumonia, marked congestive heart failure, and pulmonary hemorrhage. Although the onset of congestive heart failure in the immediate newborn period is unusual, when present it is usually accompanied by other evidence of cardiac disease. An exception to this is the often normal cardiac size of the infant with infradiaphragmatic total anomalous pulmonary venous drainage. In such instances the radiographic picture of pulmonary vascular engorgement and the findings of marked right sided hypertrophy on the electrocardiogram will be of help to properly identify this as primary cardiac disease though the attendant right heart failure may also cause secondary respiratory failure.

TREATMENT

The treatment of RDS is multifaceted and requires constant attention to all of the factors noted below. It is important to guard that therapy does not become an iatrogenic source of further insult to the precariously balanced infant.

Temperature Supplement

Almost all infants under 2500 gm or hypoxic will require some method of supplemental temperature support to achieve the neutral thermal environment which permits observation or treatment unclothed at minimal heat production. The actual temperature of the neutral thermal environment varies so greatly with weight, gestational age, and postnatal age that no arbitrary rules can be given, though for most unclothed infants below 1500 gm (3 lbs, 5 oz) birth weight, neutral thermal environment will be between 90° and 94° F (32° and 35° C)[16] or some 20° F above that of delivery room or nursery. Temperature supplement for the infant can be obtained either by convection, as in the usual incubator, or from a radiant heat source, either of which can be controlled by a skin or rectal sensor. Since provision of such support is rarely adequate in the delivery room, prompt wrapping and early removal to an adequately equipped nursery is an important aspect of care. Hyperthermia, which is also a stress, may cause increased oxygen consumption, and is to be avoided.

Alkali Therapy

There are no specific or reliable clinical signs of acid-base derangements and the clinical evaluation of oxygenation[17] depends upon many variables. Thus, the physician who treats the infant with RDS or any form of respiratory failure must have access to facilities for accurate blood pH, carbon dioxide, and oxygen measurements to permit the proper choice and control of therapy.

The physician faced with respiratory failure in the delivery room must decide whether to treat the depressed infant immediately and empirically or to await laboratory results. Under such circumstances, the infant with persistent bradycardia (less than 100/min.), cardiac standstill, or unresponsiveness to adequate pulmonary resuscitation can be empirically treated with 3 to 5 ml of 7.5 per cent sodium bicarbonate solution per estimated kg of body weight. The slow (5 to 10 min.) administration of this therapy into the umbilical vein avoids the delay of umbilical artery catheterization or peripheral vein localization. Such alkali therapy will return the infant with metabolic acidosis toward normal and not excessively over-treat the infant who has no bicarbonate depletion, for there is little evidence that mild metabolic alkalosis is harmful.

In the nursery, the acute metabolic acidosis of the asphyxiated infant and the persistent uncompensated respiratory acidosis of the infant with RDS challenge the physician to accomplish that which the patient would do for himself if given time, an option infrequently granted to these infants. We use intravenous sodium bicarbonate both to repair pure metabolic acidosis (reduction in bicarbonate in the absence of carbon dioxide retention)[18, 19] and to compensate respiratory acidosis (arterial carbon dioxide >50 mm Hg) with or without metabolic acidosis. We attempt, thus, to raise the arterial pH to >7.30, which should improve pulmonary blood flow.[20] Respiratory acidosis with arterial carbon dioxide levels above 75 mm Hg usually requires some means of ventilatory support in addition to base therapy.

To calculate the bicarbonate dose required to effect base compensation for such acidosis, either mixed or pure, one determines the base line or "original" pH, $P_{a}CO_2$, and serum bicarbonate as represented in Table 2. For the purposes of such calculations, it is assumed that the pulmonary excretion of carbon dioxide will not be altered acutely and, thus, pH and bicarbonate are the only variables subject to change. Using the nomogram in Figure 1, the "compensated bicarbonate" is determined by extending a line from the $P_{a}CO_2$ value, which has remained unchanged,

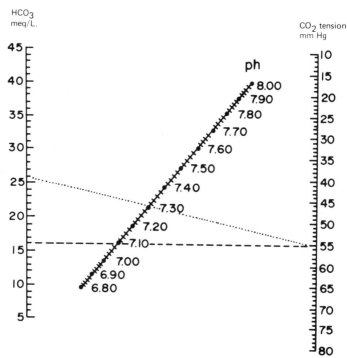

Figure 1.   Nomogram derived from the Henderson-Hasselbalch equation. (Modified from McLean Physiol. Rev., *18*:511, 1938.)

TABLE 2   DERIVATION OF THE TOTAL CORRECTING DOSE
OF BICARBONATE FROM DATA IN FIGURE 1*

Bicarbonate	*pH*	P_aCO_2 *mm Hg*	HCO_3^- *mEq/L*
Original (---)	7.10	55	16
Compensated (. . .)	7.30	55	26

*Compensated − Original   × 0.6 body wt. (kg) = correcting dose
 bicarbonate   bicarbonate   bicarbonate

$$(26 \text{ mEq} - 16 \text{ mEq}) (0.6) (3.0 \text{ kg}) = 18 \text{ mEq}$$

through the desired pH (> 7.30) to intersect with the HCO_3^- line. The difference between the "original" and the "compensated" HCO_3^- is the bicarbonate required per L total body water to repair or compensate the acidosis as indicated in the equation in Figure 1 for a 3.0 kg infant.

In asphyxiated infants, the size of the bicarbonate space appears to be smaller than that in infants with more chronic types of acidosis, so that the newborn infant with metabolic acidosis of short duration is often over-corrected by formulas assuming the bicarbonate space to relate to body weight in kilograms by a factor of 0.6.[21] To obviate this possible over-correction of such infants, we prefer to give one-half the correcting dose of alkali and repeat the acid-base measurements in 15 minutes, giving the remainder of the calculated dose if necessary to achieve a pH goal of 7.30 or greater. Chu et al.,[20] have demonstrated that below a pH of 7.32 effective pulmonary blood flow is significantly and progressively diminished.

Moderate amounts of bicarbonate therapy may be indicated during the infant's recovery from RDS. This therapy can be given effectively by mouth if renal compensation is not adequate. Blood gas and pH determinations every other day will indicate when renal compensation is adequate and supplemental bicarbonate therapy can be terminated.

The use of pH alone to interpret acidosis base derangements is inadequate since the pH is the resultant of both pulmonary and renal function. Empiric therapy based upon pH without benefit of carbon dioxide and bicarbonate levels is, therefore, capricious and may frankly complicate subsequent appropriate therapy.

The use of Tris hydroxymethyl aminomethane (Tham) to correct metabolic acidosis or the mixed acidosis of respiratory distress is warranted in infants in whom prior treatment with sodium bicarbonate has caused hypernatremia. Reportedly, Tham also has the advantage of rapid intracellular penetration and the capacity to buffer nonvolatile organic acids as well as carbon dioxide. However, carbon dioxide production renders any buffer ineffectual in the absence of adequate pulmonary function. When indicated, the formula: Body wt. (kg) × negative B.E. = ml 0.3 M Tham, taken from Strauss[22] may be used to calculate the dosage of iso-osmolar (0.3 M) Tham.

This formula considers only metabolic acidosis since base excess (B.E.) is, by definition, the titratable base at normal pH, temperature 38° C, and P_aCO_2 40 mm Hg. Therefore, alkalinization for hypercarbia with Tham must be executed in steps of treatment and acid-base assessment until the desired effect is obtained. Except in the presence of hypernatremia, Tham is used infrequently in our nursery and appears to have no significant advantage over bicarbonate.

An often neglected but important consideration in the use of such therapy is the effect of hyperosmolarity upon the capillary bed, blood pressure, and cerebrospinal fluid pressure. Recent articles by Finberg[23, 24] indicate the hazards of hyperosmolarity with specific reference to the use of bicarbonate, Tham, and hypertonic glucose so commonly used in resuscitation and the treatment of acid-base derangements. Since hypoxia, an important component of RDS, is certainly a capillary insult, the potential additive effect of hyperosmolarity must be considered.

Oxygen

As with base therapy in acidosis, oxygen is of the utmost importance in the treatment of infants with RDS and respiratory failure, though it has become increasingly apparent that this widely used therapy also has significant toxicity of which the physician must be cognizant.[25, 26] As Klaus[27] has stated, the use of mask oxygen for the infant in the immediate newborn period facilitates cardiopulmonary adaptation by reducing pulmonary arteriolar spasm and inducing closure of the patent ductus arteriosus. We advocate the use of oxygen in the delivery room for any infant who has perioral cyanosis or requires resuscitation. The continuation of such therapy for more than the immediate postpartum period of a few hours requires good justification, as it is imperative that no infant be given supplemental oxygen indiscriminately, especially for nonpulmonary respiratory distress, i.e., intracranial hemorrhage, sepsis, or hypoglycemia.

The adequacy of oxygen therapy must be judged by whether sufficient oxygen is available at the cellular level to permit aerobic metabolism. Tissue hypoxia results in anaerobic metabolism and a precipitous fall in pH as lactic acid is incompletely buffered. Moreover, anaerobic glycolysis derives only approximately 20 per cent of the potential energy (adenosine triphosphate) from glucose oxidation, and the significant quantity of waste heat ordinarily a by-product of the Krebs cycle is no longer available for temperature maintenance.

Oxygen therapy is, thus, basically oriented toward the prevention of anaerobic metabolism and the maintenance of the circulation without reversion to right $\rightarrow$ left shunting and venous admixture through the foramen ovale and patent ductus arteriosus. The exact arterial or inspired oxygen level which will accomplish these objectives without causing oxygen toxicity is not known. Usher[28] has recently suggested that arterial oxygen tensions in excess of 55 mm Hg in infants with RDS cause more severe x-ray findings and right $\rightarrow$ left shunting. Nelson[29] has found little justification to exceed 50 mm Hg in oxygen therapy for RDS. We are not convinced that the primary pulmonary pathology of RDS is likely to result from or be increased by oxygen toxicity and, thus, would prefer to have a larger margin of safety against central nervous system hypoxia. We, therefore, attempt to keep the arterial oxygen tension (P_aO_2) of infants under therapy for RDS between 50 and 70 mm Hg.

Since cyanosis often presents the significant dilemma of cardiac

TABLE 3   DIFFERENTIATION OF CAUSES OF HYPOXEMIA*

Defect	Inspired Gas		Oxygen
	Air		
	P_aO_2	P_aCO_2	P_aO_2
Hypoventilation	↓ ↓ ↓	↑ ↑ ↑	→
Diffusion	↓	↓	→
Venous admixture (Veno-arterial shunting)	↓ ↓ ↓	→	↓

*All indications are illustrative, approximate, and refer to pure (rare) rather than mixed (common) defects.

P_aO_2 = Arterial oxygen tension

P_aCO_2 = Arterial carbon dioxide tension

↑,↓,→ = increase, decrease or no change with respect to normal values.

versus pulmonary disease, Table 3, modified from Nelson,[29] may be of value in this differential. As Dr. Nelson so aptly points out, the pathology is rarely pure and most often a mixed cardiopulmonary malfunction.

We believe the drying effect of unhydrated oxygen may be disastrous for the infant with RDS whose cough is often compromised and in whom even the largest airway may be obstructed with inspissated bronchial secretions. Thus, oxygen should be administered fully hydrated at room temperature, preferably with an ultrasonic mist generator. Warming the hydrated oxygen has the advantage of reducing cold stress to the infant and decreasing the additional hydration required by the infant. Warming the inspired gas, however, may produce restlessness and hyperpyrexia in the mature infant, especially beyond the newborn period.

Inspired oxygen levels should be determined on each nursing shift and the P_aO_2 determined daily. Where P_aO_2 determinations are not available, the inspired oxygen can be reduced daily until clinical cyanosis is evident, and the oxygen percentages then increased by 10 per cent. Oxygen therapy should, obviously, be terminated as early as possible, i.e., as soon as P_aO_2 is greater than 50 mm Hg in room air, or the infant is acyanotic in room air.

Fluids and Glucose

The infant with respiratory distress requires thoughtful deliberation before oral feedings are attempted. Not only may there be paralytic ileus as part of the infant's response to his attendant metabolic derangements, but also a predisposition for poorly coordinated swallowing and aspiration of stomach contents. Even the tachypnea of the infant with delayed resorption of alveolar fluid or low grade metabolic acidosis may compromise the use of the intestinal tract as a route for hydration and caloric intake.

Depending on maturity and the degree of respiratory failure, we maintain the infant with more significant RDS during the first days of life on 10 to 15 per cent glucose in water at 75 to 100 ml/kg (approximately 60 cal/kg) as a fat-sparing caloric provision,[30] which may be inadequate with the increased work of breathing. Such fluids, infused either through an umbilical artery catheter or peripheral vein, are usually begun within 4 hours after birth. With the establishment of good renal function after the first day of life, sodium (20 mEq/L per day), potassium (20 mEq/L per day), and chloride (40 mEq/L per day) should be added to the infusate.

If respiratory distress persists, and especially if ventilatory assistance is to be employed, consideration should be given to intravenous hyperalimentation with the use of hypertonic glucose and amino acids.[31, 32] Such therapy can abort the inanition and cachexia of patients who recover from their pulmonary disease only to be challenged by the threat of starvation. We have treated a small number of infants with RDS and respiratory failure with hyperalimentation beginning as early as 2 days and continuing for 21 days and have been impressed with this approach. The hyperalimented infant who sustains or actually gains weight escapes the early and sometimes disastrous transition to oral feedings. Hyperalimentation is difficult and not without a significant incidence of complications and morbidity from hyperosmolarity, infections, and thrombosis. It should not be undertaken without agreement of the surgeon, pediatrician, nurse, and pharmacist to coordinate their efforts.

Monitoring

Many different kinds of equipment are now available for cardiorespiratory, temperature, blood pressure, and inspired oxygen monitoring. In our experience, these adjuncts are important and of significant help to the nurse and physician in the provision of factual information and second-to-second assessment of the sick infant. Intradermal electrodes have been used in our nursery to provide low impedance signals for cardiorespiratory monitoring without the troublesome skin problems or the false alarms characteristic of surface electrodes. Laboratory support is also required for the frequent micromeasurements of oxygen, acid-base parameters, and electrolytes. While an alert and sufficient staff can take the place of monitors, the physician who does not have immediate and constant access to such laboratory support should transfer the patient to a medical center with these facilities.

Personnel

When physicians must relinquish the care of the distressed infant to the nursing staff, their ability and number become a pivotal issue. It is imperative that the physician responsible for such infants be informed as to the competence of the personnel and the specific coverage to be provided for the infant in question. Lucey's assessment of the Intensive Care Nursery as a place where "people care intensely" epitomizes this consideration and appropriately relegates facilities and equipment to their proper, necessary, but subordinate role.[33]

Miscellaneous

Antibiotics. The characteristic ground-glass radiographic appearance of the lungs in infants with RDS does not permit the exclusion of infection; moreover, the findings at necropsy of significant pulmonary infection have prompted us to place all such infants on antibiotics. When possible, the choice of antibiotics is dictated acutely by the results of gram stain of the tracheal aspirate subsequently modified by culture reports. When this is not feasible, we empirically initiate penicillin G (100,000 units/kg/day) and kanamycin (15 mg/kg/day) therapy for all infants with RDS.

Jaundice. The appearance of hyperbilirubinemia in infants with RDS is a complicating factor of significant magnitude since immaturity, asphyxia, and reduced serum albumin markedly increase the risk of kernicterus in this group of patients. The use of phototherapy in our nursery has significantly reduced the number of infants coming to exchange transfusion during or after RDS. Nevertheless, because of their special susceptibility, serum bilirubin of these babies must be frequently measured and exchange considered when any sharp rise indicates the threat of CNS damage, whatever the current bilirubin level. Stern has recently emphasized the importance of individualizing each icteric patient relative to those factors which predispose to kernicterus.[34]

Ventilatory Assistance

The above therapeutic approach, which represents that employed by many infant care facilities, is sufficiently aggressive to be followed by (and probably responsible for) survival in most infants capable of recovery from RDS. The next level of commitment in the care of these infants is to provide ventilatory assistance, a form of therapy whose advocates believe significantly increases the rate of recovery.[35] Responsibility for a ventilatory assistance program is much more demanding of staff, equipment, and time than the care program outlined above. The 24-hour availability of well trained personnel familiar with the ventilator to be used and possessing a thorough awareness of the complications of this mode of therapy, is an indispensable requirement. Therefore, before deciding upon this course, it again behooves the physician to assess carefully the need of his patient for ventilatory assistance, and to consider whether referral to a better equipped and staffed intensive care nursery is indicated.

The decision to embark upon ventilatory support is prompted by periods of sustained apnea, rising arterial carbon dioxide tension in excess of 75 mm Hg, arterial oxygen levels less than 40 to 50 mm Hg and falling (in 100 per cent oxygen), and/or persistent pH below 7.20. We share with Reynolds[36] the opinion that ventilatory assistance should be postponed until it is apparent that the infant will die without such support. At times in marginal patients, respirator therapy can be postponed by judicious tracheal suctioning and gentle hand ventilation using a bag and mask. There appears to be no totally satisfactory infant ventilator at present and no general preference for either pressure or volume limitation. Moreover, it must be considered that most if not all present modes of ventilatory support impose some risk or morbidity upon the patient.

At the outset, the method for attaching the ventilator to the patient is critical. The nasal adaptor, face mask, naso- or orotracheal tube and tracheostomy each have virtues and vigorous proponents. We use oral or nasotracheal tubes for the first few weeks of ventilatory support, and change subsequently to a tracheostomy if respiratory failure persists. Certainly, the most significant problem with endotracheal tubes is their fixation to prevent extubation or inadvertent passage into one of the main stem bronchi with collapse of the contralateral lung. Since right bronchial intubation is the most frequent misplacement, decreased ventilation on auscultation of the left upper lobe or an acute rise in arterial carbon dioxide should alert one to this complication. Not only does this complication worsen respiratory failure but it also exposes the ventilated lung to significant increased ventilatory pressures with the risk of lung rupture and pneumothorax. Therefore, the fixation of the endotracheal tube must be accomplished by taping, suturing, or whatever means necessary to guarantee its stability. There appears to be little justification for the use of cuffed endotracheal tubes in infants.[37] We have not had any experiences with nasal adaptors or face masks although the latter methods have received support in recent publications.[38, 39]

Though not suitable for infants under 1500 gm because of the buffeting imposed upon the patient, the negative pressure type respirator reportedly has been more successful than those using positive pressure in larger infants with respiratory failure. Reports by Stern[40] and Linsao[41] indicate that many infants can be so ventilated without intubation and that bacterial contamination of the upper respiratory tract by opportunistic organisms is greatly reduced. The effect of negative pressure ventilation upon intrathoracic structures appears to be significantly different from that derived from positive pressure ventilators in that it promotes venous return to the right heart. In addition, there is a significant reduction in lung parenchymal complications as compared with positive pressure respirators using similar oxygen concentrations. Beyond these observations, there are few hard data to support one type of ventilator over another.

The recent studies by Gregory[42] have indicated the therapeutic value of positive and expiratory pressures in the therapy of infants with RDS. Subsequent studies by Vidyasagar and Chernick[43] have shown that continuous negative pressure around the thorax has the same efficacious result with significant improvement in neonatal morbidity. These encouraging results appear to indicate that positive end expiratory pressure is a major innovation in the care of the infant with RDS and warrants active considerations by all who undertake the ventilatory support of infants with RDS.

In the choice of a ventilator, the method of humidification must also be assessed. Hydration of the inspired gas frequently is limited by the small tidal volume in the immature infant with RDS. Ultrasonic nebulization in our experience is a satisfactory method for hydration with either volume or pressure-limited respirators. Most ultrasonic units warm the inspired gas moderately and approach 48 mg of water per L of air which is characteristic of alveolar air 100 per cent saturated with water at $38°$ C. Since high levels of water content are possible with ultrasonic nebulizers, care must be taken that condensation in the respirator tubing does not inadvertently drown the patient. Recent reappraisals of the contribution of mist therapy to bronchial hydration suggest that systemic fluid maintenance is a more important variable in minimizing the increased viscosity of secretions than the type of hydration unit or water particle size.[44]

Other Proposed Modes of Therapy

While the treatment presented above is admittedly aimed only at supporting the patient without further insult until spontaneous recovery takes place, various theories of pathogenesis have led to other proposed therapy. To the reader considering such possibilities, we recommend the review of etiological theories and comprehensive bibliography recently collected by Nelson.[45] It is sufficient to say that such specific therapies as aerosolized surfactant[20] and pulmonary vasodilators such as acetylcholine[20, 46] and tolazoline hydrochloride (Priscoline) have not been encouraging. Recovery, which appears to be dependent upon restoration of a normal oxygen and acid-base environment for the lung, adequate pulmonary perfusion, and the recovery of surfactant synthesis, cannot be hastened by known therapy. Pulmonary recovery is usually complete though the persistent morbidity of some infants who have survived RDS suggests that the ischemic insult may have permanent anatomical effects.

References

1. Rudolph, A. M.: The changes in the circulation after birth: their importance in congenital heart disease. Circulation, 41:343, 1970.
2. Brumley, G. W., Hodson, W. A., and Avery, M. E.: Lung phospholipids and surface tension correlations in infants with hyaline membrane disease, and in adults. Pediatrics, 40:13, 1967.
3. Sinclair, J. C.: Prevention and treatment of the respiratory distress syndrome. Pediat. Clin. N. Amer., 13:711, 1966.
4. Stahlman, M. T.: What evidence exists that intensive care has changed the incidence of intact survival? Problems of Neonatal Intensive Care Units, 59th Ross Conference on Pediatric Research, Columbus, Ohio, 1969, p. 17.
5. Rawlings, G., Reynolds, E. O. R., Stewart, D., and Strang, L. B.: Changing prognosis for infants of very low birth weight. Lancet, 1:516, 1971.
6. Drillen, C. M.: Prognosis of infants of very low birth weight (Letter). Lancet, 1:697, 1971.
7. Fisch, R. O., Gravem, H. J., and Engel, R. R.: Neurological status of survivors of neonatal respiratory distress syndrome. A preliminary report from the collaborative study. J. Pediat., 73:395, 1968.
8. Fedrick, J., and Butler, N. R.: Certain causes of neonatal death. I. Hyaline membranes. Biol. Neonat., 15:229, 1970.
9. James, L. S.: Complications arising from catheterizations of the umbilical vessels. Problems of Neonatal Intensive Care Units, 59th Ross Conference on Pediatric Research, Columbus, Ohio, 1969, p. 36.
10. Albert, M. S., and Winters, R. W.: Acid-base equilibrium of blood in normal infants. Pediatrics, 37:728, 1966.
11. Oliver, T. K., Jr., Demis, A. J., and Bates, G. D.: Serial blood-gas tensions and acid-base balance during the first hour of life in human infants. Acta Paediat. 50:346, 1961.
12. Murdock, A. I., Kidd, B. S. L., Llewellyn, M. A., Reid, M. McC., and Swyer, P. R.: Intrapulmonary venous admixture in the respiratory distress syndrome. Biol. Neonat., 15:1, 1970.
13. Edelman, C. M., Jr., Soriano, J. R., Boichis, H., Gruskin, A. B., and Acosta, M. I.: Renal bicarbonate reabsorption and hydrogen ion excretion in normal infants. J. Clin. Invest., 46:1309, 1967.
14. Capitano, M. A., and Kirkpatrick, J. A.: Roentgen examination in the evaluation of the newborn infant with respiratory distress. J. Pediat., 75:896, 1969.
15. Avery, M. E., Gatewood, O. B., and Brumley, G. W.: Transient tachypnea of newborn. Possible delayed resorption of fluid at birth. Amer. J. Dis. Child., 111:380, 1966.
16. Hey, E. N., and Katz, G.: The optimum thermal environment for naked babies. Arch. Dis. Child., 45:328, 1970.
17. Lees, M. H.: Cyanosis of the newborn infant: Recognition and clinical evaluation. J. Pediat., 77:484, 1970.
18. Usher, R.: The respiratory distress syndrome of prematurity. Clinical and therapeutic aspects. Pediat. Clin. N. Amer., 8:525, 1961.
19. Russell, G., and Cotton, E. K.: Effects of sodium bicarbonate by rapid injection and of oxygen in high concentrations in respiratory distress syndrome of the newborn. Pediatrics, 41:1063, 1968.
20. Chu, J., Clements, J. A., Cotton, E. K., Klaus, M. H., Sweet, A. Y., and Tooley, W. H.: Neonatal pulmonary ischemia. Pediatrics (Suppl.), 40:709, 1967.

21. Palmer, W. W., and Van Slyke, D. D.: Studies on acidosis. IX. Relationships between alkali retention and alkali reserve in normal and pathological individuals. J. Biol. Chem., *32*:499, 1917.
22. Strauss, J.: Tris (hydroxymethyl) amino-methane (Tham): a pediatric evaluation. Pediatrics, *41*:667, 1968.
23. Finberg, L.: Dangers to infants caused by changes in osmolal concentration. Pediatrics, *40*:1031, 1967.
24. Kravath, R. E., Aharon, A. S., Abal, G., and Finberg, L.: Clinically significant physiological changes from rapidly administered hypertonic solutions: acute osmol poisoning. Pediatrics, *46*:267, 1970.
25. Haugaard, N.: Cellular mechanisms of oxygen toxicity. Physiol. Rev., *48*:311, 1968.
26. Shanklin, D. R.: A general theory of oxygen toxicity in man. Perspect. Biol. Med., 80, Autumn 1969.
27. Klaus, M., and Meyer, B. P.: Oxygen therapy for the newborn. Pediat. Clin. N. Amer., *13*:731, 1966.
28. Usher, R. H.: Liberal versus restricted indications for oxygen in RDS: a controlled trial (abst.). Combined Program and Abstracts, 80th Annual Meeting, The American Pediatric Society and the 40th Annual Meeting, Society for Pediatric Research, Atlantic City, New Jersey, April 29–May 2, 1970, p. 83.
29. Nelson, N. M.: Compromised convalescence from hyaline membrane disease. Pediatrics, *44*:158, 1969.
30. Krauss, A. N., and Auld, P. A. M.: Metabolic requirements of low-birth-weight infants. J. Pediat., *75*:952, 1969.
31. Michener, W. M., and Law, D.: Parenteral nutrition: the age of the catheter. Pediat. Clin. N. Amer., *17*:373, 1970.
32. Filler, R. M., and Eraklis, A. J.: The critically ill child: intravenous alimentation. Pediatrics, *46*:456, 1970.
33. Lucey, J. F.: Closing remarks. Problems of Neonatal Intensive Care Units, 59th Ross Conference on Pediatric Research, Columbus, Ohio, 1969, p. 95.
34. Stern, L.: Temperature control, hydration and feeding, bilirubin and calcium metabolism. Biol. Neonat., *16*:92, 1970.
35. Swyer, P. R.: An assessment of artificial respiration in the newborn. Problems of Neonatal Intensive Care Units, 59th Ross Conference on Pediatric Research, Columbus, Ohio, 1969, p. 25.
36. Reynolds, E. O. R.: Indications for mechanical ventilation in infants with hyaline membrane disease. Pediatrics, *46*:193, 1970.
37. Sinclair, J. C.: Problems associated with prolonged nasotracheal intubation. Problems of Neonatal Intensive Care Units, 59th Ross Conference on Pediatric Research, Columbus, Ohio, 1969, p. 69.
38. Gruber, H. S., and Klaus, M. H.: Intermittent mask and bag therapy: an alternate approach to respirator therapy for infants with severe respiratory distress syndrome. J. Pediat., *76*:194, 1970.
39. Helmrath, T. A., Hodson, W. A., and Oliver, T. K., Jr.: Positive pressure ventilation in the newborn infant: the use of a face mask. J. Pediat., *76*:202, 1970.
40. Stern, L., Ramos, A. D., Outerbridge, E. W., and Beaudry, O. P.: Negative pressure artificial respiration: use in treatment of respiratory failure of the newborn. Canad. Med. Ass. J., *102*:595, 1970.
41. Linsao, L. S., Levinson, H., and Swyer, P. R.: Negative pressure artificial respiration: use in treatment of respiratory distress syndrome of the newborn. Canad. Med. Ass. J., *102*:602, 1970.
42. Gregory, G. A., Kitterman, J. A., Phibbs, R. H., Tooley, W. H., and Hamilton, W. K.: Treatment of the idiopathic respiratory distress syndrome (IRDS) with continuous positive airway pressure (CPAP). New Eng. J. Med., *284*:1334, 1971.
43. Vidyasagar, D., and Chernick, V.: Continuous positive transpulmonary pressure in hyaline membrane disease: a simple device. Pediatrics, *47*:295, 1971.
44. Parks, C. R.: Mist therapy: rationale and practice. J. Pediat., *76*:305, 1970.
45. Nelson, N. M.: On the etiology of hyaline membrane disease. Pediat. Clin. N. Amer., *17*:943, 1970.
46. Moss, A. J., Emmanouilides, G. C., Rettori, O., and Adams, F. H.: Acetylcholine in the treatment of idiopathic respiratory distress syndrome. J. Pediat., *69*:817, 1966.

14

Diabetic Ketoacidosis and Coma

Robert Schwartz, M.D.

Diabetic acidosis, even with coma, may not be so alarming in implications as are some other critical problems discussed in this book. Yet it certainly belongs among the critical illnesses, demanding as it does prompt action to restore a delicate physiological balance. Because the therapeutic response is very sensitive to precise management, improper therapy may be all the more dangerous. Management of diabetic coma therefore confronts the pediatrician with a more dramatic challenge than either the early recognition of diabetes in the previously normal child or the prevention of ketoacidosis in those with known diabetes, both of which should be more common problems. The mortality rate in diabetic acidosis and coma is admittedly very low. It should be nonexistent.

The frequency of presentation with ketoacidosis in children with diabetes mellitus has been variously reported as low as 18 per cent by Danowski[1] and as high as 52 per cent by Jackson.[2] Knowles indicated

From the Department of Pediatrics, Case Western Reserve University School of Medicine at Cleveland Metropolitan General Hospital, Cleveland, Ohio.

that 45 per cent of diabetic children had serum carbon dioxide concentrations of less than 20 mM/L at the initial episode of diabetes.[3] In his observations, recurrence of attacks varied widely; no subsequent acidosis occurred in 46 per cent of the children, whereas 13 per cent had 10 attacks or more each to account for almost half of all attacks tabulated. Knowles found acidosis most prevalent in the first 5 years of known diabetes, regardless of age at diagnosis, and in the teen years, regardless of duration.[3] Severe ketoacidosis (serum CO_2 < 10 mM/L and coma) occurs in less than 20 per cent of intial admissions.[1]

While the fundamental common biochemical basis for hereditary juvenile diabetes mellitus remains to be elucidated, the nonvascular metabolic derangements can in large measure be attributed to defective insulin secretion.

The metabolic derangements which result concern: (1) volume depletion, both extracellular and intracellular; (2) osmotic alterations between volume compartments; (3) acid-base disequilibrium with acidosis and buffer depletion; and (4) caloric deficiency, i.e., "metabolic starvation."

Immunoreactive insulin measurements indicate low normal values in plasma which fail to rise in response to several stimuli (glucose, arginine, tolbutamide).[4] Although a physiological recovery may occur after initial treatment, permanent deficiency of insulin secretion follows within weeks to months after onset. The several resultant physiological disturbances are well shown by the two diagrams (Figs. 1 and 2), reproduced by courtesy of Dr. Rachmiel Levine.

Insulin deprivation (Fig. 1) is associated with impairment of peripheral utilization of carbohydrates, caused in part by defective glucose uptake in insulin sensitive tissues, especially muscle and adipose tissue. In addition, decreased synthesis of glycogen in the liver and increased synthesis of glucose from amino acids (gluconeogenesis) raise the hepatic glucose output. These two factors, coupled with a continuing and sometimes increased dietary intake of carbohydrate, result in hyperglycemia. Since glucose contributes to the effective osmotic pressure of the extracellular fluid, hyperglycemia is associated with cellular dehydration as cell water shifts to the extracellular compartment. In the kidney the hyperglycemia results in a filtered glucose load exceeding the reabsorptive mechanism of tubular transport, thus producing an "osmotic" or "solute" diuresis. This in turn obligates both water and electrolyte (sodium and chloride) loss and results in extracellular fluid depletion when there is also a failure of intake. As the derangement progresses, additional solute for excretion is derived from protein catabolism (urea) and the ketoacidosis (organic acids), both of which require water and cation loss.

In the peripheral adipose tissue cells (Fig. 2) decreased lipogenesis and increased lipolysis occur. The latter produces an excess of non-esterified or free fatty acids (NEFA) which, bound to albumin, are trans-

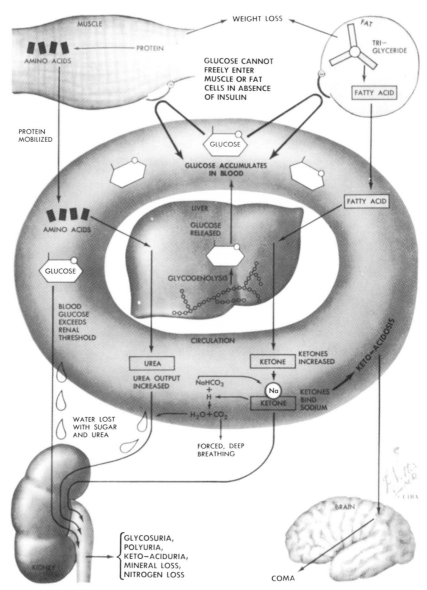

Figure 1. Pathophysiological effects of insulin deprivation. Not shown is the production of hydrogen ions due to organic acids (including "ketones"). Ketones do not "bind sodium" but are associated with cation at physiological pH, and to a large extent appear in the urine in this form. (© Copyright 1965, CIBA Pharmaceutical Company, Division of CIBA-Geigy Corporation. Reproduced with permission from The CIBA Collection of Medical Illustrations, by Frank H. Netter, M.D. All rights reserved.)

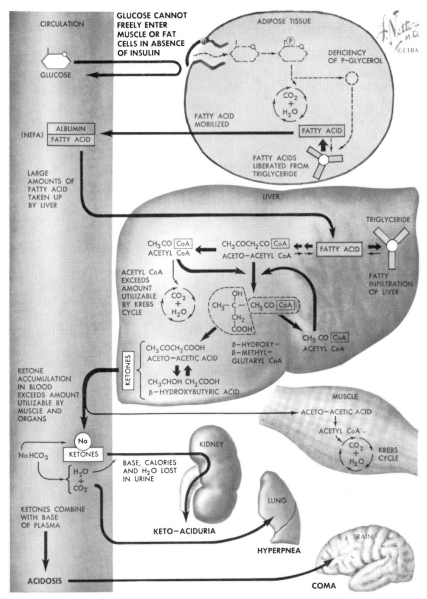

Figure 2. Ketoacidosis in diabetes. Substitution of ketone acids for "ketones" and cation for "base" would clarify terminology concepts. (© Copyright 1965, CIBA Pharmaceutical Company, Division of CIBA-Geigy Corporation. Reproduced with permission from The CIBA Collection of Medical Illustrations, by Frank H. Netter, M.D. All rights reserved.)

ported in the plasma to the liver and other tissues for further metabolism. In the liver, increased degradation of fatty acids to two carbon fragments (acetyl coenzyme A) is associated with increased formation of organic acids, especially "ketone acids" (β-hydroxybutyric and acetoacetic acids). The latter, as relatively strong organic acids (pK's approximately 4.7), interact with cellular and extracellular buffers and, at physiological pH's, exist principally in ionized form rather than as free organic acid.

The magnitude of systemic metabolic acidosis is dependent upon the rate of organic acid synthesis and metabolism coupled with renal compensatory mechanisms for excreting hydrogen ion. Three factors, urinary pH gradient, titratable acidity (determined by concentration of organic acids and phosphate), and ammonium production, particularly affect the rate at which systemic buffers are depleted. When hydrogen ion production exceeds the total of these three limiting mechanisms, acidosis proceeds inexorably toward an unphysiological state no longer compatible with cellular function.

Buffer depletion in metabolic acidosis is evident in part in the measured bicarbonate concentration of plasma. The so-called plasma anion gap is an approximation of organic acid accumulation in the plasma. This is derived by determining the difference in the sum of measured cations and anions. The measured cations are sodium and potassium, while the anions are chloride, bicarbonate, and protein. Protein equivalents are equal to 2.43 times the serum protein concentration in grams per 100 milliliters.

$$\Sigma \text{ cations} - \Sigma \text{ anions} =$$
$$\Sigma \left([Na]_p + [K]_p\right) - \Sigma\left([Cl]_p + [HCO_3] + 2.43[Pr]_p\right)$$

The total buffer deficit of the body is the resultant of two major components. One, represented by the loss of volume including osmolar (Na, K, Cl) and buffer (HCO_3) components, requires replacement from exogenous sources; the other, represented by organic "ketone" acids within the body, is a measure of potential buffer. When lipogenesis is increased and lipolysis decreased by administration of insulin and glucose, not only is organic acid (hydrogen ion) production diminished, but also the "ketone acids" in peripheral tissues are metabolized to CO_2 and H_2O, and the regeneration of some buffer occurs. However, the initial bicarbonate concentration alone cannot be relied upon to predict quantitatively the buffer regeneration with therapy.

While the principal alterations expressed above relate primarily to extracellular volume depletion and metabolic acidosis, hypertonicity and loss of cellular volume are accompanied by depletion of potassium. Though such depletion is frequent and significant, it may not be reflected in the initial serum potassium concentration, which may even be elevated. Electrolyte deficits previously measured by balance techniques in children[5, 6] and adults[7, 8] with severe diabetic acidosis were found by Darrow[9] to be (per kilogram body weight):

H_2O	Na	Cl	K
100 gm	8 mEq	6 mEq	6–10 mEq

CLINICAL AND LABORATORY FINDINGS

The onset of symptoms associated with juvenile diabetes mellitus itself may vary in duration from one to two days to as long as several months before the appearance of clinically significant ketoacidosis, although in most instances the duration is less than one month. Polyuria and polydipsia are, of course, the most common symptoms; polyphagia, nocturia, and weight loss may be somewhat less evident. Infections and emotional upsets may be contributing factors. The rapidity of progression from carbohydrate intolerance to ketoacidosis is so unpredictable that continuous medical surveillance is recommended once the diagnosis of diabetes mellitus is suspected, with laboratory studies initially not only to establish the diagnosis but also to assess the degree of metabolic derangements, especially in those aspects which require emergency therapy. The diagnosis of diabetes mellitus is confirmed by the identification of glucosuria and ketonuria in the presence of a blood sugar (glucose) above 150 mg per 100 ml.

Vomiting, with the attendant absence of fluid and calorie intake, is an ominous symptom which signals rapid deterioration and progression to serious acidosis and coma. The early phases of acidosis may produce no gross changes in the character of respiration; however, by the time moderate acidosis (serum CO_2 < 15 mM/L) supervenes definite increase in depth and rate is apparent. With severe acidosis (serum CO_2 < 10 mM/L), the characteristic Kussmaul acidotic breathing is grossly and alarmingly obvious.

Acid-base derangement is evident in a serum pH which may be as low as 6.85 to 7.00 and a decreased carbon dioxide content reaching 2.5 to 10 mM/L in severe acidosis.* Under these circumstances, there is marked depression of the actual bicarbonate concentration, while the tension of carbon dioxide is also depressed (values of 10 to 20 mm Hg) in presence of compensatory hyperventilation. Plasma ketones are elevated and approximate the bicarbonate depression. A rapid bedside test has been described by Lee and Duncan[10] which quantifies plasma ketone levels by serial dilution of plasma (1:1, 1:2, 1:4, 1:8, and so forth) and re-

---

*For those laboratories using the micro pH electrodes and the Astrup technique, familiarity with terminology and concepts such as buffer base (excess or deficit) and standard bicarbonate is indicated.

action with nitroprusside reagent. Since the latter does not react with β-hydroxybutyrate (which may account for 35 to 50 per cent of plasma ketones), the test is semiquantitative at best, but serves as a useful guide to adequacy of therapy. Diminution in the concentration of plasma ketones is usually reflected in a lessening of the metabolic acidosis and an improvement in the bicarbonate concentration.

In diabetic ketoacidosis, hyperglycemia may vary from 150 to as high as 2000 mg glucose/100 ml. Most frequently, a range of values from 250 to 600 mg/100 ml is observed. While the concentration of sodium in plasma is usually normal or slightly decreased, marked elevations of blood glucose are associated with a reciprocal decrease in sodium concentration. The value of chloride tends to parallel that of sodium. As already noted, plasma potassium initially is normal or even slightly elevated (5.5 to 6.0 mEq/L) in association with dehydration and metabolic acidosis. In the rare case of abnormally decreased plasma potassium, particular attention to early therapy with potassium is indicated.

Signs of dehydration (decreased skin turgor, softened eyeballs, dry mucous membranes) are not obvious until acute weight loss of at least 5 per cent has occurred. In diabetic acidosis occurring a month or more after the onset of unsuspected diabetes, signs of under-nutrition predominate and weight loss alone is not a valid measure of fluid deficit. When dehydration is severe (15 per cent body weight loss), signs of circulatory insufficiency with hypotension and tachycardia may be present. Azotemia may reflect circulatory inadequacy and decreased renal perfusion as well as the additional urea production from increased protein catabolism.

Hyperlipidemia, including hypercholesterolemia, may be very marked (15 to 25 gm total lipids per 100 ml plasma), especially in patients with prolonged onset. Lactescence (milky plasma) should be recognized when drawing the initial blood sample or suspected by finding lipemia retinalis on physical examination. Hyperlipemia not only interferes with spectrophotometric analysis of hemoglobin but also results in falsely low laboratory measurements of electrolytes and other aqueous phase substances because of volume displacement.[11] Thus markedly but deceptively low serum sodium values ($\pm$ 100 mEq/L) may be reported in the presence of very high blood glucose levels associated with hyperlipemia.

The state of consciousness may be as varied as other signs; however, in advanced ketoacidosis, semicoma or coma is evident. Differential diagnosis is seldom a problem. In rare instances, similar findings may occur following a head injury or in salicylate intoxication in young children, and the change in respiratory character sometimes is mistaken for a sign of primary respiratory disease such as pneumonia in young children. But once diabetes mellitus is thought of, the only possible diagnostic problem may arise from the occasional abdominal pain of acidosis and the question of appendicitis in a known diabetic.

THERAPY

Treatment of the child with diabetic acidosis is always urgent, perhaps more so than in some of the other "critical illnesses" discussed in this book, but the degree of urgency must be determined from clinical and laboratory assessment at admission, with particular emphasis on circulatory sufficiency and the extent of metabolic acidosis. Once the diagnosis has been confirmed (rapid blood glucose assessment may be made at the bedside with Dextrostix*), initial fluids, given primarily to expand circulatory volume, should consist of isotonic sodium in a balanced anion solution ($Cl + HCO_3$ at a ratio of 2:1) at a rapid rate of 20 ml/kg of body weight in the first 30 to 60 minutes.

If severe acidosis is present (pH < 7.15 and/or carbon dioxide content, combining power, or actual bicarbonate concentration less than 8 mM/L), sodium bicarbonate should then be given in a dose of 2 mEq/kg of body weight. This is easily accomplished with the 7.5 per cent sodium bicarbonate solution which contains 44.6 mEq in 50 ml (approximately 1 mEq/ml). Direct administration of this solution, with its osmolar load of 892×2 mOs/L may raise the effective osmotic pressure of extracellular fluid enough to dehydrate brain cells and other cells further. Therefore dilution with distilled water is recommended: 50 ml of 7.5 per cent sodium bicarbonate to 250 ml distilled water results in a solution of 149 mEq/L (isotonic sodium bicarbonate). Initial therapy should avoid glucose administration, especially if marked hyperglycemia (> 300 mg per 100 ml) is present.

Correction of the ketoacidosis and hyperglycemia is dependent upon reversal of the pathophysiological mechanisms by insulin administration, which is given simultaneously with therapy for circulatory insufficiency and severe acidosis. This begins with an empiric administration of crystalline or regular insulin in a dosage of 3 to 4 units per kilogram of body weight for patients with severe acidosis and coma; lesser doses to 1 unit/kg are administered to patients less critically ill. Initial insulin is given by two routes: approximately half intravenously, the remainder subcutaneously.

Urgency in attention to circulatory insufficiency and acidosis should not lead to neglect of requirements for free water, necessary in the presence of hyperosmolality as well as for correction of the significant negative water balance from hyperventilation and renal excretion. Such water may be provided by dilution of the electrolyte solution.

A program of therapy must be devised once initial emergency treatment has commenced. A detailed flow chart or data sheet containing critical clinical observations (especially body weight, blood pressure, pulse, respiration) and laboratory data (pH, CO_2, blood glucose, ke-

---

*Ames Company.

tones, Na, K, BUN, Hb) is essential to management. The frequency of observations depends upon the degree of critical concern; thus, while circulatory insufficiency is present or potential, blood pressure, pulse, and respiration are observed at least every 10 to 15 minutes. While acidosis is present, respiration is observed every 15 minutes and pH, CO_2, and ketones observed every 3 hours until significant improvement, whereupon the interval is increased. Blood sugar may be followed at 1- to 3-hour intervals at the bedside until stabilization at normoglycemia is assured. Body weight, Hb, and BUN need not be observed more frequently than every 12 hours. The recording of fluid balance must be meticulous and initially includes only intravenous fluids and urine; other volumes must subsequently be recorded. In addition, a balance of electrolytes, sodium, potassium, bicarbonate and glucose should be ascertained every 6 hours. Urine volumes may be collected separately, but cumulative periods of 6 hours are more practical. After the initial 24 hours of therapy, daily cumulative balances suffice.

The details of therapy are similar to those for other derangements of electrolyte physiology and are calculated from (1) previous deficit, (2) maintenance needs, and (3) continuing abnormal losses.

1. Previous Deficit. Since rapid restoration of the cellular deficit is not possible because of limitations of potassium administration, initial treatment is directed toward extracellular fluid restoration. According to the data of Darrow,[9] approximately half the estimated previous deficit may be restored as isotonic solution of sodium salts in the initial 24 hours.

2. Maintenance Needs. Specific maintenance requirements may be determined by a variety of techniques (based on surface area, calories metabolized, weight, or age), with an approximately similar range of values. Each physician must recognize the virtues and limitations of that system which he prefers. They may be summarized to include: (a) 1500 to 1800 ml/M^2/24 hours; or (b) 150 ml/100 cal metabolized/24 hours; or (c) insensible water losses, 10 to 50 ml/kg/24 hours + urine losses 10 to 50 ml/kg/24 hours, with a total of 20 to 100 ml/kg/24 hours; (d) $100 - 3X$ (X = age in years) ml/kg/24 hours. Maintenance fluids preferably contain $\frac{1}{5}$ volume of isotonic solution of sodium salts and $\frac{4}{5}$ free water (as 5 to 10 per cent glucose solution). Potassium in a concentration of 20 to 30 mEq/L is also included.

3. Continuing Abnormal Water Losses. Such losses due to hyperventilation and urinary output are highly variable and best assessed from acute changes in body weight relative to fluid balance.

The preceding recommendations may be summarized in an example for a 30 kg (1 M^2) child in severe ketoacidosis (Table 1). This results for the first 24 hours of therapy (when no glucose is to be given) in a solution which is approximately half isotonic sodium solution plus supplemental potassium. Practically, the initial hour of therapy must be subtracted from the above to determine remaining requirements. Thus, assuming the patient just discussed had circulatory insufficiency and severe acidosis and was treated promptly and adequately, see Table 2 for the amounts he would have received in the first hour.

Under these circumstances, and to avoid acute fluid overloads, the volume of isotonic sodium chloride should be reduced to 10 ml/kg and should be replaced in part by the isotonic sodium bicarbonate solution. If the total volumes (maximal) are as just noted, then the fluids to be given by the end of the first 24 hours will include those already administered plus the remainder in Table 3.

The remainder now represents approximately one-third isotonic sodium and two-thirds water instead of the half isotonic sodium for the total first 24 hours of therapy. The second phase of therapy (1 to 6 hours post admission) is directed primarily toward expansion of extra-

TABLE 1   WATER AND SODIUM REQUIREMENTS FOR FIRST 24 HOURS OF THERAPY

Data	Volume (ml/day)	Isotonic Na Solution (ml/day)	Na (mEq/day)	Electrolyte Free Water (ml/day)
Maintenance	1500	300	45.0	1200
Abnormal losses up to				
50 per cent maintenance	750	150	22.5	600
ECF deficit 50 ml/kg	1500	1500	225.0	0
Total	3750	1950	292.5	1800

TABLE 2   INITIAL EMERGENCY THERAPY

Data	Volume (ml)	Isotonic Na Solution (ml)	Na (mEq)	Electrolyte Free Water (ml)
Isotonic NaCl 20 ml/kg	600	600	90	0
and/or				
Na HCO_3 2 mEq/kg	400	400	60	0
Total	1000	1000	150	0

TABLE 3   CONTINUING THERAPY AFTER EMERGENCY PHASE

Data	Volume (ml/day)	Isotonic Na Solution (ml/day)	Na (mEq/day)	Electrolyte Free Water (ml/day)
First 24 hours, total	3750	1950	292.5	1800
Minus first hour	1000	1000	150.0	0
Remainder	2750	950	142.5	1800

cellular volume and correction of acidosis (insulin and sodium bicarbonate).

Total fluids of the first day of therapy may be planned so that one-half to two-thirds of the remainder are administered in the initial 12 hours and the rest in the second half day. Thus in the above example, 1375 ml total fluid remains for the first 12 hours (including 475 ml isotonic sodium solution). In the initial 6 hours (excluding first) the amounts would be: 688 ml fluid, 238 ml isotonic sodium solution. The remaining solution must contain some additional solute; otherwise it is dangerously hypotonic. Since glucose is not recommended in presence of very high glucose concentrations, this may be achieved with 5 per cent fructose (450 ml). If not, an exception must be made to the 24 hour requirements given above and only 238 ml (an equal volume) of free water administered; the requisite additional free water administration is deferred for a later phase of therapy when glucose solution may be provided.

Once blood glucose concentration has fallen to 300 mg/100 ml or less (initially hourly determinations are suggested), then the appropriate vehicle is glucose as 5 or 10 per cent solution in place of either fructose or free water alone, with appropriate electrolyte.

Serial electrocardiograms are checked every 2 hours for (1) depression of the ST segment and lowering, flattening, or inversion of the T wave; (2) prolongation of the Q-T interval; (3) presence of an elevated, broad, or diphasic U wave which may be responsible for the impression of a prolonged Q-T interval; (4) occasional prolongation of the P-R interval, as indication of hypokalemia. Since potassium therapy is not usually recommended for the first 4 to 6 hours of treatment because of initial hyperkalemia, at approximately 4 hours post therapy, potassium chloride or phosphate is added in a concentration of 30 to 40 mEq/L. If symptoms of hypokalemia (muscle weakness or ileus) or very low serum values are observed (< 3.0 mEq/L), higher concentrations of potassium may be indicated. If concentrations exceeding 40 mEq/L are administered, careful monitoring of plasma potassium concentration is necessary, in addition to the electrocardiograms taken every two hours, to avoid cardiotoxicity.

Regular insulin must be administered subcutaneously at least every 3 hours in a decreasing amount until ketosis is cleared, which may require 12 to 24 hours. When presenting findings are severe, the initial dose may be repeated once and then decreased by 50 per cent each subsequent period. At low levels of insulin (<5 U), a small 3 to 6 hourly dosage should still be maintained to avoid rebound ketonuria. A decrease in blood glucose is not sufficient reason alone for discontinuing insulin administration; rather, the amount of glucose administered parenterally should be increased from 5 to 10 per cent or greater solution. Monitoring of blood glucose at the bedside will serve to anticipate and correct hypoglycemia with glucose therapy.

Parenteral fluids are continued until the patient is free of ketones and aglycosuric. Even in the absence of vomiting, oral fluids should not be begun in the initial 12 hours, or even then if the sensorium is uncleared. Once consciousness is fully restored, fluids containing potassium may be introduced by mouth. Orange juice contains 40 mEq/L potassium and 10 per cent carbohydrate. Amounts of fluids and dosages of insulin during the second 24-hour period are dependent upon rate of repair of the estimated deficit and continuing losses. By this time, the extracellular deficit is usually minimal and beginning repair of cellular deficit through oral introduction of higher calories and protein may proceed. Regular insulin is preferred for an additional 24-hour period at regular intervals preceding oral intake. Periods exceeding 6 hours duration without insulin are to be avoided. By the third day, a planned dietary regimen may be introduced with long-acting insulin. Further management is dependent upon many factors other than those just considered—especially upon the education and adjustment of the patient and family. Nevertheless, the efficiency and skill with which the preceding more critical illness has been managed will remain significant factors in the subsequent course and care of the patient.

References

1. Danowski, T. S.: Diabetes Mellitus, with Emphasis on Children and Young Adults. Baltimore, Williams and Wilkins, 1957, p. 128.
2. Jackson, R. L., Hardin, R. C., Walker, G. L., Hendricks, A. B., and Kelly, H. G.: Degenerative changes in young diabetics in relation to level of control. Proc. Amer. Diabetes Ass., 9:307, 1949.
3. Knowles, H. C., Jr., Guest, G. M., Lampe, J., Kessler, M., and Skillman, T. G.: The course of juvenile diabetes treated with unmeasured diet. Diabetes, 14:239, 1965.
4. Parker, M. L., Pildes, R. S., Chao, K. L., Cornblath, M., and Kipnis, D. M.: Juvenile diabetes mellitus, a deficiency of insulin. Diabetes, 17:27, 1968.
5. Butler, A. M., Talbot, N. B., Barnett, C. H., Stanbury, J. B., and MacLachlan, E. A.: Metabolic studies in diabetic coma. Trans. Ass. Amer. Physicians, 60:102, 1947.
6. Darrow, D. C., and Pratt, E. L.: Retention of water and electrolyte during recovery in a patient with diabetic acidosis. J. Pediat., 4:688, 1942.
7. Atchley, D. W., Loeb, R. F., Richards, D. W., Jr., Benedict, E. M., and Driscoll, M. E.: On diabetic acidosis: a detailed study of electrolyte balances following the withdrawl and re-establishment of insulin therapy. J. Clin. Invest., 12:297, 1933.
8. Nabarro, J. D. N., Spencer, A. G., and Stowers, J. M.: Metabolic studies in severe diabetic ketosis. Quart J. Med., N. S., 21:225, 1952.
9. Darrow, D. C.: A Guide to Learning Fluid Therapy. Springfield, Ill., Charles C Thomas, 1964.
10. Lee, C. T., and Duncan, G. G.: Diabetic coma: the value of a simple test for acetone in the plasma; an aid to diagnosis and treatment. Metabolism, 5:144, 1956.
11. Albrink, M. J., Hald, P. M., Man, E. B., and Peters, J. P.: The displacement of serum water by lipids of hyperlipemic serum. A new method for the rapid determination of serum water. J. Clin. Invest., 34:1483, 1955.

15

Hypoglycemia

Robert E. Greenberg, M.D.,
and Robert O. Christiansen, M.D.

Hypoglycemia represents a significant emergency situation in pediatrics. Although recent studies indicate that cerebral tissue can utilize substrates other than glucose, especially in the newborn period and during prolonged fasting,[1] no substrate can successfully correct the neurophysiologic sequelae of glucose deprivation on the central nervous system. Since permanent neurologic effects of hypoglycemia correlate with the duration of time that cerebral tissue is deprived of glucose, early recognition and treatment of hypoglycemia is essential.

The diagnosis of hypoglycemia obviously depends on demonstration of a significant reduction in blood glucose concentration. Diagnostic criteria, similar to those developed by Cornblath and Schwartz,[2] have been widely accepted: two or more blood glucose values of less than 30 mg/100 ml in full-term infants; concentration of blood glucose less than 20 mg/100 ml in the neonate weighing less than 2,500 gm; blood glucose values of less than 40 mg/100 ml in the older infant and child. Since hypoglycemia is defined in terms of the concentration of blood glucose, it is essential to utilize analytic methods which are specific for

From the Department of Pediatrics, Stanford University School of Medicine, Stanford, California.

Supported in part by Grants HD 03150 and HD 02147 from the National Institutes of Health and 2K3HD-7263 from the Career Development Review Branch (R.E.G.), National Institutes of Health.

glucose. The most common method utilizes glucose oxidase, although other methods provide appropriate specificity. A rapid modification of the glucose oxidase method is represented by Dextrostix,* although accurate application of this diagnostic aid to hypoglycemia requires considerable training and experience.[3] Recently, a modification of the Dextrostix method has been reported, enabling reproducible measurement of values in the range of 20 to 40 mg/100 ml.[4] Confirmation of results obtained by Dextrostix with reliable laboratory methods should be effected upon recognition of hypoglycemia.

Focusing on practical approaches to the infant or child with hypoglycemia, this discussion will consider the following areas: hypoglycemia in the newborn infant; hypoglycemia in the older infant and child; mechanisms underlying hypoglycemia, and approach to diagnosis; therapy of the severely affected.

NEONATAL HYPOGLYCEMIA

The neonatal period presents a particularly difficult problem with respect to the regulation of blood glucose. Under normal conditions, the concentration of blood glucose declines during the first 24 hours after birth. Symptoms of hypoglycemia are often vague, nonspecific, and subtle. The incidence of asymptomatic hypoglycemia remains ill defined; equally obscure is the question of permanent sequelae, if any, of transient neonatal hypoglycemia, with or without attendant symptoms. Accordingly, careful attention to the symptomatology of neonatal hypoglycemia and to newborn infants at risk is essential.

Although irritability and convulsions were the first signs of hypoglycemia to be recognized, it is now well known that a myriad of other clinical findings should lead the clinician to suspect hypoglycemia. Such signs include tremor, cyanosis, apnea, listlessness, poor feeding, rotating eye motions, change in muscle tone, shrill cry, and instability of temperature regulation. Hypoglycemia may occur without clinical manifestations, a fact which has led some investigators to question the correlation between clinical signs and documented reductions in blood glucose concentration;[5] presence of clinical signs or symptoms has been found to correlate, however, with the duration of hypoglycemia.[6]

It has been possible, in recent years, to define a high risk population of newborn infants. Two major predisposing factors are apparent: (1) placental dysfunction and (2) postnatal illness. Neonates predisposed to hypoglycemia as a consequence of intrauterine events often present as dysmature (small for dates) infants, the smaller of discordant twins, and infants born of mothers with toxemia. Newborn infants with neonatal asphyxia, respiratory distress, hypothermia, or erythroblastosis fetalis exhibit an increased frequency of hypoglycemia. In addition, infants of

*Ames Company.

diabetic mothers often develop hypoglycemia during the first 6 hours after birth. Severe and prolonged hypoglycemia has also been reported in infants of mothers treated with oral hypoglycemia agents.[7] Recognition of hypoglycemia in the neonate can be enhanced by routine determination of blood glucose concentration in high risk infants, and by prompt attention to previously described signs and symptoms.

Prompt and effective treatment should accompany recognition of hypoglycemia, regardless of the associated clinical findings. Recommended initial therapy consists of rapid intravenous infusion of 1 gm glucose/kg (2 ml/kg of 50 per cent glucose), followed by a constant infusion of glucose at a rate of 10 mg/kg/minute (75 ml/kg/24 hours of 20 per cent glucose). It must be remembered that the above represents only approximate dosage; it is imprudent to assume that therapy is successful in maintaining a blood glucose concentration above 50 mg/100 ml without immediate and repetitive monitoring. Although neonatal hypoglycemia is usually transient, intravenous glucose administration should be maintained for at least 24 hours after the blood glucose concentration has been stabilized. Subsequently, the glucose infusion should be slowly decreased in conjunction with increasing oral feedings, since abrupt cessation of intravenous glucose may be associated with a recurrence of hypoglycemia. Prolonged infusion of concentrated glucose solutions may be complicated by thrombotic phenomena and excessive fluid administration; accordingly, the dangers of concentrated glucose solutions must be related to the ability of the newborn to handle fluid loads in an attempt to titrate therapy. The availability of infusion pumps applicable to intravenous therapy has markedly improved establishment of stabilized blood glucose concentrations.

If hypoglycemia cannot be successfully controlled by glucose infusion, empirical use of hydrocortisone in divided doses of 5 mg/kg/24 hours has been recommended by many investigators. Glucagon has recently been demonstrated to be capable of precociously inducing an increase in activity of phosphoenolpyruvate carboxykinase, an enzyme unique to the gluconeogenic pathway, in fetal, premature, and newborn rats.[8] Since neonatal hypoglycemia is probably related, in many instances, to relative inability to effect appropriate hepatic glucose output, utilization of intramuscular glucagon injections, 50 μg/kg every 4 hours, is, at least, based on a rational theoretical framework. As previously indicated, all therapy is empirical and the concentration of blood glucose must be closely monitored.

HYPOGLYCEMIA IN THE OLDER INFANT AND CHILD

Permanent neurologic sequelae result with greater frequency when repetitive episodes of hypoglycemia occur prior to 6 months of age. Fortunately, recognition of hypoglycemia in the older infant and child is easier than in the newborn infant. The signs and symptoms of hypoglycemia are a function of the rate of fall in blood glucose and the neurologic sequelae of prolonged glucose deprivation. Pallor, sweating, and tremulousness accompany the adrenergic response to a rapid reduction in blood glucose concentration. The development of marked and persistent reductions in blood glucose results in listlessness, apathy, irritability, headache, visual disturbances, mental confusion, bizarre behavior, and, finally, convulsions and coma. Delineation of the relationship between symptoms and previous ingestion of food, time of day, and ingestion or administration of drugs aids in the detection of hypoglycemia. Hypoglycemia, in the older infant and child, may be defined by a concentration of blood glucose less than 40 mg/100 ml associated with suggestive signs and symptoms which disappear following restoration of normal blood glucose values. Signs and symptoms accompanying prolonged hypoglycemia, however, may not be immediately obviated by intravenous glucose administration.

Treatment of the severe, acute episode involves rapid intravenous administration of 2 ml/kg of 50 per cent glucose, followed by a constant infusion of glucose at a rate of 5 to 10 mg glucose/kg/minute, sufficient to maintain a blood glucose level above 50 mg/100 ml. After the concentration of blood glucose has been stabilized for 6 hours or longer, the rate of infusion can be progressively reduced unless the child is incapable of oral alimentation. Subsequent therapy depends on the severity and frequency of hypoglycemia and the nature of causative mechanisms.

MECHANISMS UNDERLYING HYPOGLYCEMIA, AND APPROACH TO DIAGNOSIS

The concentration of blood glucose is, essentially, a resultant of two interacting processes: peripheral glucose utilization and hepatic glucose production. Application of diagnostic methods to the study of the etiology of hypoglycemia in an affected child should attempt to estimate rates of these processes in as direct and rapid fashion as possible. A distinction should be made between procedures utilized in the investigation of physiologic mechanisms and those that may lead to specific therapy. Hypoglycemia in infancy and childhood almost always occurs under conditions of fasting, in contrast to the greater frequency of post-prandial hypoglycemia in adults. A classification of etiologic factors associated with hypoglycemia is outlined in Table 1. Utilizing the framework of this classification, the history can serve as an extremely important component in diagnosis.

TABLE 1   CAUSES OF HYPOGLYCEMIA IN CHILDHOOD

I. Lack of available glucose or its precursors
Malnutrition, severe
Impaired absorption
    chronic diarrhea
    intestinal disaccharidase deficiency
    malabsorption of unknown etiology
    "dumping syndrome"

II. Increased peripheral glucose utilization
Hyperinsulinism
    pancreatic tumors
    pancreatic hyperplasia
    "prediabetic" syndrome
    excessive exogenous insulin
Tumors of mesothelial origin
Defects in hormonal regulation
    growth hormone deficiency

III. Defects in glycogenolysis
Glucose 6-phosphatase deficiency hepatorenal glycogenosis
Hepatophosphorylase deficiency glycogenosis
Amylo-1,6-glucosidase (debrancher) deficiency glycogenosis

IV. Defects in hepatic glucose formation and release
Enzymatic defects in hepatic intermediary metabolism
    hereditary fructose intolerance
    galactosemia
    pyruvate carboxylase deficiency
    fructose-1, 6-diphosphatase deficiency
Hepatic disease
    hepatitis
    cirrhosis
    malignant growth
Defects in hormonal regulation
    adrenocortical insufficiency
        idiopathic adrenocortical atrophy
        destructive lesions
        enzymatic defects in hydrocortisone biosynthesis
        unresponsiveness of adrenal to ACTH
    hypopituitarism (selective or multiple defects in ACTH, TSH production)
    hypothyroidism
    glucagon deficiency
    adrenomedullary insufficiency (?)
Defects in integrative function of the central nervous system
    congenital abnormalities, tumors, hemorrhage, injury, infection
Pharmacologic or toxic alterations in glucose homeostasis
    salicylates, biguanides, sulfonylureas, antihistamines, ethanol

V. Unknown etiology
Ketotic hypoglycemia
Leucine-induced hypoglycemia
Idiopathic hypoglycemia of childhood
Neonatal hypoglycemia
    infants of mothers with toxemia of pregnancy
    "small for dates" infants
    infants with erythroblastosis
    infants with neonatal asphyxia or respiratory distress syndrome

Our approach to diagnosis emphasizes several concepts: diagnostic procedures should be used which, with least danger to the patient, lead to specific therapy; procedures which facilitate inclusion of the patient in clinical classifications which, in turn, are not indicative of specific pathophysiologic mechanisms are of little practical value; diagnostic procedures should be based on an understanding of the physiology of prolonged fasting; and the extent of diagnostic procedures must be determined, in part, by the severity and rate of recurrence of hypoglycemia and the age of the patient.

Recent studies have clarified the specific changes that accompany fasting, and provide insight into the changing pattern of hormonal control.[9, 10] In the absence of dietary carbohydrate, endogenous glucose production must increase in order to provide sufficient glucose to maintain a normal concentration of glucose in blood and, in turn, cerebral function. While enhancement of gluconeogenesis is appreciable, a marked reduction in the rate of glucose utilization occurs in prolonged fasting, such that very little glucose is utilized by any tissues except the formed elements of blood and brain. Protein catabolism is largely obviated by a marked increase in hydrolysis of triglycerides, with resultant release of free fatty acids and glycerol into the circulation. While overall glucose utilization is sharply reduced, the brain continues to consume glucose.

As a corollary to these events, the concentration of insulin falls to low but persistent levels in blood, while that of glucagon increases. Markedly enhanced rates of lipolysis lead to increased ketone body formation, so that absence of ketonuria during a prolonged fast may be regarded as an abnormal finding.

Based on these considerations, an approach to the diagnosis of the cause(s) of hypoglycemia might proceed as follows.

Response to Prolonged Fasting

Under careful observation, the child should be studied while fasting, with regular measurements of blood glucose, free fatty acids and/or glycerol, plasma insulin, and urinary ketone bodies. If one uses Dextrostix, when hypoglycemia occurs the fast can be discontinued without endangering the child.

This study gives evidence regarding: the rapidity of development of hypoglycemia; whether insulin secretion appropriately decreases as hypoglycemia develops; whether enhanced rates of lipolysis accompany development of hypoglycemia.

In our experience, this single approach is most helpful in defining abnormalities in the control of insulin secretion. If the child fails to develop hypoglycemia after an 18- to 24-hour fast, no further studies are probably indicated since, regardless of etiology, the process is likely to be mild, although quite possibly recurrent.

Response to Consecutive Glucose Infusions

If hypoglycemia does occur, further information can be obtained by infusing glucose for 60 to 90 minutes at successive rates of 4, 8, and 12 mg/kg/minute and measuring the concentration of blood glucose during the last 15 minutes of each infusion period. Adam et al.[11] have developed a useful infusion protocol which allows one to make inferences regarding the magnitude of glucose utilization. For example, if excessive rates of glucose must be infused to maintain a blood glucose concentration in the low normal range, a rapid rate of peripheral glucose utilization may be inferred. On the other hand, maintenance of euglycemia with low rates of glucose infusion in a child who develops hypoglycemia during fasting suggests that the defect is inadequate hepatic glucose production.

Utilization of Specific Diagnostic Procedures

Specific procedures should be utilized based on information derived from the history and physical examination. For example, the child with marked hepatomegaly should be considered as possibly having glycogen storage disease or some form of intrahepatic pathology. Further, the child who develops postprandial hypoglycemia after taking a meal containing fructose should then be challenged with a fructose load.

Assessment of Hormonal Regulation

In the child with fasting hypoglycemia, the causative mechanism may reside in deficient secretion of hormones which are antagonistic to the action of insulin. Accordingly, appropriate techniques for measurement of growth hormone, thyroxine, and adrenal glucocorticoids should be employed.

MAINTENANCE THERAPY

Whenever possible, therapy should be directed toward causative mechanisms. In our hands, a specific diagnosis of the cause of infantile hypoglycemia is not possible in three quarters of affected patients. If excessive or inappropriate insulin secretion is demonstrated, direct surgical intervention is advisable. In the usual situation, recurrent but infrequent episodes of hypoglycemia during fasting should be managed by frequent feedings, especially during the night. In spite of numerous assertions, there is little evidence that the composition of such frequent feeding is of major importance. In severely affected infants, use of adjunct therapy with epinephrine-like agents or adrenal glucocorticoids may assist in stabilizing blood glucose concentration. An antihypertensive, hyperglycemic sulfonamide (diazoxide) has been extensively used in the management of hypoglycemia. Since its principal mechanism of action depends on a diminution of insulin secretion in response to various physiologic stimuli, effective control of hypoglycemia may not occur under conditions of prolonged fasting, when insulin secretion is already reduced. Hypertrichosis, edema, and hyperuricemia have been encountered as side effects of diazoxide administration.[12,13]

References

1. Owen, O. E., Morgan, A. P., Kemp, H. G., Sullivan, J. M., Herrera, M. G., and Cahill, G. F., Jr.: Brain metabolism during fasting. J. Clin. Invest., 46:1589, 1967.
2. Cornblath, M., and Schwartz, R.: Disorders of Carbohydrate Metabolism in Infancy. Philadelphia, W. B. Saunders, 1966.
3. Chantler, C., Baum, J. D., and Norman, D. A.: Dextrostix in the diagnosis of neonatal hypoglycemia, Lancet, 2:1395, 1967.
4. Swiatek, K. R., Luebben, G., and Cornblath, M.: Screening method for determining glucose in blood and cerebrospinal fluid. Amer. J. Dis. Child., 117:672, 1969.
5. Griffiths, A. D.: Association of hypoglycemia with symptoms in the newborn. Arch. Dis. Child., 43:688, 1968.
6. Raivio, K. O.: Factors affecting the development of symptoms in neonatal hypoglycemia. Ann. Paediat. Fenn., 14:105, 1969.
7. Zucker, P., and Simon, G.: Prolonged symptomatic neonatal hypoglycemia associated with maternal chlorpropamide therapy. Pediatrics, 42:824, 1968.
8. Yueng, D., and Oliver, I. T.: Factors affecting the premature induction of phosphopyruvate carboxylase in neonatal rat liver. Biochem. J., 108:325, 1968.
9. Cahill, G. F., Jr., Herrera, M. G., Morgan, A. P., Soeldner, J. S., Steinke, J., Levy, P. L., Reichard, G. A., Jr., and Kipnis, D. M.: Hormone-fuel interrelationships during fasting. J. Clin. Invest., 45:1751, 1966.
10. Cahill, G. F., Jr., and Owen, O. E.: Some observations on carbohydrate metabolism in man. In Dickens, F., Randle, P. J., and Whelan, W. J., ed.: Carbohydrate Metabolism and Its Disorders. New York, Academic Press, 1968, p. 497.
11. Adam, P. A. Jr., King, K., and Schwartz,, R.: Model for the investigation of intractable hypoglycemia: Insulin-glucose interrelationships during steady state infusions. Pediatrics, 41:91, 1968.
12. Baker, L., Kaye, R., Root, A. W., and Prasad, A. L. N.: Diazoxide treatment of idiopathic hypoglycemia of infancy. J. Pediat., 71:494, 1967.
13. Koblenzer, P. J., and Baker, L.: Hypertrichosis lanuginosa associated with diazoxide therapy in prepubertal children: A clinicopatholgic study. Ann. N.Y. Acad. Sci., 150:373, 1968.

16

Acute Metabolic Disease in Infancy and Early Childhood

Donough O'Brien, M.D., F.R.C.P.,
and Stephen I. Goodman, M.D.

The infant or young child who becomes acutely and seriously ill with or without a preliminary period of "failure to thrive" and who shows marked and sometimes intractable metabolic acidosis with anorexia, lethargy, convulsions, and perhaps coma represents an infrequent but important problem. It is increasingly apparent that a significant proportion of patients with this clinical picture are accounted for by inborn errors of intermediary metabolism, although from the standpoint of the practicing pediatrician, these still remain a group of individually rare and complex conditions, much discussed and rarely seen. There are certain exceptions, it is true; but for the most part, these are diseases in which additional, more definitive physical signs offer some specific clue to diagnosis. For example, severe neonatal edema with hypoproteinemia may suggest cystic fibrosis; an odd smell may suggest branched-chain ketoaciduria; a large heart and macroglossia may suggest acid maltase deficiency; an electrolyte disturbance in the male

From the B. F. Stolinsky Research Laboratories, Department of Pediatrics, University of Colorado Medical Center, Denver, Colorado.

may suggest the adrenogenital syndrome, and jaundice and hepatomegaly may suggest galactosemia.

The special purpose of this article is to call attention to that group of inborn errors which may be associated with sudden, severe, and perhaps fatal illness in early life. Individually rare but collectively worth recognition, they can often be promptly, accurately, and inexpensively diagnosed and, as important, can usually be successfully treated. Some typical case histories are presented as illustrations, together with a table of currently recognized diseases in this category and a second table listing some screening tests useful in diagnosis. The whole is intended as an *aide-mémoire* for the pediatrician, to assist him with the practicalities of diagnosis and initial management in this field.

CASE HISTORIES

Branched-Chain Ketoaciduria

D. D. was the product of an uncomplicated pregnancy and delivery. He appeared normal at birth and was discharged from the hospital at 3 days of age. At 5 days of age he became listless and began to feed poorly and was admitted to hospital two days later. A previous male sibling had died at 13 days of age with what was described as aspiration pneumonia.

Physical examination was completely normal except for moderate flaccidity, poor Moro and tonic neck reflexes, and a slight increase of deep tendon reflexes.

A hemogram and routine urinalysis were normal. The cerebrospinal fluid was normal and sterile; blood and urine cultures were negative. Serum pH, PCO_2, CO_2, Na, Cl, K, BUN, and glucose measurements were all normal. Chest x-ray revealed minimal bronchopneumonia at the right base.

On the second hospital day a sweetish urinary odor led to an examination of serum amino acids and the increased concentrations of leucine, isoleucine, and valine characteristic of branched-chain ketoaciduria were observed. Treatment with a diet low in branched-chain amino acids was promptly instituted. At the age of $3\frac{1}{2}$ years, the child was developmentally normal. This outcome is in sharp contrast to the prognosis for the untreated case, in which there is usually progressive neurological deterioration followed by death within the first two months of life.

Methylmalonic Aciduria

D. O., also a male, was discharged from the hospital at 3 days of age, following an uncomplicated term delivery. On the fourth day of life, he developed feeding difficulties, somnolence, and respiratory grunting, which prompted his hospitalization. Family history was non-contributory. On admission he was mildly jaundiced and his respirations were labored. Other positive physical findings were a slightly bulging anterior fontanelle with no neck stiffness, extreme lethargy, no Moro, suck, or grasp reflexes, and hypoactive deep tendon reflexes. His clinical condition steadily deteriorated until assisted ventilation was required.

Hemogram and routine urinalysis were normal. Biochemical measurements included a pH of 6.99, total CO_2 of 8 mEq/L, Na of 145 mEq/L, K of 4.8 mEq,

TABLE 1 RARE INBORN ERRORS OF METABOLISM ASSOCIATED WITH SEVERE CLINICAL DISEASE IN INFANCY AND EARLY CHILDHOOD[1,2]

Disorder	Biochemical Defect	Associated Clinical Findings	Lab Test (See Table 2)	Diagnosis	Treatment
In aminoacid metabolism					
Hyperammonemia	1. Carbamyl phosphate synthetase[4]	Episodic vomiting and lethargy exacerbated by protein ingestion	1	Hyperammonemia	Protein restriction to 1 gm/kg/day
	2. Ornithine trans-carbamylase[5]		1,12	Hyperammonemia, oroticaciduria	
Citrullinemia[6]	Argino-succinic acid synthetase	Episodic vomiting, coma exacerbated by protein ingestion	1,2a,2b	Hyperammonemia Increased citrulline in blood and urine	As above
Argino-succinic[7] aciduria	Argino-succinic acid lyase	Seizures, mental, retardation, ataxia	1,2a 2b	Hyperammonemia Increased urinary argino-succinic acid	As above
Argininemia[33]	Arginase	Mental retardation seizures, spastic diplegia	1,2a,2b	Increased serum arginine, increased urine cystine, lysine, arginine, and ornithine	As above
Sulfite oxidase[3] deficiency	Defect in conversion of sulfite to sulfate	Neonatal pyramidal signs, blindness, lens dislocations	15	Increased urinary sulfite and thiosulfate, and S-sulfo-cysteine	None
Hyperprolinemia,[8] Type II	Δ¹-pyrroline-5-carboxylic acid dehydrogenase	Seizures and coma	2a,2b 14	Increased proline in blood and urine	Low proline diet, possibly
Branched-chain ketonuria					
1. Permanent[9]	Branched-chain ketoacid decarboxylase	Maple-syrup-like odor to urine, neonatal acidemia, lethargy, and feeding difficulty	2a,2b, 4,5,13, 16,19	Increased valine, leucine, isoleucine, and alloisoleucine in blood and urine	Diet low in branched-chain amino-acids. Some cases are thiamine dependent

Disorder	Biochemical Defect	Associated Clinical Findings	Lab Test (See Table 2)	Diagnosis	Treatment
2. Intermittent[22]	As above but slightly higher enzyme activity	Episodic acidemia and CNS symptoms associated with infection	2a,2b,4, 5,13,16, 19	As above (during attacks)	As above during attacks
Hypervalinemia[10]	Valine α-ketoglutarate transaminase	Neonatal vomiting, lethargy, and feeding problems	2a,2b	Increased valine in blood and urine	Valine restriction to 100 mg/kg/day
Isovaleric acidemia[11]	Isovaleryl-coenzyme A dehydrogenase	Odor of "sweaty feet," resistant metabolic acidemia, progressive neurological signs	13,16,19	Demonstration of isovaleric acid in urine	Leucine restriction
β-alaninemia[14]	β-alanine-α-ketoglutarate transaminase	Neonatal lethargy, seizures	2a,2b	Increased β-alanine in blood and urine	Low protein diet, possibly pyridoxine supplementation
Carnosinemia[15]	Carnosinase	Seizures, mental retardation	2a,2b, 18	Increased carnosine in urine, decreased serum carnosinase activity	Low meat diet
Hyperlysinemia[16]	1. Lysine dehydrogenase	Feeding difficulty, episodic vomiting	1,2a,2b	Hyperammonemia, increased lysine in blood and urine	Protein restriction to c 1.5 gm/kg/day
	2. Lysine-α-ketoglutarate reductase	As above	1,2a,2b	Increased lysine in blood and urine	As above
Tyrosyluria[17]	? p-hydroxyphenyl-pyruvic acid oxidase	Neonatal cirrhosis, renal tubular dystrophy, rickets	2a,2b 13,19.	Increased serum tyrosine	Diet low in tyrosine and phenylalanine
Hyperglycinemia 1. Ketotic[31]	? propionyl-coenzyme A carboxylase	Episodic vomiting, seizures, and ketosis exacerbated by protein ingestion	2a,2b 13,19.	Increased glycine in blood and urine	Protein as soy formula limited to <1.5 gm/kg/day

TABLE 1   RARE INBORN ERRORS OF METABOLISM ASSOCIATED WITH SEVERE CLINICAL DISEASE IN INFANCY AND EARLY CHILDHOOD[1,2] —Continued

Disorder	Biomechanical Defect	Associated Clinical Findings	Lab Test (See Table 2)	Diagnosis	Treatment
2. Non-ketotic	Glycine, FH[4] transferase	Seizures, microcephaly, retardation	2a,2b	Increased glycine in blood and urine	2 g sodium benzoate daily
Methylmalonic[12] aciduria					
1. Vitamin B$_{12}$ responsive	Defective conversion of Vitamin B$_{12}$ to coenzyme B$_{12}$	Episodic metabolic acidemia, ketonuria, hypoglycemia	11,13, 19	Increased urinary excretion of methylmalonic acid	Protein restriction, vitamin B$_{12}$ in doses of 1 mg i.m. daily
2. Vitamin B$_{12}$ unresponsive	Methylmalonyl-coenzyme A isomerase	As above	11,13, 19	As above	Protein restriction to <1.5 gm/kg/day
Propionic acidemia[13]	Propionyl-coenzyme A carboxylase	Severe neonatal metabolic acidemia, hypotonia, vomiting	13,19	Increased urine propionic acid	Dietary protein restriction to <1 gm/kg/day
Oast-house syndrome[18]	Unknown	Hypotonia, seizures, edema	13,16,19	Increased urine α-hydroxybutyric acid	None
Formininotransferase deficiency[19]	Defect in conversion of histidine to glutamic acid	Growth retardation, edema, hepatomegaly, seizures	6	Increased urine forminino-glutamate after histidine load	None
Pyridoxine dependency[20]	? glutamic acid decarboxylase	Neonatal irritability, hyperacusia, seizures	—	Prompt response to parenteral pyridoxine	Pyridoxine, 100 mg i.m. daily × 3, then 50 mg daily p.o.
In carbohydrate metabolism					
Galactosemia[22]	UDP-galactose transferase	Vomiting, growth retardation, hepatomegaly, jaundice	7,8	Demonstration of enzyme defect in red cells, urine galactose increased	Galactose restricted diet
Glucose-galactose malabsorption[23]	Enteric and renal epithelial transport defect	Failure to gain, diarrhea, vomiting and severe dehydration	7	Glucose and galactose in stools	Galactose and glucose restricted diet

Disorder	Biochemical Defect	Associated Clinical Findings	Lab Test (See Table 2)	Diagnosis	Treatment
Fructose intolerance[24]	Absence of hepatic aldolase for fructose-1-P; reduction in aldolase for fructose-1:6-diphosphate	Anorexia, lethargy, failure to thrive. Hypomagnesemia, hypoglycemia, and hypophosphatemia with seizures and coma	7,18	Fructosuria, hypoglycemic response to oral fructose load 0.6 gm/kg	Exclusion of all cane sugar from the diet
Lactic and pyruvic acidosis[25,34]	Not known	Obesity, hypotonicity, retardation, severe acidosis	9,13	Elevated blood lactate and pyruvic levels	Continuing alkali therapy; thiamine supplements may be of value
In lipid metabolism Green acyl dehydrogenase deficiency[26]	Failure to convert butyryl to crotonyl coenzyme A	Convulsions, lethargy, hepatomegaly, leukopenia, thrombocytopenia, distinctive odor	13,16	Increased urine butyric and hexanonic acids	None
Miscellaneous Hyperuricacidemia[27]	Hypoxanthine-guanine, phosphoribosyl transferase deficiency	Spasticity, athetosis, developmental retardation after first 6 months	17,18	Blood uric acid >9 mg/100 ml	Probenecid 100 mg/kg/24 hr. Adenine 10 mg/kg/24 hr. Sodium glutamate 6 gm/day
Familial hypomagnesemia[28]	Specific enteric transport defect for magnesium	Seizures, tetany, progressive neurological deterioration. Responsive to Mg^{++} but not Ca^{++} therapy	10	Low serum calcium with normal serum phosphorus. Serum magnesium <1.4 mEq/L	Initially, 1 mEq/kg/day of magnesium i.v. Later 4-5 mEq/kg/day p.o. until serum normal
Acid phosphatase deficiency[29]	Lysosomal acid phosphatase deficiency in brain, liver, spleen, and kidney	Vomiting, lethargy, opisthotonos, terminal bleeding	18	Low lysosomal acid phosphatase in liver biopsy	None

TABLE 2 SCREENING AND CONFIRMATORY TESTS FOR INBORN ERRORS OF METABOLISM CAUSING SEVERE CLINICAL DISEASE IN INFANCY[2,30]

Test	Availability*	Conditions Detected
1. Ammonia in plasma	B	Carbamylphosphate synthetase deficiency,[4] ornithine transcarbamylase deficiency,[5] citrullinemia,[6] argininemia,[33] and arginosuccinic aciduria.[7]
2. Amino acids a. Paper chromatography	A	Citrullinemia,[6] argino-succinic aciduria,[7] hyperprolinemia,[8] maple syrup urine disease,[9] hypervalinemia,[10] β-alaninemia,[14] argininemia,[33] carnosinemia,[15] hyperglycinemia,[21,31] hyperlysinemia,[16] and tyrosyluria.[17]
b. Column chromatography	C	Confirmatory for above. Request if any possibility of abnormality on paper chromotography.
3. Carnosinase in serum	B	Carnosinemia.[15]
4. Dinitrophenylthydrazine test for keto acids	A	Branched-chain ketoaciduria. Not diagnostic.[9,32]
5. Ferric chloride test	A	α-ketobutyric acid in Oast-house syndrome[18]–purple going brown[15] to brownish red. Branched-chain keto acids[9]–gray green. Pyruvic acid–yellow brown.[25]
6. Formiminoglutamic acid in urine	C	Formiminotransferase deficiency.[19]
7. Paper chromatography of sugars	B	Fructose intolerance,[24] galactosemia,[22] glucose-galactose malabsorption.[23]
8. Galactosemia screening test RBC enzyme	B	Galactosemia,[22] G-6-P-D deficiency.
9. Lactic and pyruvic acid in serum	B	Lactic and pyruvic acidosis.[25]
10. Magnesium in serum	A	Familial hypomagnesemia.[28]

TABLE 2 SCREENING AND CONFIRMATORY TESTS FOR INBORN ERRORS OF METABOLISM CAUSING SEVERE CLINICAL DISEASE IN INFANCY[2, 30]—*Continued*

Test	Availability*	Conditions Detected
11. Methylmalonic aciduria screening test	A	Methylmalonic aciduria.[12] However, this test is erratically negative in the acute case and organic acid chromatography should always be carried out as well.
12. Oroticaciduria screening test	A	Indicative of ornithine transcarbamylase deficiency.[5]
13. Organic acids by gas chromatography	C	α-hydroxybutyric acid in Oast-house syndrome,[18] butyric and hexanoic acids in green acyl dehydrogenase deficiency,[26] propionic-acidemia,[13] methylmalonic aciduria,[12] branched-chain ketoacids in maple syrup urine disease[9] and isovaleric acidemia,[11] and lactic and pyruvic acids.[28]
14. Proline in serum	B	Hyperprolinemia due to Δ pyrolline carboxylic acid dehydrogenase deficiency.
15. Sulfite in urine and thiosulphate in urine	A	Sulfite oxidase deficiency.[3]
16. Presence of an unusual smell in sweat, breath, urine	—	Branched-chain ketoaciduria,[9] isovaleric acidemia,[11] short chain fatty acids in green acyl dehydrogenase deficiency,[26] α-hydroxybutyric acid in the Oast-house syndrome.[18]
17. Uric acid in serum	A	Hyperuricacidemia.[27]
18. Specific enzyme assays	C	Carnosinemia.[15] Lyosomal acid phosphatase deficiency.[29]
19. Mass spectroscopy	C	Definitive tests not required for treatment or specific diagnosis.

*A—could be carried out by any clinical laboratory.
B—likely available only in a major medical center.
C—probably available through specialized laboratories.
Serum or heparinized plasma samples should be separated from red cells and dispatched to the laboratory by the quickest route. Urine should be brought to <pH 3.0 for amino acids and pH 7.6 for organic acids. Except for ammonic, lactic, and pyruvic acid assays, which should be processed immediately, other tests can be carried out on mailed samples of 0.5 ml serum or 1.0 ml urine.

BUN of 14 mg/100 ml, and a blood sugar of 3 mg/100 ml. The spinal fluid was clear, contained no cells, 210 mg/100 ml protein, and no detectable glucose. Cultures of blood, CSF, and urine were sterile. Chest x-ray showed diffuse infiltration, compatible with either infection or aspiration. Paper chromatography of amino acids in blood and urine were normal.

Severe metabolic acidemia suggested either renal tubular acidosis or organic acidemia. Gas chromatography of urinary organic acids revealed a large amount of methylmalonic acid characteristic of methylmalonic acidemia. A low protein diet and parenteral Vitamin B_{12} in large doses, which might have been effective if given earlier, were instituted on the seventh day of life. They had no clinical effect and he died the next day.

Galactosemia

S. A., born in a small country hospital after a normal pregnancy and delivery, weighed 6 pounds, 6 ounces at birth and was discharged on the fifth day of life. On the eighth day he was noted to be moderately jaundiced, and this increased up to the twelfth day when he was first seen by a pediatrician, at which time the serum total bilirubin measured 16.8 mg/100 ml. The liver edge was palpated 4 cm below the costal margin. There was also some pyuria and an umbilical discharge containing coagulase-positive staphyloccocci. Understandably, these observations led to a diagnosis of septicemia and treatment with antibiotics; his general condition then improved and the jaundice disappeared. On the twenty-eighth day the infant was again seen by the pediatrician. At this time, neonatal hepatitis was considered to be the most probable diagnosis. One week later the child had deteriorated clinically. A spinal fluid sugar at that time was 400 mg/100 ml and a blood sugar 300 mg/100 ml by a method that measured total reducing substances. Galactosemia was tentatively diagnosed and the infant placed on a galactose-free regimen. UDP galactose transferase activity was found to be < 8 ImU/gHb, but treatment was ineffectual, and the infant died on the thirty-third day of life.

DISCUSSION

Children's physicians are already accustomed to the idea of screening for inborn errors of metabolism in certain specified circumstances: for hyperphenylalaninemia and perhaps hypertyrosinemia in the newborn; for Wilson's disease in patients with liver disease, and for a more extended array of conditions among the mentally retarded. The idea that sudden acute serious illnesses in infancy and early childhood may, in certain cases, be engendered by inborn errors of metabolism has been less accepted. Nonetheless, it is apparent both from the frequency of cases similar to those described here and from the descriptions of early infant deaths in the relatives of identified index cases that this danger exists. The purpose of this memorandum is to call attention to these conditions and to provide an introduction to and reference source for their diagnosis and initial management.

Table 1 is a compendium of the diseases now recognized that fall into this category; it is not all-inclusive in that certain conditions such as cystic fibrosis have been omitted which are already well described and long recognized. The list is primarily intended to include those states in which there are non-specific signs, usually neurological, which may or may not be accompanied by severe acidosis. Distinguishing features such as special odors, in so far as they exist, are listed; but in general, identification will depend on the laboratory. Few of these conditions are well described in standard pediatric texts.

The appropriate biochemical determinations are given in Table 2, where tests have been divided into three categories: those that can be completed in any hospital clinical laboratory; those like one-dimensional amino acid chromatography that should be available in a group hospital clinical chemistry laboratory; and others, including organic acid chromatography, that need to be carried out in special centers. It is usually wise not to presume that a laboratory can carry out these tests and to check in advance their preparedness for a given test.

Sample collection and delivery is another consideration. Ideally, urine samples should be aliquots of a known 24-hour volume. Such accuracy is not always possible, and random specimens that have been stored frozen at a pH of 3 or less for amino acids or pH 7 for organic acids are satisfactory. Five-milliliter samples can be sent air express in standard containers. Blood samples are sometimes hard to obtain from small infants except by heel prick. Thus, whole blood in heparinized capillaries, which can be protected in the mail by insertion into the folds of corrugated paper, is quite adequate, although plasma alone is always preferable.

References

1. Stanbury, J. B., Wyngaarden, J. B., and Fredrickson, D. S.: The Metabolic Basis of Inherited Disease, 2nd ed. New York, Blakiston Division, McGraw-Hill, 1966.
2. O'Brien, D.: Rare Inborn Errors of Metabolism in Children with Mental Retardation, 2nd ed. Department of Health, Education, and Welfare, U.S. Children's Bureau Publication No. 429–1965. Washington, D.C., U.S. Government Printing Office, 1970.
3. Irreverre, F., Mudd, S. H., Heizer, W. D., and Laster, L.: Sulfite oxidase deficiency: studies of a patient with mental retardation, dislocated ocular lenses and abnormal urinary excretion of S-sulpho-L-cysteine, sulfite and thiosulfate. Biochem. Med., 1:187, 1967.
4. Hommes, F. A., DeGroot, C. J. E., Wilmink, C. W., and Jonxis, J. M. P.: Carbamylphosphate synthetase deficiency in an infant with severe cerebral damage. Arch. Dis. Child., 44:688, 1969.
5. Levin, B., Oberholzer, V. G., and Sinclair, L.: Biochemical investigations of hyperammonaemia. Lancet, 2:170, 1969.
6. McMurray, W. C., Rathbun, J. C., Mohyuddin, F., and Koegler, S. G.: Citrullinuria. Pediatrics, 32:347, 1963.
7. Carton, D., DeSchrizver, F., Kint, J., Van Durme, J., and Hooft, C.: Argininosuccinic aciduria. Neonatal variant with rapid fatal course. Acta Paediat. Scand., 58:528, 1969.
8. Berlow, S., and Efron, M.: A new cause of hyperprolinemia associated with the excretion of Δ′ puroline-5-carboxylic acid. Program and Abstracts, Thirty-fourth An-

nual Meeting, Society for Pediatric Research, Olympic-Western Hotel, Seattle, Washington, June 18–20, 1964 (abst.), p. 43.

9. Goodman, S. I., Pollack, S., Miles, B. A., and O'Brien, D.: The treatment of maple syrup urine disease. J. Pediat., 75:485, 1969.

10. Dancis, J., Hutzler, J., Tada, K., Wada, Y., Morikawa, R., and Arakawa, T.: Hyperva-linemia. Pediatrics, 39:813, 1967.

11. Tanaka, K., Budd, M. A., Efron, M. L., and Isselbacher, K. J.: Isovaleric aciduria: a new genetic defect of leucine metabolism. Proc. Nat. Acad. Sci., 56:236, 1966.

12. Morrow, G., Barness, L. A., Auerbach, V. H., DiGeorge, A. M., Ando, T., and Nyhan, W. L.: Observations of the coexistence of methylmalonic acidemia and glycinemia. J. Pediat., 74:680, 1969.

13. Hommes, F. A., Kuipers, J. R. G., Elema, J. D., Jansen, J. F., and Jonxis, J. N. P.: Propionicacidemia. Pediat. Res., 2:519, 1968.

14. Scriver, C. R., Uesche, S., and Danes, E.: Hyper-β-alaninemia associated with β amino aciduria and α-aminobutyric aciduria, somnolence and seizures. New Eng. J. Med., 274:635, 1966.

15. Perry, T. L., Hansen, S., and Lore, D. L.: Serum carnosinase deficiency in car-nosinaemia. Lancet, 1:1229, 1968.

16. Colombo, J. P., Richterich, R., Donath, A., Spahr, A., and Rossi, E.: Congenital lysine intolerance with periodic ammonia intoxication. Lancet, 1:1014, 1964.

17. Scriver, C. R., Partington, M., and Sass-Kortsak, A.: Conference on hereditary tyrosinemia. Canad. Med. Ass. J., 97:1045, 1967.

18. Smith, A. J., and Strang, L. B.: An inborn error of metabolism with urinary excretion of α-hydroxybutyric and phenylpyruvic acid. Arch. Dis. Child., 33:109, 1958.

19. Arakawa. T., Ohara, K., Kudo, Z., Tada, K., Hayashi, T., and Mizuno, T.: Hyperfolic-acidemia with forminoglutamicaciduria following histidine loading. Tohoku J. Exp. Med., 80:370, 1963.

20. Rosenberg, L. E.: Inherited aminoacidopathies demonstrating vitamin dependency. New Eng. J. Med., 281:145, 1969.

21. Ziter, F. A., Madsen, J. A., and Nyhan, W. L.: The clinical findings in a patient with nonketotic hyperglycinemia. Pediat. Res., 2:250, 1968.

22. Isselbacher, K. J.: Galactosemia. In The Metabolic Basis of Inherited Disease, 2nd ed. J. B. Stanbury, J. B. Wyngaarden, and D. S. Fredrickson, editors. New York, Blakiston Division, McGraw-Hill, 1966, p. 178.

23. Meeuwisse, G. W., and Melin, K.: Studies in glucose-galactose malabsorption. Acta Paediat. Scand., Suppl. 188, 1969.

24. Levin, B. Oberholzer, V. G., Snodgrass, G. J. A., Stimmler, L., and Wilmers, M. J.: Fructosemia: an inborn error of fructose metabolism. Arch Dis. Child., 38:220, 1963.

25. Erickson, R. J.: Familial lactic acidosis. J. Pediat., 66:1004, 1965.

26. Sidbury, J. B., and Harland, W. R.: An inborn error of short-chain fatty acid metabo-lism. J. Pediat., 70:8, 1967.

27. Nyhan, W. L., Oliver, W. J., and Lesch, M.: A familial disorder of uric acid metabolism and central nervous system function. II. J. Pediat., 67:257, 1965.

28. Stromme, J. H., Nesbakken, R., Norman, T., Skjorten, F., Skyberg, D., and Johannes-sen, B.: Familial hypomagnesemia: biochemical, histological and hereditary aspects; studies in two brothers. Acta Paediat. Scand., 58:433, 1969.

29. Nadler, J. L., and Egan, T. J.: Deficiency of lysosomal acid phosphatase. New Eng. J. Med., 282:302, 1970.

30. O'Brien, D., Ibbott, F. A., and Rodgerson, D. O.: Laboratory Manual of Pediatric Micro-biochemical Techniques, 4th ed. New York, Hoeber, 1968.

31. Soriano, J. R., Taitz, L. S., Finberg, L., and Edelmann, C. M.: Hyperglycinemia with ketoacidosis and leukopenia. Pediatrics, 39:818, 1967.

32. Dancis, J., Hutzler, J., and Rokkones, T.: Intermittent branched chain ketoaciduria. New Eng. J. Med., 276:84, 1967.

33. Terheggen, H. G., Schwenk, A., Lowenthal, A., van Sande, M., and Colombo, J. P.: Argininaemia with arginase deficiency. Lancet, 2:748, 1969.

34. Brunette, M. G., Hazel, B., Scriver, C. R., Mohyuddin, F., and Dallaire, L.: Thia-mine-dependent neonatal lactic acidosis with hyperalaninemia. Meeting of the American Pediatric Society and The Society for Pediatric Research, Atlantic City, New Jersey, May 2, 1970 (abst.). Pediat. Res., 4:451, 1970.

17

Salicylate Intoxication

William E. Segar, M.D.

Salicylate is a potent pharmacologic agent, and the rational therapy of salicylate intoxication must be based on an understanding of its pharmacologic actions and consequent pathophysiologic effects.[1] Because it acts to uncouple oxidative phosphorylation in a manner analogous to that of 2,4-dinitrophenol, salicylate is, first of all, a general metabolic stimulant.[2] Oxygen consumption, carbon dioxide formation, and heat production are increased by its action; consequently, oxygen requirement, blood CO_2 concentration, and the need to eliminate heat are also increased. Respiration, heart rate, and cardiac output must increase to satisfy the demands imposed by the acceleration of metabolic processes. Increased heat production causes an increase in evaporated water losses from skin surfaces. Sweating usually occurs.

Second, salicylate interferes in a complex manner with the normal metabolism of carbohydrate.[3] Many factors seem to be involved, some tending to decrease and others to increase the blood glucose concentration, and, clinically, either hyperglycemia or hypoglycemia may be observed. Hyperglycemia may be partially explained by the release of epinephrine due to activation of hypothalamic sympathetic centers. However, large doses of salicylate also decrease aerobic metabolism and

From the Department of Pediatrics, University of Wisconsin Medical Center, Madison, Wisconsin.

increase glucose-6-phosphatase activity, effects which tend to increase the blood glucose level. Hypoglycemia, on the other hand, may be caused by an increased utilization of glucose by peripheral tissues or by interference with gluconeogenesis by salicylates. Recent studies suggest that brain glucose concentration may be decreased despite minimal alterations in blood glucose level.[4]

As a result of these salicylate-induced alterations in carbohydrate metabolism, organic acids, particularly lactic, pyruvic, and acetoacetic, accumulate.[5] Infants appear to be particularly susceptible to the toxic effects of salicylate on carbohydrate metabolism and are more likely to have disturbances in blood glucose concentration and severe metabolic acidosis than are older children.

Salicylate also is a known stimulant of the respiratory center of the central nervous system, and increased salicylate levels produce an increase in ventilation.[6] This effect, which occurs promptly after the ingestion of a toxic amount of salicylate, results in a net decrease in Pco_2 and a respiratory alkalosis despite the fact that the hypermetabolic action of salicylate would increase Pco_2. In turn, the renal excretion of sodium, potassium, and bicarbonate is increased, a known response to respiratory alkalosis. As a result of the loss of sodium and potassium bicarbonate, the patient's ability to compensate for the metabolic acidosis, which, in severely intoxicated children, is superimposed on the pre-existing respiratory alkalosis, is significantly compromised.

Dehydration, particularly in the infant or in the child with chronic salicylate intoxication, is an important and, often, an inevitable consequence of the pathophysiologic processes noted. Both hyperventilation and sweating result in increased water and electrolyte expenditure. Vomiting and diarrhea occur frequently and contribute to the development of dehydration. Initially, the volume of urine will be increased by the increased solute load characteristic of any state of hypermetabolism and ketosis. It might be noted that once body water stores are depleted, salicylate can no longer induce effective sweating, and the hyperpyretic action of the drug is no longer balanced by effective defenses. Thus, hyperpyrexia accelerates dehydration, and dehydration potentiates hyperpyrexia. The magnitude of the water losses cannot be precisely quantitated. To our knowledge no balance studies have been performed on children recovering from salicylate intoxication. However, one might assume that the water losses are comparable to those observed in diabetic acidosis[7-9] and would, in the severely intoxicated child, approximate 80 to 120 ml per kilogram of body weight.

DIAGNOSIS AND TREATMENT

The symptoms and clinical findings exhibited by the child with salicylate intoxication will vary depending on the age of the child, the amount of salicylate consumed, and whether the poisoning is a result of accidental ingestion or therapeutic overdosage. The severity of the illness often correlates poorly with the blood salicylate level and may be more severe than predicted from the salicylate concentration alone, particularly in infants and in children poisoned by therapeutic overdosage.

Mild Intoxication

Hyperventilation is frequently the only symptom of mild intoxication in a child 2 years old or older. Respiratory alkalosis is usually present. After emptying the child's stomach by the use of syrup of ipecac or by mechanical means, the physician need only be sure than the child receives an adequate fluid intake, either orally or parenterally. The type of fluid given is of little importance because these children recover uneventfully.

Moderate Intoxication

The infant with salicylate intoxication, the child poisoned by therapeutic overdosage, or the older child with any disturbance in sensorium or hydration probably should be hospitalized and given parenteral fluid therapy. These moderately ill patients are not, by definition, significantly hypernatremic or hyperthermic. Recovery will be complete if the child is given adequate fluid therapy. Assuming that no significant dehydration exists, these children require maintenance therapy plus replacement of the concurrent abnormal losses that are the result of hyperventilation and diaphoresis. This additional fluid requirement can be provided by increasing maintenance therapy by 30 to 50 per cent. Because large amounts of potassium are lost in the urine as a response to the respiratory alkalosis, adequate potassium, usually at a concentration of 40 mEq/liter, should be included in the intravenous fluids.

Severe Intoxication

The child with severe salicylate intoxication presents a major therapeutic challenge. Many will be small infants who have received chronic overdosage and, despite plasma salicylate levels as low as 15 mg/100 ml, are gravely ill. Severe hyperthermia is common in this group and is an important cause of death. It is a result of the increase in heat production coupled with decreased efficiency of cooling mechanisms.

Severe hyperthermia cannot develop unless the normal heat-regulating mechanisms are impaired. Since these mechanisms depend, in part, upon the evaporation of water from the skin and lungs, as well as the loss of body heat by radiation and convection, they are compromised by dehydration. When the environmental temperature and humidity remain constant, an increase in the heat production must be compensated for by an increase in the evaporation of water or hyperthermia results. In circumstances in which normal body temperature cannot be maintained, sweat is formed, and its evaporation augments the cooling processes. This regulation of body heat requires a delicate balance between heat production and heat loss.

The central nervous system, especially the hypothalamic nuclei, plays an essential part in regulating the peripheral mechanisms concerned with the conservation or loss of body heat. Because of this action the hypothalamus has been termed the "thermostat" of the body. In fever the balance between heat production and heat loss persists, except that the "thermostat" is set at a higher level. Salicylate acts to reset the "thermostat" at a normal temperature. Heat production is not inhibited by salicylates; rather, it is, as noted above, increased. However, heat dissipation is also increased by means of increased insensible expenditure of water, as well as by the expenditure of large quantities of sweat. Salicylate, then, can reduce body temperature, but only through the loss of sizable quantities of water. This ability of salicylate to reduce body temperature to normal is undoubtedly due to its action on the central nervous system, for it can be prevented by the experimental production of hypothalamic lesions.[10] In any event, this combination of events can rapidly lead to lethal hyperpyrexia.

Moderate to severe dehydration is usually noted in the child seriously ill with salicylate intoxication. Shock and, rarely, acute renal failure may occur. The large respiratory and cutaneous water losses represent loss of water without equivalent loss of electrolyte. Hypernatremia occurs when the child's ability to excrete electrolyte, particularly sodium, is impaired by dehydration or when the renal transport of sodium is affected by the toxic action of salicylate. Significant hypernatremia is not infrequent, occurring in 5 of 25 severely intoxicated children reported by Segar and Holliday.[1] Severe hyperpyrexia and convulsions were observed in the same patients.

The infant with severe salicylate intoxication may be hypoglycemic or hyperglycemic. Glucosuria and ketonuria are present in the latter, and the clinical picture may be confused easily with that of diabetic acidosis. A history of salicylate ingestion and a blood salicylate determination are needed to establish the proper diagnosis. Hypoglycemia may be a more important physiologic disturbance than hyperglycemia since seizures and damage to the central nervous system are possible consequences. A blood sugar determination should be performed on all children with salicylate intoxication and if hypoglycemia exists prompt therapy with a glucose-containing solution is essential.

Finally the child with severe salicylate intoxication may display alarming evidence of central nervous system dysfunction, including stupor, coma, convulsions (either focal or generalized), and, rarely, paralysis. The central nervous system symptoms can usually, but not always, be attributed to hyperpyrexia, disturbances in carbohydrate metabolism, hypernatremia, or severe acidosis and ketosis.

Metabolic acidosis may be a serious and life-threatening complication of salicylate intoxication. Although the abnormalities in the chemical composition of the plasma can be readily corrected, the symptomatic recovery of the patient is, in our experience, less rapid than that of the child with diabetic acidosis of comparable severity.

The acidosis of salicylate intoxication is the end result of several pathologic processes. Initially, during the stage of hyperventilation, respiratory alkalosis occurs as a result of the increased pulmonary excretion of carbonic acid. This decrease in plasma carbon dioxide tension produces, in turn, a decreased renal reabsorption of bicarbonate and increased excretion of both sodium and potassium bicarbonate.[11, 12] The loss of carbonic acid and of sodium bicarbonate diminishes the buffer capacity of the extracellular fluid to a measurable degree. Loss of potassium similarly leads to a decreased buffer capacity of intracellular fluid. Therefore, pH may change in either direction more readily than before.

The primary cause of the acidosis of salicylate intoxication, however, is the derangement of carbohydrate metabolism. Fat is mobilized and converted in the liver to ketone bodies, which are then utilized by cells for energy purposes. Since the ketone bodies are produced in excess of the capacities of tissue utilization and renal excretion, they accumulate as unmeasured anions in the body fluids. The bicarbonate and other buffer anions are further reduced by this accumulation of organic anions. The concentrations of lactic and pyruvic acids also increase in the body fluids as a result of faulty aerobic carbohydrate metabolism. Salicylate itself is an acid, and its ingestion will increase fixed cation excretion and, because it may displace some bicarbonate in plasma (2 or 3 mEq per liter), will increase acidosis. Finally, impairment of renal function may augment the development of acidosis.

The metabolic acidosis of salicylate intoxication is therefore the result of the increased production of various organic acids in an organism whose defenses against acidosis are impaired by a pre-existing depletion of buffering capacity and are further compromised by inadequate renal function. Laboratory evidence of the metabolic acidosis includes a low serum pH and total Pco_2 content. The child will exhibit Kussmaul respirations and, indeed, hyperventilation is needed for survival. If respiratory rate decreases, the Pco_2 increases and the blood pH, which is already low, may decrease to a level incompatible with life. Finally, myocardial performance may be inadequate—impaired as a result of acidosis, potassium deficiency, hyperthermia, and inefficient myocardial metabolism—and thus may lead to congestive heart failure.

Although adequate intravenous administration of fluids is the sine qua non of effective therapy, other important aspects of treatment should not be overlooked.

Hyperpyrexia must be attacked intelligently. Sponging the patient with tepid water is usually adequate. Ice-water sponging should be used judiciously, if at all, because this procedure may cause cutaneous vasoconstriction and interfere with heat loss, or cause shivering and thereby increase heat production. Convulsions may be treated with short-acting barbiturates. Intravenous injection of calcium gluconate is sometimes beneficial.

Care must be taken to avoid procedures and medications that depress respiration since, as noted, hyperventilation is required to increase CO_2 elimination and to prevent a further decrease of blood pH. Oxygen should be used only if the child is cyanotic or in heart failure. If respiratory depression occurs, artificial ventilation is needed and the pattern of hyperventilation must be maintained. Measurements of pH and Pco_2 should be made frequently to guide the rate and depth of artificial ventilation.

Tetany, should it occur, can usually be controlled by decreasing the amount of alkali administered and by the intravenous administration of calcium gluconate. Congestive heart failure also merits an attempt to correct the serum pH rapidly by the judicious administration of alkali because myocardial function may not improve until the serum pH exceeds 7.20.

Intravenous fluid therapy must (1) provide the child with his daily maintenance requirements of water and electrolytes, (2) correct pre-existing body fluid deficits, and (3) allow extra water to meet the abnormally great insensible water losses. The usual maintenance requirements are 100 ml of water, 3 mEq of sodium, 2 mEq of potassium, and 2 mEq of chloride per 100 kcal of caloric expenditure per day[13] (or 1500 ml of water, 45 mEq of sodium, 30 mEq of potassium, and 30 mEq of chloride per m^2/day). These amounts should be increased by 25 to 50 per cent to meet the increased requirements for water and electrolytes caused by hyperventilation and sweating.

The additional amount of intravenous fluids required to correct the pre-existing deficit in body fluids is determined by the degree of dehydration. If severe, 100 ml of water, 9 mEq of sodium, 6 mEq of potassium, and 6 mEq of chloride should be given per kilogram of body weight. If dehyration is not severe, proportionately lesser amounts of fluid are needed. As is always the case, deficit fluid therapy should be given in addition to that required for maintenance therapy and for the replacement of ongoing losses. An example of the recommended therapy per 24 hours for a child weighing 10 kg with severe dehydration due to salicylate intoxication is shown in Table 1.

If the serum sodium concentration is more than 155 mEq/liter, the amount of sodium and chloride given as deficit therapy should be reduced by 25 to 50 per cent. Potassium is added to the intravenous

TABLE 1   RECOMMENDED INTRAVENOUS THERAPY FOR CHILD WEIGHING 10 KG WITH SEVERE DEHYDRATION DUE TO SALICYLATE INTOXICATION

Therapy	Amounts per 24 hours			
	H_2O (ml)	Na (mEq)	K (mEq)	Cl (mEq)
Maintenance	1000	30	20	20
Deficit	1000	90	60	60
Replacement of abnormal losses	500	15	10	10
Total	2500	135	90	90

fluids as soon as urine flow is established, and all intravenous fluids should contain 5 gm of glucose per 100 ml.

Perhaps not all physicians will wish to use the system of parenteral fluid therapy described here, although it and similar systems provide a degree of flexibility not otherwise available. However, if the use of polyionic solutions is preferred, those containing approximately 50 mEq of sodium and 40 mEq of potassium and chloride per liter are appropriate. The amount needed will vary from 150 to 250 ml/kg (2250 to 4000 ml/m²), depending on the severity of the dehydration.

If the child is in shock, the initial therapy should consist of the rapid administration of Ringer's lactate solution, 20 to 40 ml/kg, given in a period of 20 to 30 minutes. Should anuria or severe oliguria persist once the child is adequately hydrated, hemodialysis or intermittent peritoneal dialysis should be instituted. The latter procedure is usually more easily accomplished and can be made more efficient by the addition of 5 per cent human serum albumin solution to the dialysis fluid.[14] However, if urinary output is satisfactory, dialytic procedures are seldom necessary.

It is well established that the renal excretion of salicylate is increased manyfold if the urine can be made alkaline. Sodium bicarbonate administration[15, 16] and the use of acetazolamide[17] or tris buffer have been recommended, and each, given properly, will increase the rate of salicylate excretion. However, both acetazolamide and tris buffer have major undesirable side effects which preclude their use except in carefully controlled experimental circumstances.[18, 19] Alkalinization of the urine by the administration of sodium bicarbonate is less dangerous. However, as noted here, the child with mild or moderately severe salicylate intoxication will recover uneventfully if he receives an adequate fluid intake, irrespective of the rapidity of salicylate excretion. The use in these children of sodium bicarbonate or of other alkalinizing agents is, therefore, unnecessary.

The severely ill child, on the other hand, would undoubtedly be helped by the more rapid elimination of salicylate and by a prompt restoration of a more normal serum pH. Hill[19] has shown that in experimental salicylate poisoning rapid alkalization causes a decrease in muscle, brain, and liver salicylate concentrations. Since one might assume that the more rapid removal of salicylate from tissue is advantageous, the temptation to use sodium bicarbonate therapy in the treatment of these children is strong. However, the large amounts of sodium bicarbonate needed to alkalinize the urine of the child with severe metabolic acidosis may increase the serum sodium concentration rapidly and significantly, thereby incurring the risk of central nervous system damage.[20] Furthermore, tetany occurs fairly frequently after the administration of alkali. It is the author's opinion that the dangers of urine alkalization outweigh the admitted benefits and, therefore, sodium bicarbonate is not recommended for this purpose.

On the other hand, if an immediate increase in serum pH is required, as it might be if the patient were in myocardial failure or had profound coma or respiratory depression due to severe metabolic acidosis (serum pH < 7.20), the intravenous administration of sodium bicarbonate would be the treatment of choice, and 3 to 5 mEq/kg should be given rapidly. These recommendations concerning the use of sodium bicarbonate represent the author's opinion, based solely on his experience; statistical data, utilizing survival rates and absence of neurologic sequelae as the criteria of successful therapy, are not available.

References

1. Segar, W. E., and Holliday, M. A.: Physiological abnormalities of salicylate intoxication. New Eng. J. Med., 259:1191, 1958.
2. Smith, M. J. H.: Salicylates and metabolism. J. Pharm. Pharmacol., 11:705, 1959.
3. Goodman, L. S., and Gilman, A.: The Pharmacological Basis of Therapeutics, ed. 3. New York, Macmillan, 1965, pp. 312–330.
4. Thurston, J. H., Pollock, P. G., and Mayer, S. K.: Effect of salicylate on the energy metabolism of the brain. Pediat. Res., 3:358, 1969.
5. Schwartz, R., and Landy, G.: Organic acid excretion in salicylate intoxication. J. Pediat., 66:658, 1965.
6. Winters, R. W., White, J. S., Hughes, M. C., and Ordway, N. K.: Disturbances of acid-base equilibrium in salicylate intoxication. Pediatrics, 23:260, 1959.
7. Darrow, D. C., and Pratt, E. L.: Retention of water and electrolyte during recovery in patient with diabetic acidosis. J. Pediat., 41:688, 1952.
8. Atchley, D. W., Loeb, R. F., Richards, D. W., Jr., Benedict, E. M., and Driscoll, M. E.: On diabetic acidosis: detailed study of electrolyte balances following withdrawal and reestablishment of insulin therapy. J. Clin. Invest., 12:297, 1933.
9. Nabarro, J. D. N., Spencer, A. G., and Stowers, J. M.: Metabolic studies in severe diabetic ketosis. Quart. J. Med., 21:225, 1952.
10. Guerra (Perez-Carral), F., and Brobeck, R.: Hypothalamic control of aspirin antipyresis in monkey. J. Pharm. Exp. Ther., 80:209, 1944.
11. Barker, E. S., Singer, R. B., Elkinton, J. R., and Clark, J. K.: Renal response in man to acute experimental respiratory alkalosis and acidosis. J. Clin. Invest., 36:515, 1957.
12. Stanbury, S. W., and Thomson, A. E.: Renal response to respiratory alkalosis. Clin. Sci., 11:357, 1952.

13. Holliday, M. A., and Segar, W. E.: The maintenance need for water in parenteral fluid therapy. Pediatrics, *19*:823, 1957.
14. Etteldorf, J. N., Dobbins, W. T., Summitt, R. L., Rainwater, W. T., and Fischer, R. L.: Intermittent peritoneal dialysis using 5 per cent albumin in the treatment of salicylate intoxication in children. J. Pediat., *58*:226, 1961.
15. Oliver, T. K., Jr., and Dyer, M. E.: The prompt treatment of salicylism with sodium bicarbonate. Amer. J. Dis. Child., *99*:553, 1960.
16. Whitten, C. F., Kesaree, N. M., and Goodwin, J. F.: Managing salicylate poisoning in children. Amer. J. Dis. Child., *101*:178, 1961.
17. Schwartz, R., Fellers, F. X., Knapp, J., and Yaffe, S.: The renal response to administration of acetazolamide (Damox) during salicylate intoxication. Pediatrics, *23*:1103, 1959.
18. Kaplan, S. A., and del Carmen, F. T.: Experimental salicylate poisoning: observations on the effects of carbonic anhydrose inhibitor and bicarbonate. Pediatrics, *21*:762, 1958.
19. Hill, J. B.: Experimental salicylate poisoning: observations on the effects of altering blood pH on tissue and plasma salicylate concentrations. Pediatrics, *47*:658, 1971.
20. Kravath, R. E., Aharon, A. S., and Finberg, L.: Effect of hypertonic saline infusions on blood and cerebrospinal fluid. Pediat. Res., *3*:352, 1969.

18

Dehydration Secondary to Diarrhea

Laurence Finberg, M.D.

Diarrhea, a symptom of a variety of disorders affecting infants, often leads to marked physiologic disturbances. Vomiting, a common accompanying symptom, adds to and modifies the disturbances produced by diarrheal diseases. Enteric infections cause these symptoms more often than all other diseases combined, but noninfectious causes may occasionally also occur. The discussion here will deliberately limit consideration of the management to the physiologic disturbances that accompany excessive loss of water and salts from the gastrointestinal tract. Etiologic considerations, however important they may be, will not be further pursued. This emphasis is appropriate since survival following critical dehydration depends far more upon the correction of the physiologic disturbance than upon the removal of the cause.

From the Department of Pediatrics, Montefiore Hospital and Medical Center and the Department of Pediatrics of the Albert Einstein College of Medicine, Bronx, New York.

A critical stage in diarrheal disease may be defined as that which occurs when a volume of fluid equal in mass to about 10 per cent of the body weight has been lost over a period of a day or two. Clinically this usually occurs shortly after the illness, through anorexia or vomiting, has precluded oral intake. At this stage of illness parenteral fluid therapy should be employed. Oral intake should be curtailed during the early hours of therapy. The use of milk or other foods high in calories and solute markedly increases stool water losses and thus complicates management. Even if severe undernutrition coexists with the diarrhea, the first few hours nonetheless should be a period of brief starvation; the parenteral glucose will provide emergency calories.

Although such routes of administration as intragastric drip and subcutaneous infusion have been employed successfully, their usage should be restricted to places where a deficiency of supplies or trained personnel interdicts the preferred parenteral route—continuous intravenous infusion. With modern equipment, skilled house officers and pediatricians should be able to use venipuncture technique with only rare recourse to venesection (cutdown).

CLINICAL EVALUATION

The plan for therapy begins with clinical assessment of the patient. When available, laboratory analyses add valuable complementary assistance. Even if chemical analyses cannot be performed for many hours, an initial blood sample to be analyzed for urea N, Na^+, CO_2 content, Cl^-, and K^+ should be obtained. If enough blood and a sufficiently versatile laboratory are available, tests for Ca^{++}, pH, and Pco_2 are also of interest. The role of each of these determinations will be discussed as the areas of assessment are further delineated. Since weight of the patient (accurately determined and repeated at intervals) constitutes the most important and useful measurement, as much attention should be paid to the technique of weighing as to the laboratory procedures.

Clinical evaluation may be divided into five useful parameters, in decreasing order of immediate importance: volume, osmolality, hydrogen ion status, intracellular ion deficits, and calcium ion homeostasis (Table 1). Each of these may be profitably discussed in terms of the method of clinical evaluation, usefulness of laboratory measurements, and calculation for physiological correction during each of the three phases of critical therapy: emergency, initial repletion, and early recovery. First, a 24-hour period of therapy will be considered: this will be followed by a breakdown for the first hour, the next 6 to 8 hours, and the remaining hours of the first 24. For the more seriously ill infants, a plan for the second day will be outlined, thus completing the critical therapy of dehydration.

TABLE 1   CLINICAL APPRAISAL OF PROBLEMS OF HYDRATION*

Point of Appraisal	Clinical Symptoms and Signs*	Laboratory Determination of Greatest Value
Volume	Circulatory impairment, skin changes, eye and fontanelle changes, oliguria.	Body weight, urea N in serum
Osmolality	For hypernatremia: CNS signs—disturbance of consciousness, hypertonicity of muscles, increased reflexes, marked thirst, "inapparent dehydration" with good circulation for degree of loss. For hyponatremia: Exaggeration of the signs listed under *Volume*.	Na$^+$ in serum
Hydrogen ion status	Hyperpnea in acidemia.	CO$_2$ content (HCO$_3^-$) in serum
Intracellular ion deficits	Abdominal distension, muscle weakness, diminished reflexes.	K$^+$ in serum (limited use), ECG
Calcium homeostasis	Tetany, convulsions.	Ca^{++} in serum (complex interpretation), ECG

*Only the symptoms and signs of dehydration have been given in this table. A companion group of signs for the corresponding disturbances of overhydration have been omitted for simplicity. The same points of appraisal and the same laboratory examinations may be advantageously used.

Volume

Water volume repletion and maintenance constitute the most important facet of the care of dehydration.* The therapeutic volume needs are threefold: (1) the deficit, (2) the ongoing usual requirements for normal maintenance, and (3) continuing abnormal losses.

The Deficit. Deficit refers to a loss of volume or mass of water from the hydrated state. When diarrhea causes loss of water and salt in physiologic proportions (about two thirds of the time in North American experience), clinical signs first appear when about 5 per cent of the body mass (7 per cent of the body fluid) has been lost over a 1- or 2-day

---

*Dehydration to the physiologist and clinician ordinarily means loss of water plus solute rather than the literal meaning of loss of water alone usually intended in other usages of the word.

period. Tachycardia and dryness of the mucous membranes appear as the earliest signs. Earlier symptoms, such as thirst and a dry feeling in the mouth, are not useful in infants; moreover, thirst may be obscured by nausea. Next in order of appearance are evidences of advancing circulatory insufficiency and changes in the elasticity of the skin and subcutaneous tissue. Thus, by the time the deficit has progressed to the order of 10 per cent of the weight, the extremities show cyanosis or mottling and diminished temperature. The pulse rate may be very rapid, even for the fever which may also be present. Oliguria becomes manifest. The fontanelle, if open, will be depressed, and the eyeballs appear sunken. The skin and subcutaneous tissue of the abdomen in the infant will show loss of elasticity by sustaining folds when pinched and loss of turgor by the slow return of color after pressure. After the age of about 2 years subcutaneous tissue composition differs from that of the infant and these last signs are not usually elicitable. When losses of water exceed 10 per cent of body weight, the circulatory failure becomes more pronounced so that, at an acute weight loss of about 15 per cent, a moribund irreversible state may occur.

From the preceding discussion, the repeated reference to weight makes it evident that this measurement delineates the deficit. Because pre-illness weights are seldom known, a clinical estimate by the criteria discussed may be usefully employed with reasonable accuracy. When by good chance the previous weight is known, use it. A clinical axiom, applicable without significant error, states that changes in body weight within any 24-hour period may be considered to be water. However, one must remember not to extend this period of time because clinically insignificant deviations within 24 hours may be cumulative and highly significant over longer intervals.

Normal Maintenance. Though weight constitutes the direct measure of a water deficit, normal maintenance requirements of water are not a simple function of mass but rather of energy expenditure. Since the infant and the young child have a higher rate of metabolism per unit of mass than older, larger individuals,[1] their obligate water losses, hence maintenance requirements, are also greater per unit of mass. One hundred calories expended result in 100 ml of water loss through skin, lungs, urine and stool. This relationship, in which obligate water losses directly follow energy expenditure, roughly parallels the surface area relation to mass, a fact which has led some to use surface area in calculation. In fact, neither surface area nor caloric expenditure measurements are made on clinical services. Either system requires for practical application that a table of estimates, such as Table 2, or a nomogram be used to derive from the weight a quantity of water per unit mass appropriate for age and size. The weight remains the practical measurement available.

The fact that two distinct bases, namely the metabolic expenditure and the loss in weight, are necessary for the volume calculation remains

TABLE 2   APPROXIMATE BASAL WATER REQUIREMENTS IN RELATION TO AGE, WEIGHT, AND SURFACE AREA

Age	Weight (kg)	Surface Area (M²)	Minimal Basal Water Requirement		
			ml/kg or cal/kg	ml/M²	ml/24 hrs
Newborn	2.5–4.0	0.20–0.23	50	750	125–200
1 week–6 months	3.0–8.0	0.20–0.35	65–70	1000–1100	200–520
6 months–12 months	8.0–12.0	0.35–0.45	50–60	1000–1050	500–600
12 months–24 months	10.0–15.0	0.45–0.60	45–50	1000–1050	500–750

the most fundamental contribution by pediatric clinicians to the field of hydration therapy.[1] No single reference base may be used; weight, calories, or surface area alone will not be accurate over a range of ages and sizes. The author prefers for two reasons to use calories rather than surface area for maintenance calculations: (1) for clarity of thinking in terms of physiology to stress the fundamental relationship, and (2) because the newborn and a few other states (edematous and obese patients) are exceptions to a simple surface area relationship. If these matters are understood, surface area nomogram enthusiasts may use their nomograms with results equal to those obtained by the scheme proposed here.

Using a value for caloric expenditure at basal conditions from a table requires an additional interpretation of the patient's actual state. Allowing for usual activity, temperature variation, and rate of breathing, coupled with observed urine formation, energy expenditure may ordinarily be assumed to be one and one half times the basal rate. Persistent high fever warrants doubling the basal figure; and the extreme combination of persistent high body temperature, hyperventilation, and convulsive muscular activity might triple the basal allotment.

Abnormal Losses.   Continued abnormal losses, the third factor in assessing volume requirements, are measured or estimated by direct collection or observation, including any tube drainages as well as stool losses.

In addition to weight, though much less useful, a measure of the urea nitrogen concentration in the serum helps in assessing volume depletion. The level of this determination depends upon the duration as well as the quantity of deficit, since it reflects the effect of failure of glomerular filtration, roughly indicating the degree of severity of extracellular fluid loss. Since that compartment sustains most of the loss in volume when water and sodium salts are lost together in physiologic proportion, in the absence of complicating primary renal disease the urea nitrogen level may be used for retrospective and prognostic estimates.

To illustrate the application of the foregoing, consider a 6-month-old infant weighing 5000 gm in the dehydrated state with clinical features suggesting a loss of 10 per cent of body weight. This leads to an estimate of a 500 ml (gm) deficit. (For convenience the dehydrated rather than the hydrated weight may justifiably be used by ignoring the water of oxidation which would, at the age in the example, constitute an arithmetical quantity of similar magnitude in the opposite direction.) Estimating the usual requirement figure at this age and size ($5 \times 65 \times 1\frac{1}{2}$) adds about another 500 ml/day (Table 2). Together these total 1000 ml, if the volume of the deficit is to be repaired in one day. Continued abnormal losses are observed and added. Details concerning rate of administration and solute content at the various time segments are best considered after the remainder of the appraisal is completed. In general, however, except as noted, a volume of water roughly equal to the deficit (500 ml) will have been administered in 6 to 8 hours; the remaining 500 ml plus the volume of any abnormal losses will have been administered by the end of 24 hours.

Osmolality

Osmolality of body fluids is the second most important general element in evaluation. In a somewhat simplified sense, the content of sodium salts in the body determines the physiologically signifcant osmolality because Na^+ and Cl^-, owing to their relative exclusion from intracellular fluid, determine, by their content, the distribution of body water into its two main compartments — extracellular fluid (ECF) and intracellular fluid (ICF). Therefore, sodium concentration constitutes a more clinically relevant determination than the actual osmolality because those solutes which are evenly distributed in body water do not affect the relative size of the compartments.

This knowledge, together with the clinical appearance and course, has led to a classification of dehydration on the basis of sodium concentration in serum. In North America, isonatremic dehydration accounts for about 65 per cent of patients, hypernatremic for 20 to 25 per cent, and hyponatremic for about 10 per cent of those admitted to hospitals with dehydration. These incidence values vary from one region to another and also vary with the season and the prevailing feeding practices.

A high sodium concentration, defined as > 150 mEq/L of serum, implies relative cellular desiccation and relative preservation of ECF volume; conversely, a low sodium, < 132 mEq/L denotes relatively greater ECF depletion per unit volume lost. Hypernatremic dehydration then has, for a given degree of loss in volume, less than the expected evidence of circulatory failure and subcutaneous tissue changes, frequently justifying the description "deceptively inapparent" dehydration. The cellular desiccation produced by hypernatremia leads to a preponderance of central nervous system symptoms, signs, and pathologic damage. These manifestations usually occur at about the same volume loss as do the circulatory signs of classic or isonatremic dehydration.

Certain features from the history and physical findings enable one to recognize hypernatremia prior to laboratory confirmation. Younger infants have a higher incidence. Intake usually has abruptly stopped fairly early in the course of the disease. Less constant features which suggest the possibility include a high solute intake (e.g., full-strength skim milk) just before cessation of intake, persistent high fever, a hot dry environment (e.g., heated apartment in winter), and hyperventilation. On examination, disturbance of consciousness is usually manifested by a peculiar combination of marked lethargy or somnolence, coupled with hyperirritability when the infant is stimulated by touch, noise, or light. Hypertonicity of muscles, often producing mild nuchal rigidity, may occur. More extreme manifestations of central nervous system involvement include muscle twitchings, tremors, and frank convulsions. The abdominal skin has a velvety feel and inconstantly a "doughy" consistency. Circulation is usually maintained, but, if the dehydration exceeds 10 per cent weight loss or if the hypernatremia is very severe ($Na^+ > 180$ mEq/L), shock may complicate even this variety of dehydration.[2]

Hyponatremic dehydration is most likely to appear when protracted stool losses have produced large electrolyte losses, and especially when this circumstance is accompanied by an ample water intake very low in solute (i.e., water without electrolyte). The clinical manifestations consist of an increase of circulatory failure per unit of volume lost. Thus extreme shock may appear at an earlier stage of volume deficit. The low sodium concentration in patients with kwashiorkor represents a different and more complex phenomenon requiring an approach not applicable in this discussion of a better nourished population.

The most common osmolal occurrence in dehydration, a normal concentration of sodium (isonatremia), produces the well-known picture of extracellular depletion with moderate circulatory deficit when about 10 per cent of body weight has been lost over a day or two. In isonatremic dehydration, balance studies have shown losses of Na^+ in the order of 8 to 15 mEq/kg.[3] Patients with hypernatremic dehydration have lost as little as 2 to 5 mEq/kg; hyponatremic patients may have deficits up to 20 mEq/kg.

With regard to solute loss, hence osmolality, treatment should take into account not only the magnitude of sodium loss but also the important fact that brain swelling results when dilute solutions of electrolyte are administered rapidly. Therefore, in hypernatremic dehydration, when the solute requirement is low, to avoid central nervous system insult on the one hand or edema from excessive isotonic ECF expansion on the other, the deficit replacement should be spread evenly over at least 48 hours.

Except as noted in hypernatremic dehydration, the sodium salt replacement should be planned to take place during the first 24 hours of therapy. During this period, the deficit of sodium so exceeds that necessary for normal maintenance that no provision need be made for sodium "requirement." In the 5 kg infant not thought to have hypernatremia in our previous example, the sodium deficit of about 12 mEq/kg (range, 8 to 15 mEq/kg) would be 5 × 12 or 60 mEq (or a range of 40 to 75). Administering this amount of sodium to the infant would produce the necessary expansion of ECF to carry out life functions, including urine formation. The average concentration of sodium in the first day's therapy would thus be 60 mEq/L (range, 40 to 75 mEq/L). If the hypothetical patient was diagnosed as hypernatremic, the recommended average concentration would be lower, e.g., 25 to 40 mEq/L. The sodium administered to patients with hypernatremia may even have to exceed the deficit slightly in order to avoid too rapid infusion of water without electrolyte, a circumstance which produces brain swelling.

If restoration of volume and sodium replacement are achieved in patients with reasonably intact functioning renal and pulmonary systems, the remaining three points of assessment will require little or no attention other than the provision of the intracellular ions by mouth.

Hydrogen Ion Status

Patients with diarrhea usually have a primary excess of H^+ for three reasons: (1) stool water may contain a relatively large amount of HCO_3^-; (2) starvation and dehydration lead to increased production of keto acids (nonvolatile acid production); and (3) perhaps most importantly, progressive reduction of renal function leads to retention of nonvolatile acids (H^+). In spite of compensatory blowing off of CO_2 reducing the Pco_2, pH may fall. The CO_2 content of the serum will be low, and, for reasons beyond the present scope of discussion, Cl^- ion concentration is usually increased in this type of acidosis.

Unless these changes are very severe (CO_2 content < 3 mEq/L) or some persistent impairment of kidney or lung exists, no specific administration of alkali will ordinarily be required. The physiologic proportion of basic anions to the total in extracellular fluid is about 1:5 or 1:4. Thus, all deficit repair solutions for acidotic states and all maintenance solutions should have from a fifth to a quarter of the anions as base. While this may be safely increased slightly in diarrheal disease, experience shows that this extra base is not usually necessary so long as volume and osmolality needs are met and, very important, urine formation occurs. For this reason, the emergency phase of therapy will be optimal if it promotes urine formation.

Intracellular Ion Deficits

The loss of potassium from cells, first demonstrated more than 20 years ago, has proved to be an important cause of the physiologic disturbance of severe diarrheal disease.[4] All infants with severe diarrheal disease will sustain potassium loss, and replacement is necessary during the phases of repletion and early recovery. Clinical signs often not seen until unmasked by initial hydration include hypotonia of muscles, abdominal distention, and weakness. The level of K^+ in serum may be high because of poor glomerular filtration, even in severe K^+ deficit. Because the myocardium is quite sensitive to small (absolute) changes in K^+ levels in serum, caution is required in administration, particularly prior to the establishment of urine output. Even afterwards, parenteral K^+ must be given carefully, and experience has shown that the safer oral route may be employed in most instances. The magnitude of the deficit may be as much as 10 mEq/kg.[3] This does not necessarily represent a corresponding volume of loss of ICF, because probably not all the K^+ is osmotically active.

Generally, 3 mEq/kg per day is a reasonably effective and safe rate of replacement. If parenteral K^+ must be given, concentrations greater than 40 mEq/L should be avoided and rates greater than 4 mEq/hour may be risky for small infants.

Correcting Mg^{++} and $PO_4^=$ deficits has not been shown to be clinically important.

Homeostasis

Calcium homeostasis occasionally goes awry during dehydration, especially with hypernatremia, with resultant hypocalcemia. However, this rarely leads to tetany.[2] For this reason, during the management of hypernatremic dehydration, the addition of 10 ml of 10 per cent calcium gluconate to every 500 ml of intravenous solution has seemed a wise precaution.

IMPLEMENTATION OF THERAPY

Having presented the principles, let us return to the example. At this point a volume of 1000 ml has been tentatively established for administration during the first 24 hours of treatment. The sodium content will be approximately 60 mEq and the potassium content will be about 15 mEq. The 75 mEq of anions should be apportioned approximately 55 mEq as chloride and 20 mEq as base, e.g., bicarbonate, lactate, or acetate. The solution should also include glucose to supply calories.

As previously stated, this therapy should be considered in three phases: emergency, repletion, and early recovery.

Phase 1 — Emergency

Immediate infusion of a volume of fluid over a 10- to-15 minute period to expand the intravascular compartment and thus restore circulation should begin therapy for every patient in circulatory distress. The following fluids have been used successfully: whole blood, single donor plasma, 5 per cent albumin, and a 10 per cent glucose solution with a sodium concentration of 75 mEq/L, bicarbonate of 20 mEq, and chloride of 55 mEq/L. Blood and plasma have fallen into mild disfavor because of suspected problems with hepatitis and actual problems of availability. The albumin solutions are not available everywhere but have proved particularly useful for the coincidence of shock and hypernatremia, a potentially deadly combination. The author prefers hypertonic glucose (10 per cent) to plain electrolyte solutions (e.g., Ringer's lactate) because of the more immediate expansion of the intravascular space and the empiric impression of more rapid urine formation.

The volume of these rapid infusions should be 20 ml/kg of body weight for blood, plasma, or 5 per cent albumin and 40 ml/kg for the solution of 10 per cent glucose with 75 mEq/L of sodium. The larger volume (40 ml/kg) will require 30 to 40 minutes for administration.

Phase 2 — Repletion

The remaining water volume with electrolytes may now be combined as a single solution for the rest of the 24 hours, with the rate adjusted appropriately. The glucose concentration now should be reduced to 5 per cent. In the example of the 5 kg infant, with estimated deficit of 500 ml, if the amount already administered in Phase 1 was 40 ml/kg, then 200 ml subtracted from 1000 ml leaves 800 ml to be infused. Fifteen milliequivalents of sodium have been given, leaving 45 to be given. Potassium will be added after urine formation has been assured by clinical observation; 15 mEq will be added in a concentration not to exceed 40 mEq/L. The anions for Na^+ and K^+ combined should be approximately one-quarter base (HCO_3^-, acetate$^-$, or lactate$^-$) and three-quarters chloride. The rate of administration should be adjusted to deliver the remaining estimated volume of deficit, 300 ml (500 − 200 = 300), by the time 8 hours have elapsed from the onset of therapy. Even though body composition remains abnormal, the circulation and renal function will be adequately restored, enabling physiologic mechanisms to operate maximally in the final recovery phase. Because ongoing losses have occurred, the patient's water volume remains somewhat less than the estimated normal.

Note that all of the plan outlined has been based on clinical observations and general principles. Should laboratory values be available during this phase of therapy, suitable adjustments may be made—if, for instance, the Na^+ concentration is in an unexpected range or the acidosis is more severe than supposed. Only occasionally will such adjustments be truly necessary, since the model permits treatment of a fairly wide latitude of disturbances narrowed by decisions derived from clinical data.

In hospitals where only commercial polyionic solutions are available, they may be readily modified to the compositions indicated herein. Small differences, even up to 20 per cent in concentration values, need not be adjusted. The author does not use these solutions because of the inflexibility their exclusive use imposes.

If the example had been a patient suspected to have hypernatremia, the rate of fluid administration would have been slower during repletion, which would then have been planned for a 48-hour period. In that event, the Na^+ concentration of the intravenous infusion would be at the lower level (25 to 40 mEq/L), and K^+ salts would be added at the earliest safe moment. The rate should then deliver the deficit volume plus 2 days' maintenance volume added together in equal hourly increments over 48 hours.

Phase 3—Early Recovery

After 8 hours many patients may take fluids by mouth, and their therapy may be continued with an oral electrolyte-glucose solution containing sodium and potassium salts. Those more severely ill will remain on the same infusion, now slowed in rate to deliver the rest of the calculated volume by the end of 24 hours. Observed abnormal losses will be quantitatively added to the infusion as 120 mEq/L sodium chloride for gastric drainage and 40 mEq/L sodium chloride plus 40 mEq/L of potassium acetate for intestinal loss. Several interim weighings will give valuable information about success of therapy. The example given and the use of solutions described in the preceding text may be summarized as shown in Table 3.

Ideally, the patient should show a 7 to 9 per cent gain in weight at 24 hours. Too little or too much suggests an error in appraisal or technique. Except as previously noted for hypernatremic dehydration, the next 24 hours will, in most instances, be calculated as maintenance plus any continuing abnormal losses; the deficit will usually have been overcome. The same five-point analysis should be repeated, and individual variation should be managed accordingly. In most patients, recovery from the critical phases of the illness will be indicated by ability to take fluid and solute by mouth. On the second day, whether oral feeding contain-

TABLE 3   SUMMARY OF THERAPEUTIC MEASURES USED IN
THE EXAMPLE IN THE TEXT

Phase	Time	Water (ml)	Na⁺ (mEq)	K⁺ (mEq)	Cl⁻ (mEq)	Base (mEq)	Glucose (gm)
1	0–20 min	200	15	0.0	11.0	4.0	2.0
2	20 min–8 hr	300	15	5.6	16.5	4.1	1.5
3	8–24 hr	500	30	9.4	27.5	11.9	2.5
TOTAL	24 hr	1000	60	15.0	55.0	20.0	6.0

ing calories as carbohydrate and protein may be added or whether high caloric parenteral feedings should be used depends upon the state of nutrition, the etiology and duration of the disorder, and a number of other factors. These matters have become increasingly important as the problems of hydration have yielded to understanding and techniques.

References

1. Darrow, D. C.: The significance of body size. Amer. J. Dis. Child., *98*:416, 1959.
2. Finberg, L.: Hypernatremic dehydration. Adv. Pediat., *16*:325, 1969.
3. Darrow, D. C., Pratt, E. L., Flett, J., Jr., Gamble, A. H., and Wiese, H. F.: Disturbances of water and electrolytes in infantile diarrhea. Pediatrics, *3*:129, 1949.
4. Govan, C. D., and Darrow, D. C.: The use of potassium chloride in the treatment of diarrhea in infants. J. Pediat., *28*:541, 1946.

Additional Reading

Darrow, D. C.: A Guide to Learning Fluid Therapy. Springfield, Ill., Charles C Thomas, 1964.
Welt, L. G.: Clinical Disorders of Hydration and Acid-Base Equilibrium, 2nd ed. Boston, Little, Brown, 1959.
Winters, R. W.: Disorders of Electrolyte and Acid-Base Metabolism. *In* Pediatrics, edited by H. Barnett. New York, Appleton-Century-Crofts, 1968.

19

Intravenous Alimentation

Robert M. Filler, M.D., Angelo J. Eraklis, M.D.,
and John B. Das, M.D., Ph.D.

Insufficient caloric intake over a long period contributes appreciably to mortality in infants and children with lesions of the gastrointestinal tract. Not uncommonly, patients with persistent intestinal obstruction, bowel fistulas, short-bowel syndrome, and chronic nonspecific diarrhea die solely from inanition and its complications before curative treatment can be completed.

Four years ago, Dudrick and co-workers[1] first demonstrated that the intravenous infusion of a fat-free amino acid, glucose solution could support normal growth and development. Filler and co-workers[2] reported the successful long-term use of this solution in 14 critically ill infants, and as of May, 1971, 109 infants and children had been so treated at the Children's Hospital Medical Center. This experience and

From the Department of Surgery, Children's Hospital Medical Center, and the Harvard Medical School, Boston, Massachusetts. Supported in part by USPHS Grants No. FR00128 and 5S01Fro5482–07.

reports from other institutions confirm the contention that satisfactory total intravenous nutrition is possible even in the very small infant.

The success of this new method depends on the infusion of glucose for calories and a protein hydrolysate as a source of nitrogen. Special equipment is required to administer this hypertonic solution at a uniform rate into the vena cava. Because of problems not ordinarily seen with routine intravenous therapy, intelligent use of this life-sustaining system requires the careful selection of patients for therapy, constant surveillance for the development of complications, and persistent attention to the minute details of procedures which minimize the dangers.

INDICATIONS

Total intravenous alimentation is reserved for those infants and children whose lives are threatened because feeding by means of the gastrointestinal tract is impossible, inadequate, or hazardous. The goal of treatment depends on the patient's underlying condition. In some instances, such as in those infants with chronic nonspecific diarrhea, placing the gastrointestinal tract at rest for a prolonged period is curative. In others, the restoration and maintenance of adequate nutrition will permit corrective surgery.

The common conditions for which this treatment has been used include chronic intestinal obstruction due to adhesions or peritoneal sepsis, complicated omphalocele and gastroschisis, bowel fistulae, inadequate intestinal length, chronic nonremitting severe diarrhea, extensive body burns, and enteritis arising during tumor therapy (Table 1). Although total intravenous alimentation is used to replete the malnourished child, it may be started prophylactically in clinical situations where prolonged starvation is expected.

As confidence and experience with the method have grown, new indications have developed. For example, with certain modifications we

**TABLE 1.   INDICATIONS FOR LONG-TERM INTRAVENOUS
ALIMENTATION IN 109 CHILDREN**

Diagnosis	Number of Patients
Chronic Intestinal Obstruction	20
Intraperitoneal Sepsis and Bowel Fistulae	6
Omphalocele and Gastroschisis	13
Complicated Esophageal Abnormalities	12
Chronic Diarrhea	17
Enteritis during Tumor Therapy	13
Prematurity (less than 1000 gm.)	3
Miscellaneous	25

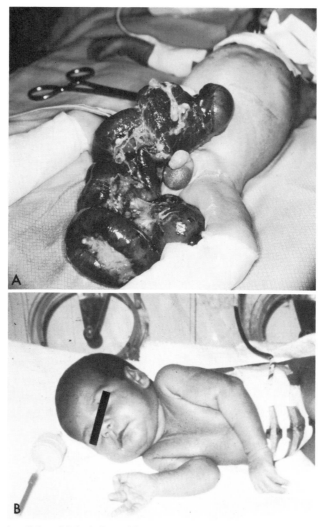

Figure 1.   C.D., a 1.9-kg infant with antenatal rupture of omphalocele, repaired in six stages over 19 days. Total parenteral nutrition was started on the first day of life and was maintained for 23 days. *A*, Infant at admission showing the obstructed densely adherent, edematous dilated intestinal loops. *B*, Infant after completion of abdominal closure on the 23rd day of life. Good wound healing occurred and satisfactory nutrition is apparent.

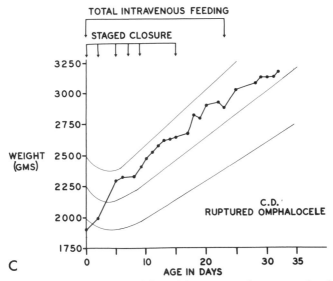

Figure 1 *Continued.* *C,* Infant's daily weights compared to expected weight curve. Sustained weight gain during the period of total intravenous alimentation paralleled expected growth pattern.

have employed this method of total intravenous nutrition in very small premature infants (less than 1 kg) who, despite an apparently normal gastrointestinal tract, constantly regurgitate feedings placed in the stomach either by gavage or by gastrostomy. Dudrick[3] has successfully treated the uremia and hyperkalemia of acute renal failure with intravenous infusions of purified amino acids and glucose, thus completely eliminating the need for dialysis.

The decision to begin a program of total intravenous alimentation requires mature clinical judgment. Such a decision can be made readily in an infant with complicated omphalocele (Fig. 1) or in one in whom a large portion of the midgut has been resected because of volvulus. In others, the decision may be more difficult. For example, in a child with chronic diarrhea and malnutrition, one must be certain that customary therapy has failed before beginning total intravenous therapy (Fig. 2). Although anorexia, vomiting, and diarrhea commonly accompany irradiation and chemotherapy, only the occasional patient becomes so markedly debilitated that treatment is required (Fig. 3).

One must cautiously weigh the need for improved nutrition to save life and reduce morbidity against the possibility of serious complications. Intravenous alimentation should not be employed in those children in whom nutrients can be safely delivered and absorbed from the gastrointestinal tract by careful oral feedings, gavage, or gastrostomy.

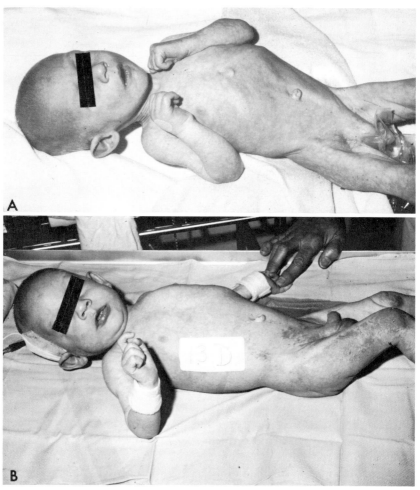

Figure 2. C.S., an 11-week-old child who developed explosive diarrhea with associated projectile vomiting two weeks prior to admission. No specific cause of diarrhea could be found and symptoms did not improve with routine treatment, which included intravenous fluids and drugs to decrease intestinal motility. Attempts to administer even clear fluids by mouth increased the diarrhea. Because of life-threatening unremitting starvation, all oral feedings were withheld and total nutrition was provided by vein for 21 days. Thereafter oral feedings were progressively increased and IV feedings eventually terminated 10 days later. *A*, The appearance of patient just prior to institution of total parenteral alimentation. Weight, 3.6 kg. *B*, After 13 days the patient's nutrition has improved markedly. Weight, 4.20 kg.

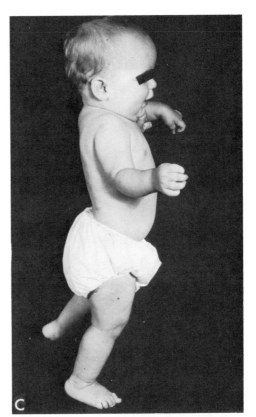

Figure 2 *Continued.* *C*, Patient at 18 months of age, tolerating a normal diet with no evidence of persistent bowel dysfunction.

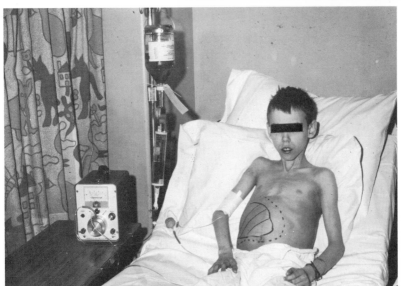

Figure 3. F.H., a 13-year-old boy with very large Wilms' tumor and pulmonary and groin metastases. Because of the massive tumor and the boy's poor general condition, x-ray therapy and chemotherapy were administered prior to surgical excision. Concurrent vomiting and diarrhea caused further deterioration in this boy's general condition. Oral feedings were withheld and nutrition was improved by parenteral alimentation during preoperative anti-tumor therapy. Surgery three weeks later was well tolerated.

TABLE 2.   CONTENT OF INFUSATE USED IN INTRAVENOUS ALIMENTATION

Constituent	Content (per Liter)	
Protein Hydrolysate	30	gm
Glucose	200	gm
Sodium*	15	mEq
Potassium*	16	mEq
Chloride*	11.7	mEq
Calcium	27	mEq
Magnesium	7.6	mEq
Phosphorus	19	mEq
Multivitamin Infusion†	5	ml
Vitamin B_{12}	6.6	mcg
Phytonadione (AquaMephyton)	0.2	mg
Folic Acid	0.5	mg

*Further adjusted at bedside.
†U.S. Vitamin & Pharmaceutical Corp., N.Y., N.Y.

METHODS

The fat-free infusate which is prepared in the hospital pharmacy by mixing 50 per cent glucose and 5 per cent protein hydrolysate (Aminosol* or Hyprotigen†) contains 20 per cent glucose, 3.0 per cent protein (as amino acids and polypeptides), and 0.80 calorie per millimeter. Vitamins and minerals are added as noted in Table 2. Details of preparation have been previously described.[2] The sodium, potassium, and chloride concentrations in the infusate are further adjusted to the needs of the individual patient at the bedside. In general, sodium chloride and potassium chloride are added to raise the concentration of sodium to 40 mEq/L, of potassium to 40 mEq/L, and of chloride to 60 mEq/L. These quantities supply maintenance electrolytes without overloading the normal infant kidney or cardiovascular system. An infusion of 135 ml/kg/day provides 110 calories per kilogram of body weight per day, the amount necessary to meet the normal infant's need for tissue repair and growth. In the older child whose basic caloric requirements are somewhat less, 135 ml/kg/day may be administered safely.

Other amino acid solutions are also commercially available and we have employed a solution containing 4.2 per cent purified amino acids (FreAmine†) and 25 per cent glucose in 15 children. With the more concentrated solutions lesser volumes are needed to supply the same number of calories. In addition, the electrolyte content of the stock solu-

*Abbott Laboratories, 14 Sheridan Boulevard, North Chicago, Illinois 60064.
†McGaw Laboratories, 1015 Grandview Ave., Glendale, California 91201.

tion is different for each amino acid preparation, a factor which must be considered before final electrolyte adjustment at the bedside.

Plasma (10 cc/kg) is given twice weekly to provide trace elements and essential fatty acids which are not present in the mixture. In general, plasma infusions are not necessary during the first 2 weeks of therapy. Iron requirements are met either by weekly intramuscular injections of iron dextran or by blood transfusions. Daily requirements of all vitamins are supplied in the mixture.

This hypertonic infusate must be delivered through a central venous catheter to avoid peripheral venous inflammation and thrombosis. For this purpose, a silicone rubber catheter is passed through the internal or external jugular vein to the superior vena cava. This procedure is best carried out in an operating room or cardiac catheterization laboratory, where adequate exposure, proper instruments, and strict aseptic conditions are available. To minimize blood stream contamination, the venous catheter is tunneled from the vein entry point to a skin exit site which is placed 2 to 4 inches away. In the infant it is brought out on the scalp, whereas in the older child the exit site may be the neck or upper extremity. Central venous intubation by percutaneous subclavian vein puncture has also been used.[4] The silicone rubber venous line may be left in place until the completion of therapy unless it becomes accidentally dislodged or septic complications develop. We have had a single catheter in place for as long as 90 days.

The proper position of the catheter in the vena cava must be confirmed. This is easily accomplished radiographically by the use of a radiopaque catheter or one filled with contrast material.

An antibacterial ointment and sterile dressing are applied to the skin exit site and, to avoid accidental displacement, a coil of catheter is included in the dressing. Every 3 days the dressing is removed aseptically, the skin cleansed with an antiseptic, and a sterile dressing and antibacterial ointment reapplied. Povidone iodine (Betadine) ointment is now used routinely for its effectiveness against both bacteria and fungi. Before the infusion is started, a Millipore Filter* (0.22μ) is placed in line to remove particulate matter or microorganisms which may have contaminated the solution. A calibrated burette is placed in the circuit to monitor accurately the volume delivered. An injection tubing† may also be added to the circuit so that antibiotics or other intravenous drugs can be administered aseptically beyond the filter.

The infusate must be delivered at a slow uniform rate to insure proper utilization of the glucose and amino acids. In the small infant, this is most readily accomplished by the use of a constant infusion pump,‡ which functions by compressing a section of disposable tubing.

---

*Millipore Corporation, Bedford, Massachusetts.
†"T" Connector manufactured by Abbott Laboratories.
‡Sigmator Pump, TM 20–2 and appropriate tubing. Manufactured by Sigmamotor Incorporated, 3 North Main Street, Middleport, New York.

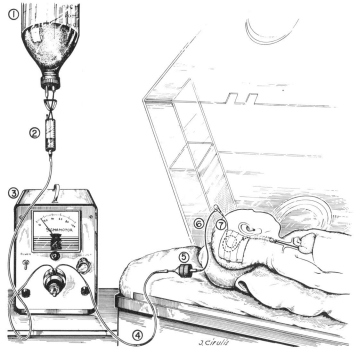

Figure 4. System for long-term intravenous alimentation ("Lifeline"). (1) Amino acid-glucose infusate. (2) Calibrated burette. (3) Constant infusion pump. (4) Disposable tubing with a compressible section which adapts to pump head. (5) Millipore filter. (6) "T" connector. (7) Silicone rubber intravenous catheter.

The particular pump we employ avoids frequent uncoupling of the tubing. In some centers, infusion to the older patients has been accomplished by gravity drip. The entire system, locally referred to as the "Lifeline," is shown in Figure 4.

Outline of Technique for Use of Central Venous Lifeline

A. Purpose
   To provide adequate protein and calorie intake to sustain life and growth in the absence of adequate gastrointestinal tract function.
B. General Information
   1. Insertion of Lifeline
      The Central Venous Lifeline is a silastic catheter inserted through one of the jugular veins in the neck and threaded down to the superior vena cava to the level of the right atrium. The catheter is secured subcutaneously with a silastic wing at the level of the neck incision.

The end of the catheter is then tunneled subcutaneously from the venous entry site to exit at the temporal area of the scalp, where it is secured exteriorly.

In older patients any arm vein may be used.

The procedure is performed in the operating room.

2. Major Considerations

   a. Lifeline solution is usually ordered at a rate of 135 to 150 cc/kg/day (approx. 104 to 115 calories/kg/day). Given at the constant ordered rate the solution allows the metabolic system to function at full capacity at all times. The flow rate cannot be increased to compensate for interruption or slowing of the infusion without risk of glycosuria with osmotic diuresis, which, if untreated, can lead to dehydration, seizures, and coma. Variations in flow may not exceed 10 per cent of the ordered rate per hour. If variations do occur notify nurse in charge.

   b. As solutions administered are rich in life supporting nutrients, they are excellent culture media for yeast and bacteria. Sepsis is the most serious and common complication of hyperalimentation therapy and in most cases is probably preventable. Two nurses or a nurse and physician must participate in any procedure involving entering Lifeline tubing or dressing. (Aseptic procedure is fully described below.)

   c. Young patients must be properly restrained at all times to avoid the possibility of contamination or withdrawal of the Lifeline. Older patients must be well instructed not to manipulate the Lifeline or equipment.

   d. Many studies are required on these patients. Accuracy and attention to detail are of utmost importance.

3. Routine patient procedures

   a. Accurate daily weight is recorded on a graphic sheet with the day of catheter insertion in red.

      The weight curve will serve as a guide to the physician as to the patient's progress.

   b. Daily 24° intake and output is totaled each morning at 7:00 a.m.

      Responsibility of the night nurse.

   c. Urine sugar content is determined on each voided specimen (Clinitest) for the first 4 days. Thereafter test one specimen per shift unless otherwise ordered.

      Sugar is usually spilled. 0 to 3 plus can be expected. Consistent 4 plus tests are to be reported to the physician.

      If a Foley catheter is in place, check with the physician as to the frequency of testing.

      Continuous use of pedi bags, metabolic beds for collection of urine may be discontinued after 4 days.

I. To change or set up Lifeline Solution and Administration Tubing

A. *Equipment Needed*   *Points of Emphasis*

1. Bottle of Lifeline solution as ordered.

2. Additives as ordered by physician.

3. I.V. administration set and burette.

4. Appropriate size Sigmamotor administration set.

   Not necessary if IVAC pump is used.

5. Millipore filter.

6. 2½ cc syringe filled with sterile saline.

7. 20″ or 30″ extension tubing if necessary for added length.

   At times Lifeline tubing is short, leaving no room between patient and pump.

8. Betadine ointment and solution.

9. 2×2 sterile gauze sponges.

10. Paper tape.

11. Alcohol sponges (prepackaged).

12. "T" connection if ordered.

13. Infusion pump.

14. Restraints.

B. *Special Considerations*

1. Bottle, all tubing, and filter are to be changed daily.

   See #2 of General Information.

   If transfusion is to be administered on any given day, defer procedure until after transfusion is finished to avoid changing setup twice.

2. Equipment should be entirely set up and ready to function before disconnecting system already running.

   No prolonged disconnection of system is indicated.

3. When actual changing of solutions is carried out, two people should participate.

   See #2 of General Information.

C. *Procedure*

1. Prepare Lifeline solution according to orders in Doctor's Order Book and label bottle appropriately.

   Although many nutrients, electrolytes, and vitamins are provided in the standard solutions, individual modifications are necessary, according to patient needs.

   Be careful not to contaminate fluid in bottle when making additions.

2. Insert I.V. administration set into bottle.
3. Connect Sigmamotor administration set.
4. Fill burette with 20 to 30 cc of Lifeline solution and allow to run through burette and Sigmamotor tubing.
5. If "T" connector is ordered, attach at this point.

If a "T" connector is ordered it must go above the filter.

6. Prepare Millipore filter.
   a. Remove cover from package.

The Millipore filter has an air space which must be filled—filling by gravity often takes 10 to 15 minutes.

   b. Attach 2½ cc syringe with saline to female adaptor.
   c. Hold filter with male end toward ceiling and fill filter until saline comes through male adaptor.
   d. Carefully remove cover from male end of filter.
7. Connect Millipore filter to Sigmamotor tubing.
8. Connect extension tubing.
9. Allow Lifeline solution to fill extension tubing.
10. Clamp tubing when all air is expelled.

Replace sterile cap on male end of extension tubing until ready to connect to Lifeline adaptor.

11. Disengage tubing to be disconnected from pump.
12. Disconnect tubing to be discarded from Lifeline adaptor.

Two nurses are needed to avoid contamination.

13. Clean end of administration tubing and Lifeline adaptor with Betadine solution and 2×2 sponge.

If crusts of blood or Lifeline solution are present around the Lifeline adaptor, remove carefully with Betadine solution.

If clotted blood is present inside the adaptor or tubing, follow procedure for flushing a Lifeline.

14. Connect new administration set to Lifeline adaptor.

Allow no air to enter system.

15. Attach appropriate infusion pump.

See Section II.

16. Unclamp tubing, turn on pump, and adjust rate if necessary.
17. Wipe burette and all tubing with alcohol sponge

Solution on tubing may be a site of bacteria or yeast growth.

to remove all trace of Life-line solution that may have dripped when setting up administration set.

	In cleansing burette be aware that numbers and lines on scale will be eradicated by vigorous rubbing.
18. Wipe all tubing with Betadine solution.	Only a small amount need be applied, as a large amount will leave a sticky residue.
19. Apply Betadine ointment and sterile 2×2 dressing to all junctions of tubing and filter below burette. Secure with paper tape.	Connections at the Millipore filter and below are particularly important.

II. Infusion Pump
  A. *General Information*

1. Only Sigmamotor and IVAC pumps should be used.	The infusion pump controls the rate of flow of the solution, delivering the solution at a constant uniform rate.
2. One type of Sigmamotor pump is labeled according to the (approximate) minimum and maximum output the machine can deliver per hour.	The choice of the size of the pump is determined by the rate of flow of solution ordered.
a. 0.5 cc–45 cc/hr.	Use administration set #8209 with a or b.
b. 1.5 cc–120 cc/hr.	
c. 10 cc–900 cc/hr.	Use administration set #8409 with c.
3. Another type of Sigmamotor pump has a scale which equals cc/hr.	No computation is necessary.
4. The IVAC pump may be set at the desired rate.	

  B. *Procedure: Setting Up Sigmamotor Infusion Pump*

1. Place infusion pump on bedside table. Plug into electrical outlet.	Some Sigmamotor pumps run on battery as well.
2. Unscrew infusion pump head.	
3. Fit silicone rubber part of Sigmamotor administration set around pump head and secure.	Silicone rubber part of tubing is near the center of the set. Be sure the tubing encircles the pump head in the proper direction.

"In" refers to: from the bottle to the pump. "Out" refers to: from the pump to the patient.

Be certain that this is secure.

Flow rates will not be accurate if the tubing is not properly "milked" by the machine.

4. Screw the infusion pump head into place firmly.
5. Unclamp tubing.
6. Turn motor switch on.
7. If machine is not set for ordered rate, then adjust.
8. Once set at desired rate, turn the locking device.

Check accuracy of flow rate by comparison with the hourly delivery of fluid as measured from the burette. This locks the adjusting knob to prevent accidental turning.

III. Care of Lifeline Equipment
1. Check every ½ hr. to be sure the system is patent and operating.

Is there fluid in the burette?
Is the diaphragm in the burette closing the outlet?
Is one of the several clamps closed?
Is the infusion pump plugged in and turned on?
Is the tubing threaded in the pump in the proper way?
Is the pump head on firmly?
Is the tubing tense and rigid between the patient and the pump? (If so, the filter or catheter may be plugged).
Is the tubing twisted, kinked, or bent?
Is there pressure on the tubing? (bedside, patient, equipment).
Is the central joint of the filter tight?
Are the connections tight at all points?

2. Observe for signs of infiltration.

Particular notice should be paid to the site where the catheter enters the vein.
Note: Infiltration may cause airway obstruction in infants by compressing the trachea.

3. Each shift, and as needed, clean bottle, burette, and all tubing with alcohol, then wipe with Betadine solution.
4. Be sure Betadine dressings are intact.

This will deter growth of bacteria or yeast on Lifeline solution.

IV. Administration of Medications
1. All medications are given above the Millipore filter.

Medications will pass through the filter without plugging the line.

2. Follow nursing procedure for "Administration of Intravenous Medications."
3. Any medication allowed to be administered via the "side arm" of the I.V. tubing may be given through a "T" connector inserted above the Millipore filter.

V. Administration of Whole Blood and Plasma

1. Transfusions are ordered routinely and are given directly into the Lifeline.	Blood products will plug the Millipore filter.
2. Following transfusion clear all blood from silicone rubber line and adaptor.	Flush line with normal saline (see Section VI). Blood along the wall of the tubing in the adaptor will promote the growth of bacteria and yeast.
3. Resume Lifeline infusion.	Change filter, all tubing, and bottle of Lifeline solution according to procedure outlined (Section I).

VI. Procedure for Flushing Lifeline

  A. *Equipment*
    Sterile sponges
    Betadine solution
    2½ cc syringe filled with normal saline

  B. *Procedure*

1. Remove Betadine dressing from junction of administration setup and adaptor in silicone rubber catheter.	Be sure the child is adequately restrained. Two nurses or a nurse and physician must participate.
2. Turn off infusion pump.	
3. Separate administration setup from adaptor.	Maintain sterility.
4. Cleanse adaptor with Betadine solution.	
5. Insert syringe hub in adaptor and gently attempt to flush the sicicone rubber catheter.	Do not try to forcefully dislodge a clot. If Lifeline does not flush readily, notify physician. Be sure there are no crusts of solution or blood around the adaptor. (See Section V.)
6. Cleanse male end of administration setup with Betadine solution and connect to Lifeline adaptor.	
7. Turn on infusion pump.	
8. Apply sterile Betadine dressing to junction of administration setup and Lifeline adaptor.	

VII. Changing Dressing

                           To be done every third day by a surgeon. A nurse is required for assistance in this procedure.

Equipment
Razor and green soap
Betadine solution and ointment
Sterile 3×3 gauze
Dressing set
Ace adherent
Paper tape

VIII. Miscellaneous

1. Blood may be drawn through the Central Venous Line only by a physician.

   A nurse is to assist in this procedure. No trace of blood should remain in the tubing or on Lifeline adaptor.

2. The Lifeline may be used to obtain central venous pressure only by written doctor's order.

   Check with physician daily to verify continuance of order. A Lifeline open to the air runs a great risk of infection.

3. Three way stopcocks are not to be used.

   Removing traces of blood is virtually impossible.

4. When transporting the patient off the floor, the pump may be left on the division if the solution will run by gravity at the rate ordered.

IX. To Assist Doctor with a Lifeline Removal

Equipment
Cutdown tray
Betadine solution
Betadine ointment
Culture tube

A doctor must do a cutdown procedure to remove the Lifeline.
The tip of the catheter is usually cultured when removed.

METABOLIC OBSERVATIONS AND RESPONSES

Early in our experience, patients receiving all nutrients by vein were admitted to the Metabolic Unit of the Clinical Research Center at the Children's Hospital Medical Center so that careful extensive observations could be obtained. As a result of this experience, a simplified protocol of care has evolved so that patients can now be adequately cared for on general medical and surgical divisions.

Clinical measurements which have been found essential to evaluate the child's metabolic response include daily body weight, accurate volume of urine, and other body fluid losses. The important laboratory tests include qualitative urinary sugar analysis, blood sugar concentrations, and serum electrolyte content and osmolarity. The urine sugar content is monitored at each voiding. In the stable patient the other tests are obtained every 3 days for the first 2 weeks, and thereafter only as indicated. These determinations will indicate the child's nutritional progress and readily detect the occurrence of an osmotic diuresis or abnormal retention.

Weight change during the period of intravenous feeding will vary with the patient's overall clinical status. Weight gains comparable to those of normal infants may be expected in those children who are not malnourished at the time intravenous feedings are instituted or in whom sepsis is not a part of the clinical picture.[2] In the patient with other complications, such as infection or another clinical problem which increases metabolic requirements, a flatter growth curve may be observed. A significant weight gain in the first 2 weeks of therapy is not usually seen in those infants and children who are severely depleted at the start of treatment.

Despite the variations in weight curves, positive nitrogen balance has been noted in all patients studied in detail.[5, 6] On an intravenous diet providing 0.74 gm nitrogen/kg/day (equivalent to 4.4 gm protein/kg/day), persistent positive balance of nitrogen of 100 to 300 mg/kg/day has been observed. Fecal loss of nitrogen is usually negligible since stools are infrequent and scanty during periods of intravenous feeding. Urinary amino acid losses have been found to be negligible and not sufficient to produce an osmotic diuresis except in infants under 1 kg and in those children with severe renal disease.

In most patients the large quantity of intravenous glucose (27 gm/kg/day) is well tolerated without the addition of exogenous insulin. Blood sugar levels remain in the normal range, but urinary sugar content usually varies between 0 and 3+ by the Clinitest method. Quantitative glucose excretion studies have shown that this represents less than 1 per cent of the total glucose infused. Urinary sugar levels are generally highest during the first day or two of treatment. In the day-to-day management of these children, qualitative urine sugars consistently above 3+ signal the likelihood of an osmotic diuresis or early sepsis. A temporary decrease in hourly infusion rate or use of a more dilute solution usually corrects the problem if not due to septicemia.

Water balance is maintained even in infants under 2.5 kg in weight and in those following surgery, despite the infusion of this hypertonic solution (2600 mosm/L) at the rate of 135 ml/kg/day. Urinary solute excretion on this intravenous diet is usually greater than that observed during oral feeding, but this increased load does not exceed the concentrating capability of the normal infant kidney.[6]

COMPLICATIONS

The most serious complication of this method is sepsis. Long-term indwelling venous cannulae have been a well-documented source of blood stream infection.[7, 8]

Organisms may enter the blood stream along the catheter tract or with a contaminated intravenous solution. The catheter, a foreign body in the blood stream, may act as a focus for bacterial growth even if organisms enter from a distant septic site. Measures aimed at minimizing the risk of sepsis include: (1) aseptic preparation of the solution; (2) placement of the catheter under ideal conditions; (3) meticulous care of the catheter entry site with frequent dressing changes, skin disinfection, and the application of a bactericidal and fungicidal ointment; (4) the use of a Millipore Filter; and (5) prohibiting the use of the venous line for blood sampling except for blood culture when sepsis is suspected. We have not employed antibiotics in these cases unless warranted by the child's primary illness.

In spite of these precautions in our 109 patients, 16 instances of septicemia occurred between the 14th and 90th day of treatment. Fever was the one early clinical finding common to all. *Candida albicans* grew from the blood in eight patients, *S. aureus* in three, *S. fecalis* in three, *E. coli* in one, and diphtheroids in one. Infants with proved blood stream infection were treated by removal of the central venous line. In addition appropriate antibiotics were given to those with bacterial sepsis. In these 16 children with septicemia, only one death could be attributed directly to catheter sepsis. However, sepsis contributed to death in two others because nutrition could not be maintained after the catheter was withdrawn. Recovery from septicemia was generally rapid, indicating that early detection and treatment of this complication can avoid serious sequelae.

Although most patients tolerate this infusate, an occasional patient will develop hyperglycemia, glycosuria, and an osmotic diuresis in the absence of sepsis. In our series, this inappropriate response was seen in one child with several renal diseases, another with a suspected hypothalamic lesion, and in three very small premature infants. In the premature infant, the osmotic diuresis was controlled by temporarily decreasing the content of glucose and amino acids in the mixture. In the others, treatment was discontinued.

The presence of a catheter in the superior vena cava for prolonged periods adds the hazard of venous thrombosis and pulmonary embolus. In our series, thrombosis of the superior vena cava contributed to the death of one infant, who also had overwhelming Candida septicemia. The use of nonreactive silicone rubber tubes minimizes this danger.

Accidental withdrawal of the venous line has been a common problem. This complication is ordinarily recognized by the occurrence of swelling near the venotomy site. It may be confirmed by x-ray visualization of the catheter tip. If the tip is not in the superior vena cava, the catheter should be completely removed and a new line inserted at another site. This event is more frequent when using a soft silicone rubber catheter, which is difficult to secure. Perforation of the vena cava has been reported with central catheters, but we have not encountered this problem.

CONCLUSION

In the past, starvation has been the mode of death for many seriously ill children. By utilizing this new method of intravenous alimentation, these fatilities may often be prevented. In this series of 109 infants and children, 86 are alive. Four infants died of malnutrition, two because they were unable to tolerate the infusate, and two because sepsis required withdrawal of the intravenous catheter. Only one infant died because of a complication of the method. Other causes of death included extreme prematurity, pulmonary complications of cystic fibrosis, acute surgical complications, tumor metastases, extensive burns, and immune deficiency disease. Despite its effectiveness, this life-saving method of feeding should be reserved for those patients in whom satisfactory nutrition is not otherwise possible.

References

1. Dudrick, S. J., Wilmore, D. W., Vars, H. M., and Rhoads, J. E.: Long-term total parenteral nutrition with growth, development, and positive nitrogen balance. Surgery, *64*:134–142, 1968.
2. Filler, R. M., Eraklis, A. J., Rubin, V. G., and Das, J. B.: Long-term parenteral nutrition in infants. New Eng. J. Med., *281*:589–594, 1969.
3. Dudrick, S. J., and Steiger, J. M.: Renal failure in surgical patients. Treatment with intravenous essential amino acids and hypertonic glucose. Surgery, *68*:180–186, 1970.
4. Dudrick, S. J., Wilmore, D. W., Vars, H. M., and Rhoads, J. E.: Can intravenous feedings as the sole means of nutrition support growth in the child and restore weight loss in an adult? An affirmative answer. Ann. Surg., *169*:974–984, 1969.
5. Filler, R. M., Das, J. B., Rubin, V. G., Coran, A. G., and Eraklis, A. J.: Total intravenous nutrition in infants with a dextrose fibrin hydrolysate mixture. Proceedings of the Symposium on Fluid Replacement in the Surgical Patient. May 26–27, 1969, Columbia University College of Physicians and Surgeons 1970, pp. 353–364.
6. Das, J. B., Filler, R. M., Rubin, V. G., and Eraklis, A. J.: Intravenous dextrose amino acid feeding. The metabolic response in the surgical neonate. J. Ped. Surg., *5*: 127–135, 1970.
7. Smits, H., and Freedman, L. R.: Prolonged venous catheterization as a cause of sepsis. New Eng. J. Med., *276*:1229–1233, 1967.
8. Moran, J. M., Atwood, R. P., and Rowe, M. I.: A clinical and bacteriologic study of infections associated with venous cutdowns. New Eng. J. Med., *272*:554–560, 1965.

20

The Problem of Disseminated Intravascular Coagulation

William E. Hathaway, M.D.

Disseminated intravascular coagulation (DIC) is a disease process characterized by intravascular consumption of plasma clotting factors and platelets. In many clinical instances, this process results in widespread deposition of fibrin thrombi within the peripheral vascular system and a generalized hemorrhagic diathesis. As outlined in Figure 1, several events can initiate or trigger the process of DIC. Activation of the coagulation mechanism through Hageman Factor (XII) or by tissue thromboplastin leads to the formation of fibrin. During coagulation certain factors are consumed. These factors, depleted or lowered during active DIC, are antihemophilic factor (VIII), proaccelerin (V), platelets, prothrombin (II), and fibrinogen. As fibrin is deposited in the small vessels and capillaries, the fibrinolytic system is activated, and the newly formed fibrinolysin splits the fibrin into fragments. Limited action of thrombin may produce fibrin monomer which can complex with native fibrinogen or fibrin split products. These fibrin split products (FSP) and fibrin complexes are cleared from the circulation by action of the reticuloendothelial system (RES). While circulating, the FSP have several functions. They act as an anticoagulant on the initial as well as latter

From the Department of Pediatrics, University of Colorado Medical Center, Denver, Colorado. Supported in part by USPHS Grant No. HD 01965-04.

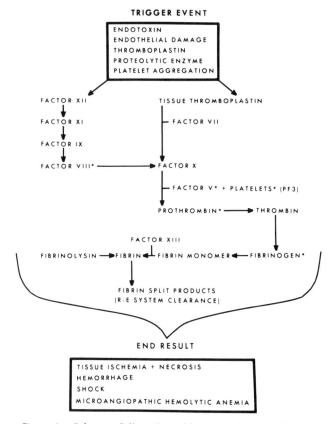

Figure 1.   Scheme of disseminated intravascular coagulation.

stages of coagulation; they decrease platelet function; and they may exhibit vasoactive properties.

The end results of this process include: (1) thrombi and emboli which produce *tissue ischemia and necrosis* in various organs (principally lungs, kidneys, gastrointestinal tract, adrenal glands, brain, liver, pancreas, and skin); (2) depletion of clotting factors plus the antihemostatic effect of FSP which lead to widespread *hemorrhage;* (3) a *microangiopathic hemolytic anemia* due to red cell fragmentation by strands of fibrin in the peripheral vasculature; and (4) finally *shock* and death. At the onset, it should be emphasized that DIC can occur with varying degrees of severity. This fact plus the variability of physiologic compensation mechanisms (fibrinolysis, clotting factor synthesis) leads to different clinical expressions of the disorder which may not always include diffuse thrombi or hemorrhagic diathesis. The emphasis in this discussion is on the problem of recognition and treatment of DIC in the ill child. Several recent articles are available for review and detailed discussion of the problem.[1-4]

In particular, the subject of chronic intravascular coagulation[5] is not discussed here.

Table 1 lists many diseases seen in children in whom DIC has been documented or suspected as an etiologic or complicating mechanism.

RECOGNITION OF DISSEMINATED INTRAVASCULAR COAGULATION

Clinical Aspects

The preceding paragraphs suggest that any severely ill child may develop the complication of disseminated intravascular coagulation.

TABLE 1   DISEASES IN WHICH DISSEMINATED INTRAVASCULAR COAGULATION HAS BEEN DOCUMENTED OR SUSPECTED

Infection:	
Bacterial sepsis:	Meningococcus, *E. coli, A. aerogenes*, Clostridia, *Pasteurella pestis, Pseudomonas aeruginosa*, B-hemolytic streptococcus, *H. influenzae*, staphylococcus
Viral infections:[6]	Varicella, vaccinia, variola, rubella, rubeola, arboviruses, herpes,[7] cytomegalic virus
Other:	Malaria, rickettsia (Rocky Mountain spotted fever)
Surgical Conditions:	Burns (thermal, electrical)
	Trauma
	Hemorrhagic shock
	Renal transplants[8]
	Liver transplants[9]
	Fat embolism
Neonatal Conditions:	Idiopathic respiratory distress syndrome[10, 11]
	Infant born to mother with toxemia, abruptio placentae, or diabetes mellitus
	Twin with dead fetus[12]
Malignancies:	Disseminated cancer: neuroblastoma, rhabdomyosarcoma
	Leukemia: acute myelocytic, acute lymphatic or stem cell
Metabolic Disorders:	Cirrhosis[13]
	Hyperthermia: heat stroke,[14] anesthesia[15]
Miscellaneous Conditions:	Snake bite
	Purpura fulminans
	Giant hemangioma
	Hemolytic transfusion reactions
	Drug ingestion and reactions[4]
	Thrombotic thrombocytopenic purpura
	Cyanotic congenital heart disease
	Acute anaphylactic reaction[16]
	Hemolytic-uremic syndrome[17, 18]

Indeed, the multiple and frequently nonspecific features may well explain why the condition may be diagnosed either too often or not often enough. Suspicious clinical signs are: (1) evidence of multiple organ involvement by thrombi and emboli, i.e., respiratory distress; hematuria and progressive renal shutdown; deterioration of consciousness, coma, and convulsions; gastrointestinal distention, ileus, vomiting, and diarrhea; and thrombotic lesions of the skin; (2) a bleeding tendency which initially may be only skin purpura or oozing from puncture sites, but which may progress to widespread hemorrhage; (3) pallor or slight jaundice due to an acute hemolytic anemia; (4) shock. Corrigan[19] and McKay[2] have emphasized the association of hypotension leading to peripheral vascular collapse in patients with DIC. Obviously, accurate diagnosis requires not only clinical suspicion but laboratory confirmation.

The multiple system involvement in DIC is illustrated by the following case report.

Case Report

R. D., a 6-year-old Caucasian male, was admitted to the University of Colorado Medical Center on May 28, 1967, with the complaints of fever, rash, and cough. He had been in good health until 8 days prior to admission when he became febrile (103 to 104°F.). Two days later he developed cough, conjunctivitis, and photophobia followed one day later by a diffuse morbilliform rash which spread from neck and face to entire body. A diagnosis of rubeola was made in the Outpatient Department one day prior to admission for increasing fever, cough, and respiratory distress. Past history revealed no significant illnesses; all immunizations had been given except measles vaccine.

Physical examination showed a well-nourished acutely ill child with a generalized fading morbilliform rash typical of rubeola. He was moderately dehydrated, extremely lethargic, and dyspneic. Blood pressure was 80/60, temperature 104°F., pulse 160/minute and respirations 40 to 50/minute. Initial laboratory studies showed hematocrit 30 per cent, hemoglobin 10.4 gm per 100 ml, WBC 26,500 with 73 segmented PMN, 8 bands, 16 lymphs, and 3 monocytes; platelets were 267,000/cu mm. Red cell morphology was described as 3+ anisocytosis and poikilocytosis. Coomb's test was negative. Lumbar puncture was negative except for 120 RBC's/cu mm. Urinalysis showed occasional cast and 1+ protein. Serum sodium was low; BUN was 44 mg per 100 ml. Blood, CSF, and throat cultures were negative for bacterial pathogens. Chest film showed bilateral pulmonary infiltrates. The initial impression was rubeola with pneumonitis and possible encephalitis; the patient was treated with parenteral fluids, antibiotics, and oxygen by tent.

Over the next 48 hours the patient became increasingly ill and was examined for complications by several consultants who reported as follows: Neurology—"alternating levels of responsiveness, hemorrhages in fundi, sustained clonus bilaterally"; Chest Service—"massive right-sided pneumonia probably secondary to interstitial pneumonia"; Cardiology—"severe congestive heart failure, myocarditis"; Hematology—"blood smear shows burred red cells, anemia, consider Shwartzman-like reaction."

Patient developed diffuse purpuric lesions over his fading rubeola rash and urine output diminished. Coagulation studies revealed platelets 132,500; bleeding time >12 minutes, kaolin partial thromboplastin time 47 seconds (C-45);

normal euglobulin fibrinolysin test, prothrombin time 17 seconds (C-12 sec.), Factor VIII 22.5 per cent, and FSP positive. Because of a low Factor VIII, slightly low platelets, and prolonged prothrombin time (low Factor V), a consumption coagulopathy was suspected.

Heparinization was instituted on the third hospital day, but the patient became anemic, hypotensive, and comatose and expired 12 hours later.

Postmortem examination revealed microthrombi in glomerular tufts and in renal arterioles, pulmonary arterioles, myocardial and pericardial small vessels, and in brain capillaries. Bilateral renal cortical necrosis and focal hepatic and brain necroses were also seen. Pulmonary interstitial pneumonitis and hyaline membranes were prominent. These findings were interpreted as being diagnostic of diffuse intravascular coagulation.

Comment. Multiple system (brain, heart, kidney, lung, red cells) involvement in a seriously ill child should have suggested DIC before the appearance of purpuric skin lesions led to the suspected diagnosis.

Laboratory Tests

The laboratory signs of DIC usually produce evidence of the following: (1) consumption of factors utilized when blood clots (fibrinogen, V, VIII, II, and platelets); (2) secondary fibrinolysis leading to fibrin split products; and (3) microangiopathic hemolytic anemia.[2] Table 2 outlines the coagulation tests which can be abnormal in DIC. Ideally, the specific factor assays should be performed; occasionally they are necessary to confirm the diagnosis in a complicated case. In our experience, Factor V levels are especially sensitive indicators of a consumption coagulopathy. Because of wide physiological fluctuations, Factor VIII levels do not appear to be as much help in the diagnosis of DIC. Also, a commonly used method for Factor VIII assay (PTT method) may give spuriously high values in cases of intravascular coagulation.[21] The determination of the degradation products of fibrin (FSP) is helpful to indicate that excessive

TABLE 2   COAGULATION TESTS WHICH MAY BE ABNORMAL IN INTRAVASCULAR COAGULATION

Test	Pathophysiologic Abnormality Detected
Bleeding time (tourniquet test)	Thrombocytopenia and platelet hypofunction due to fibrin split products (FSP)
Platelet count	Platelet consumption
Partial thromboplastin time	Factor VIII, V, II, fibrinogen consumption; anticoagulant effect of FSP
Prothrombin time	II, V, fibrinogen consumption
Thrombin time	Fibrinogen consumption; presence of FSP
Fibrinogen, II, V, VIII assays	Factor consumption
Euglobulin lysis time	Presence of fibrinolysins
Immunoassay for FSP (Cryofibrinogen test, ethanol precipitation test, protamine precipitation test)	Presence of degradation products of fibrin and complexes of fibrin monomer with fibrinogen or FSP

fibrin deposition and lysis have occurred intravascularly. The most rapid and sensitive tests for FSP are those based on hemagglutination inhibition of fibrinogen-coated, tanned red cells.[22, 23] Other immunologic methods for FSP measurement are too cumbersome or slow to be of significant clinical benefit. Rapid and simple tests for FSP or complexes of fibrin monomers and fibrinogen have recently been described as helpful in diagnosis of DIC; these tests (cryofibrin,[24] protamine precipitation,[25] and ethanol gelation[26]) will need further clinical investigation before their usefulness is proved.

Fragmented, burred, microspherocytic, and helmet-shaped erythrocytes are frequently seen in the peripheral blood in DIC.[20] These cells are the basis for the hemolytic anemia (microangiopathic anemia) noted above. Therefore, careful examination of a freshly made blood smear should be done in all suspected cases of DIC.

The laboratory diagnosis of disseminated intravascular coagulation during the neonatal period may be difficult. The physiologic alterations of the coagulation system in the newborn cause a few seconds' prolongation of the clotting tests that are most helpful in the older child, i.e., the prothrombin time, partial thromboplastin time, and thrombin time (see Table 3). Unless the screening tests are markedly abnormal, therefore, it may be necessary to do specific factor assays for fibrinogen, V, and VIII. If care is taken in collection of newborn infant blood (into tubes containing fibrinolytic inhibitors) increased amounts of FSP should be considered of pathologic significance and reflecting increased fibrinolysis.[27, 28]

When the process of DIC is interrupted (by heparin therapy), a rebound increase of the consumable factors is occasionally seen. When hepatic function is normal, this rebound can be helpful in confirmation of the diagnosis.

With so many possible laboratory approaches, the author would ad-

TABLE 3   COAGULATION TESTS IN THE NEWBORN*

Test	Normal Adult	Normal Newborns (Full Term and Premature)
1. Kaolin partial thromboplastin time	38–50 sec.	41–80 sec.
2. Prothrombin time	12–14 sec.	12–18 sec.
3. Thrombin time	7– 9 sec.	8–18 sec.
4. Platelet count	200,000–450,000/cu mm	200,000–400,000/cu mm
5. Factor assays:		
I (Fibrinogen)	190–420 mg/100 ml	157–369 mg/100 ml
II (Prothrombin)	70–120%	24– 66%
V (Proaccelerin)	70–150%	60–140%
VIII (Antihemophilic factor)	60–150%	64–147%
6. Euglobulin fibrinolysin time	90–300 min.	21–145 min.†

*Values are from the author's laboratory.
†Cord blood.

vise concentrating on the following tests for laboratory confirmation of DIC: red cell smear, platelet count, prothrombin time, thrombin time, fibrinogen, and Factors V and VIII levels. At the least, the diagnosis of a consumption coagulopathy should not be made without abnormalities of the prothrombin and thrombin times and platelet count.

Differential Diagnosis

Several conditions causing critical illness in a child may be confused on clinical grounds with DIC. Patients with massive hepatitis or acute hepatic necrosis as seen in Reye's syndrome may develop a severe bleeding diathesis with depression of fibrinogen, Factors V and II, and platelets. Even mildly increased fibrinolysins (and FSP) may be present owing to partial activation of the fibrinolytic system. Specific assay of Factor VIII levels may be necessary for the differential diagnosis. Factor VIII levels remain normal in liver disease but would be decreased in severe DIC.

Severe uremia is often seen with a bleeding diathesis which is associated with decreased platelets, prolonged prothrombin and thrombin times, and increased levels of FSP. However, fibrinogen and Factors V and VIII levels usually remain normal or even increased.

Infections, especially meningococcemia, Rocky Moutain spotted fever, and certain viral diseases, can present with thrombocytopenia, and even prolongation of the prothrombin time,[29] without other evidence of DIC. Demonstration of a prolonged thrombin time and decreased fibrinogen level would be necessary in order to confirm the diagnosis of DIC in such patients.

Patients with cyanotic congenital heart disease may have marked derangement of the coagulation mechanism without definite consumption coagulopathy. These abnormalities include prolonged bleeding times, thrombocytopenia, increased prothrombin, and euglobin lysis times.[30] However, an occasional patient with cyanotic heart disease can develop DIC as a complication during the natural course of the disorder.[31, 32]

Fibrin split products and thrombocytopenia may be present in several conditions without other evidence of diffuse intravascular coagulation. These diseases include renal disease,[33] hemolytic-uremic syndrome, and thrombotic thrombocytopenic purpura.

Rarely, primary fibrinolysis may occur in children in association with liver disease. Release of activators from the damaged liver causes pathologically increased fibrinolysis, thus resulting in decreased fibrinogen and increased FSP. Direct action of the proteolytic enzyme may cause decreased levels of Factors V and VIII as well. Platelets usually remain normal. The process may not be as severe as acute DIC, but the differential diagnosis is obviously a difficult one; often serial measurements or cautious therapeutic trials or both may be necessary to establish the diagnosis.

Since therapy with heparin may aggravate the bleeding in many of the aforementioned conditions, i.e., liver disease, renal disease, presence of a consumption coagulopathy must be proved before therapy. This may require extensive studies, including factor assays.

In these seriously ill children positive answers to the following questions should be obtained before heparin therapy is instituted:

1. Does the patient have a triggering event present (infection, tissue damage, endothelial damage, etc.)?

2. Is hypotension or multiple system involvement present?

3. Is there evidence of a consumption coagulopathy (low platelets, fibrinogen, II, V, VIII)?

TREATMENT

When DIC is established as a working diagnosis in the critically ill infant or child, the following therapeutic plan is suggested:

1. *Heparin* (sodium heparin, U.S.P.) is given in intravenous push doses of 100 to 150 units per kilogram of body weight every 4 to 6 hours (always calculate heparin dosage in units rather than mg). Heparinization is continued until the patient has improved clinically, coagulation factors have returned to normal, and the triggering event is removed — usually in 48 to 72 hours. Clinical response of patients, cessation of bleeding, and improvement of clotting tests (drawn just prior to next dose of heparin) are the important parameters to follow rather than whole blood clotting time.

2. *Replacement therapy* of depleted coagulation factors may be indicated in cases of severe DIC in which the consumable factors are nearly absent. Fresh frozen plasma (10 ml/kg) and platelet concentrates in appropriate dosage should be given when bleeding is severe and when hepatic synthesis of clotting factors may be impaired, i.e., in severe viral diseases with hepatic necrosis or cirrhosis of the liver.

3. *Supportive therapy* to correct contributing factors aggravating the DIC are indicated. Correction of severe polycythemia, metabolic acidosis, hypoxia, dehydration, and anemia are important, as well as specific measures to remove the triggering events. Indeed, a recent study[34] has suggested that heparinization of the severely ill, hypotensive, septic patient did not significantly improve the mortality rate, even though DIC was highly probable in 96 per cent of the cases. Heparin did correct the coagulation deficit in most of the cases. Support of the circulation (plasma, blood, isoproterenol) may be the most important aspect of therapy in septic patients. Adrenal steroids may be indicated in severe endotoxin shock with or without DIC.[35]

4. Antifibrinolytic agents such as epsilon amino caproic acid

(EACA, Amicar) are *contraindicated* in DIC. Rather, efforts to increase fibrinolytic activity may be a major part of future therapy.

SUMMARY

The complication of disseminated intravascular coagulation should be suspected in a critically ill child when evidence of the following signs and symptoms is present: (1) the potential of a triggering event, such as endotoxin, tissue thromboplastin (damaged tissue), endothelial damage, or proteolysis; (2) multiple system involvement producing coma, renal shutdown, respiratory disease, and shock; (3) a bleeding diathesis; and (4) a hemolytic anemia associated with fragmented and burred red cells. Laboratory confirmation should include evidence for depletion of coagulation factors consumed during clotting, i.e., platelets, fibrinogen, and Factors II, V, and VIII. Treatment consists of heparinization, replacement of depleted factors if needed, and supportive care, which includes removal of the triggering event.

References

1. Abildgaard, C. F.: Recognition and treatment of intravascular coagulation. J. Pediat., 75:163, 1969.
2. McKay, D. G.: Progress in disseminated intravascular coagulation. Part I. Calif. Med., 111:187, 1969.
3. McKay, D. G.: Progress in disseminated intravascular coagulation. Part II. Calif. Med., 111:279, 1969.
4. Merskey, C., Johnson, A. J., Kleiner, G. J., and Wohl, H.: The defibrination syndrome: clinical features and laboratory diagnosis. Brit. J. Haemat., 13:528, 1967.
5. Owen, C. A., Oels, H. C., Bowie, J. W., Didisheim, P., and Thompson, J. H., Jr.: Chronic intravascular coagulation (CIF) syndrome. Thrombos. Diathes. Haemorrh. Suppl., 36:197, 1969.
6. McKay, D. G., and Margaretten, W.: Disseminated intravascular coagulation in virus diseases. Arch. Int. Med., 120:129, 1967.
7. Miller, D. R., Hanshaw, J. P., O'Leary, D. S., and Hnilicka, J. G.: Fatal disseminated herpes simplex virus infection and hemorrhage in the neonate. J. Pediat., 76:409, 1970.
8. Starzl, T. E., Lerner, R. A., Dixon, R. J., Groth, C. G., Brettschneider, L., and Terasaki, P.: Shwartzman reaction after human renal transplantation. New Eng. J. Med., 278:642, 1968.
9. Groth, C. G., Pechet, L., and Starzl, T. E.: Coagulation during and after orthotopic transplantation of the human liver. Arch. Surg., 98:31, 1969.
10. Hathaway, W. E., Mull, M. M., and Pechet, C. S.: Disseminated intravascular coagulation in the newborn. Pediatrics, 43:233, 1969.
11. Stark, C. R., Abramson, D., and Erkan, V.: Intravascular coagulation and hyaline membrane disease of the newborn. Lancet, 1:1180, 1968.
12. Moore, C. M., McAdams, A. J., and Sutherland, J.: Intrauterine disseminated intravascular coagulation: A syndrome of multiple pregnancy with a dead twin fetus. J. Pediat., 74:523, 1969.
13. Johansson, S. A.: Studies on blood coagulation factors in a case of liver cirrhosis — remission of the hemorrhagic tendency on treatment with heparin. Acta Med. Scand., 175:177, 1964.

14. Weber, M. B., and Blakely, J. A.: The haemorrhagic diathesis of heatstroke. Lancet, *1*:1190, 1969.
15. Purkis, I. E., Horrelt, O., de Young, C. G., Fleming, R. A. P., and Langley, G. R.: Hyperpyrexia during anaesthesia in a second member of a family, with associated coagulation defect due to increased intravascular coagulation. Canad. Anaes. Soc. J., *14*:183, 1967.
16. Blombäck, M., Johansson, S.-A., and Sjöberg, H.-E.: Coagulation factors and defibrination syndrome in anaphylaxis. Acta Physiol. Scand., *69*:313, 1967.
17. Piel, C. F., and Phibbs, R. H.: The hemolytic-uremic syndrome. Pediat. Clin. N. Amer., *13*:295, 1966.
18. Gianantonio, C. A., Vitacco, M., Mendilaharzu, F., and Gallo, G.: The hemolytic-uremic syndrome. Renal status of 76 patients at long-term follow-up. J. Pediat., *72*:753, 1968.
19. Corrigan, J. J., Jr., Ray, W. L., and May, N.: Changes in the blood coagulation system associated with septicemia. New Eng. J. Med., *279*:851, 1968.
20. Baker, L. R. I., Rubenberg, M. L., Dacie, J. V., and Brain, M. C.: Fibrinogen catabolism in microangiopathic haemolytic anaemia. Brit. J. Haemat., *14*:617, 1968.
21. Niemetz, M., and Nossel, H. L.: Activated coagulation factors: *in vivo* and *in vitro* studies. Brit. J. Haemat., *16*:337, 1969.
22. Merskey, C., Lalezari, P., and Johnson, A. J.: A rapid, simple, sensitive method for measuring fibrinolytic split products in human serum. Proc. Soc. Exp. Biol. Med., *131*:871, 1969.
23. Israels, E. D., Raymer, H., Israels, L. G., and Zipursky, A.: A microhemagglutination inhibition assay for the quantitation of fibrinogen breakdown products. J. Lab. Clin. Med., *71*:333, 1968.
24. Shainoff, J. R., and Page, I. H.: Significance of cryoprofibrin in fibrinogen-fibrin conversion. J. Exp. Med., *116*:687, 1962.
25. Kowalski, E.: Fibrinogen derivatives and their biological activities. Sem. Hemat., 5:45, 1968.
26. Breen, F. A., and Tullis, J. L.: Ethanol gelation: a rapid screening test for intravascular coagulation. Ann. Int. Med., *69*:1197, 1968.
27. Ekelund, H., Hedner, U., and Nilsson, I. M.: Fibrinolysis in newborns. Acta Paediat. Scand., *59*:33, 1970.
28. Fibrin split products in serum of newborn: possible technical errors (Letters to the Editor). Pediatrics, *45*:154–158, 1970.
29. McGehee, W. G., Rapaport, S. I., and Hjort, P. R.: Intravascular coagulation in fulminant meningococcemia. Ann. Int. Med., *67*:250, 1967.
30. Ekert, H., Gilchrist, G. S., Stanton, R., and Hammond, D.: Hemostasis in cyanotic congenital heart disease. J. Pediat., *76*:221, 1970.
31. Dennis, H. L., Stewart, J. L., and Conrad, M. E.: A consumption coagulation in congenital cyanotic heart disease and its treatment with heparin. J. Pediat., *71*:407, 1967.
32. Komp, D. M., and Sparrow, A. W.: Polycythemia in cyanotic heart disease—a study of altered coagulation. J. Pediat., *76*:231, 1970.
33. Stiehm, E. R., and Trygstad, C. W.: Split products of fibrin in human renal disease. Amer. J. Med., *47*:774, 1969.
34. Corrigan, J. J., and Jordan, C. M.: Heparin therapy in septicemia with disseminated intravascular coagulation. New Eng. J. Med., *283*:778, 1970.
35. Hodes, H. L.: Care of the critically ill child: Endotoxin shock. Pediat., *44*:248, 1969.

21

Sickle Cell Disease Crises and Their Management

Howard A. Pearson, M.D.,
and Louis K. Diamond, M.D.

The population shifts which have characterized American demography during the past few generations have made it imperative that practicing physicians throughout the country learn to recognize the protean manifestations of the most common hematologic abnormality of the black race—sickling of the red cells. Because the clinical consequences and sequelae of the sickling phenomenon frequently present life-threatening emergencies, successful management requires prompt diagnosis, ready application of rational therapy, and alertness in an often rapidly changing clinical situation.

This brief review will be confined to the recognition and treatment of the acute crises seen in infants and children with sickle cell disease. The word "disease" is used rather than "anemia" since the degree of anemia may be variable, and some dangerous crises occur without an increase in the severity of the anemia.

From the Departments of Pediatrics, Yale University, New Haven, Connecticut, and University of California, San Francisco Medical Center, San Francisco, California.

TABLE 1   SELECTED LABORATORY VALUES IN SICKLE-CELL DISEASE

| | Normal Values | Values in Sickle Cell Disease | |
		Average	Range
Hemoglobin (gm/100 ml)	12	7.5	5.5–9.5
Hematocrit (%)	36	22	17–29
Reticulocytes (%)	1.5	12	5–30
Nucleated RBC/ 100 WBC	0	3	1–20
White Blood Cell Count (per mm³)	7500	20,000	12,000–35,000
Bilirubin (mg/100 ml)	<1.0	2.5	1.5–4.0

Although the child with sickle cell disease always has anemia, its severity varies in degree in different patients and even in the same individual from time to time. A well-compensated hemolytic anemia may be aggravated by infections, dietary deficiencies — especially folic acid — dehydration, and occasionally by certain drugs. In these clinical situations damage to the circulatory red cells or their precursors in the bone marrow may occur.

Sickle cell disease is associated with an accelerated hemolytic process, so that symptoms of anemia (pallor, weakness, and fatigability) are usually prominent. In addition to these features of any chronic anemia, unique clinical aspects of sickle cell disease result from occlusion of blood vessels and subsequent tissue infarction, caused by the distorted sickled red cells found in large numbers in the circulation of these patients. The clinical and hematologic manifestations of sickle cell disease thus reflect two processes: (1) severe hemolysis and the compensatory mechanisms evoked by hemolytic anemia; and (2) widespread vaso-occlusive phenomena involving many tissues and organs.

There are four types of episodic events which are usually called "crises" and which can threaten the comfort or life of the pediatric patient with sickle cell disease. These are: (1) aplastic crises; (2) hyperhemolytic crises; (3) acute splenic sequestration crises and chronic splenic dysfunction (functional asplenia) with increased susceptibility to certain bacterial infections; and (4) vaso-occlusive crises.

In order to put the laboratory findings during the episodic crises into perspective, the average values found in patients with sickle cell disease during intercritical periods are listed in Table 1. These values, rather than those of normal children, must be considered in the evaluation of these patients.

APLASTIC CRISES

In patients with sickle cell disease the red cell survival is only 15 to 20 days compared with 120 days in normal individuals. Despite this extreme hemolysis, the patient with sickle cell disease usually maintains a hemoglobin of 5.5 to 9.5 gm per 100 ml by increasing red cell production five- to eight-fold. If this maximal compensatory response is compromised, profound anemia can be explained without invoking "hyperhemolysis" as the cause. Diminished red cell production superimposed on the usual rapid destruction is the basis of the "aplastic crisis." A number of infections, usually viral in type, may in some way damage the erythroid bone marrow and result almost in a cessation of red cell production which may persist for 10 to 14 days.[1] Aplastic crises may occur in several members of a family—further evidence of their infectious origin. Although nutritional deficiencies of folic acid have been invoked in the genesis of some of these crises, other studies did not confirm a relationship.[2] During these "aplastic" episodes, reticulocytes disappear from the blood and a markedly reduced number of erythroid precursors are present in the bone marrow.

The hematologic findings during aplastic crises differ, depending on the stage at which the patient is studied. Early, the degree of anemia is progressively more extreme and the numbers of reticulocytes in the blood and nucleated red cells in the bone marrow are sharply decreased. However, platelet and white blood cell counts are not usually affected, and jaundice may even decrease. At the nadir of the aplastic crisis, the hemoglobin level may fall as low as 1 gm/100 ml and death may result from severe anemia and congestive heart failure.

Erythroid aplasia usually terminates spontaneously after 7 to 10 days and recovery is accompanied by a surge of reticulocytes and nucleated red cells in the blood. Reticulocyte count may then climb as high as 50 to 60 per cent. Shortly thereafter the hemoglobin returns to precrisis levels. If the patient is first studied early in the recovery stage from an aplastic crisis, a mistaken diagnosis of "hemolytic" crisis may be entertained because of the still present severe anemia and the marked reticulocytosis.

The treatment for an aplastic crisis is transfusion of relatively fresh packed red cells, given slowly in a dose of not more than 2 to 3 ml/kg of body weight every 8 hours until the hemoglobin level is increased by about 5 gm/100 ml. For the small child, a whole unit of packed cells (250 to 300 ml) can be divided and used sequentially, thereby reducing the risk of transfusion hepatitis associated with multiple donors. When profound anemia is present, very fresh blood should be used first to assure normal levels of 2,3-diphosphoglyceride so that oxygen transport of the transfused red cells is normal.[3] Oxygen may be administered if the patient is dyspneic, but digitalis is not recommended nor usually needed. If signs of congestive heart failure are present, venous pressure may be monitored by a central venous catheter during transfusion, and blood can be withdrawn from the patient as the donor blood is given, resulting in a partial exchange transfusion.

Parents of children with sickle cell disease should be made aware of the manifestations of the aplastic crisis. They should seek medical attention promptly if the child becomes pale or weak, especially following an infection.

HYPERHEMOLYTIC CRISES

The frequency of so-called hyperhemolytic crises is somewhat controversial, owing to the difficulty in proving a more rapid rate of hemolysis superimposed upon an already severe process.[4] Nevertheless, in association with certain drugs or acute infections, hyperhemolysis may ensue.[5] During these episodes the patient begins to feel weak, look more pale, and show more scleral icterus. There may be abdominal pain and an increase in splenomegaly. The hematocrit may fall from its usual 21 to 25 per cent to 15 per cent or less in a few days. The reticulocytes may rise to 35 per cent or more. The urine may darken with excess urobilinogen. After several days to a few weeks, the excessive hemolysis tends to subside gradually, especially if treatment is prompt.

Treatment consists of a search for sites of infection, culture of the nose and throat, sputum, blood, urine, and stools; if significant organisms are found or their presence suggested (e.g., pneumonic consolidation by x-ray), antibiotics should be given. Drugs which may produce hemolysis should be discontinued. At the same time, dehydration and acidosis must be corrected promptly and completely. Adequate blood transfusion of packed or sedimented red cells should be given to reverse or prevent incipient heart failure from anemic anoxia. Persistence of a hyperhemolytic state suggests residual infection, which must be identified and treated vigorously.

SPLENIC SEQUESTRATION CRISES, ACUTE AND CHRONIC

Acute Crises

Infants and young children with sickle cell disease whose spleens have not yet undergone multiple infarctions and subsequent fibrosis may suddenly pool vast amounts of blood in the spleen. During these sequestration crises the spleen becomes enormous, even reaching to the pelvis. The hemoglobin level may drop so precipitously that hypovolemic shock and death may occur. This is the most immediately dangerous crisis in the life of the young child with this disease; it must be recognized and treated promptly. Infants between 8 months and 5 years of age are particularly susceptible and may succumb within hours of the first signs of illness.[6]

Treatment of the sequestration crisis is directed toward the prompt correction of hypovolemia with plasma expanders and, particularly, with whole blood transfusion. If the shock can be reversed, much of the blood sequestered in the spleen appears to be remobilized and dramatic regression of splenomegaly may occur in a short time. Because of the rapidity with which a sequestration crisis can occur and even recur and because of its potential fatality in a matter of hours, we recommend splenectomy after a child has had one or two of these crises.

Chronic Splenic Dysfunction (Functional Asplenia)

Increased susceptibility to pneumococcal infection of the pharynx, lungs, meninges, and even of the blood stream has long been a puzzling occurrence in infants and children with sickle cell disease. To perhaps a lesser extent, they show diminished resistance to infections with Salmonella, often localized as osteomyelitis, and also to *H. influenzae* bacilli. Taken in conjunction with observations of nucleated red cells, Howell-Jolly bodies, and bizarre-shaped erythrocytes in peripheral blood smears, the specific immunologic deficiency involving the pneumococcus strongly resembles the changes seen in young children lacking spleens, either congenitally or post-surgery, despite the presence of considerable splenomegaly! We have recently clarified this apparent paradox by demonstrating with radioactive tagging techniques that "functional asplenia" exists in these patients, possibly as the result of temporary vaso-occlusive episodes or of puddling in the splenic circulation.[7, 8] Such an occurrence could cause shunting of the blood so as to bypass the splenic sinusoids, where defective and particle-containing red cells are ordinarily sequestered or are culled and, more important, where bacteria are removed and processed preparatory to antibody action. In essence, therefore, such patients have the handicaps and face the hazards of the asplenic infant or young child. It has also been shown that transfusion with normal blood to a level of 50 per cent or more of hemoglobin A restores the splenic circulation to its normal pathways and corrects the functional asplenia, at least for a few weeks or months.[9]

At any rate, because of this susceptibility to overwhelming pneumococcal infection, penicillin therapy is indicated in the treatment of sickle cell disease in an infant who develops unexplained significant fever.

VASO-OCCLUSIVE CRISES

These are by far the most common types and also the only painful ones. The manifestations may vary markedly, depending upon the tissues or organs involved and the extent of the ischemic damage. The basic cause of such a crisis is obstruction of blood flow by tangled masses of sickled cells and an immeasurable degree of vasospasm. There are usually few or no changes in the hematologic parameters during these episodes. The events which trigger vaso-occlusion are largely undefined, but a number of distinctive syndromes can be recognized.

"Hand-Foot Syndrome"

A common initial manifestation of sickle cell disease during infancy is dactylitis resulting from symmetrical involvement of metacarpals and metatarsals and manifested as painful swelling of the dorsa of the hands and feet. Low-grade fever may accompany this — occasionally there may be high fever — but without characteristic hematologic changes. X-ray films show no abnormalities initially, but later areas of osteolysis, periostitis, and bone reabsorption may appear. The diffuse symmetrical pattern of involvement of multiple bones and the finding of sterile blood cultures differentiate the "hand-foot syndrome" from osteomyelitis, which is so often suggested. There is no specific therapy. Repeated attacks may occur over many months but after the second or third year of life the syndrome does not usually recur. There are no permanent sequelae.

Involvement of the Joints and Extremities

Symptomatic, painful crises involving the joints and extremities usually begin during the second or third year of life. Extremity pains may be due to areas of infarction of the long bones or the bone marrow or involvement of the periosteum or of periarticular tissues of the larger joints. There is swelling and limitation of motion but no redness. Joint pain may mimic acute rheumatic fever or rheumatoid arthritis. X-ray studies may show areas of bone infarction and periostitis but may also be negative, especially at the onset, and even for the following week or so. There are, in general, no hematologic changes during these crises and significant fever is usually not observed.

Abdominal Involvement

These episodes are due to areas of infarction in abdominal structures such as liver, spleen, and abdominal lymph nodes, with stretching of their capsules. Occasionally the pain may be incapacitatingly severe and episodic in character. Signs of peritoneal irritation are sometimes present but peristalsis usually persists. This finding may differentiate the abdominal crisis from an inflammatory process, such as appendicitis or peritonitis, which requires surgical intervention. Painful abdominal crises are often associated with low-grade fever but when very severe may be accompanied by hyperpyrexia and prostration.

The duration of the painful crises averages 3 to 4 days. There may be early termination, but protracted episodes can also occur. This variability makes evaluation of any specific drug therapy or new method of treatment very difficult.

Hepatic Involvement

Some degree of hyperbilirubinemia is usual in sickle cell disease; however, an episode of severe obstructive jaundice may also occur, and may even end in death. The basis of this is extensive intrahepatic sickling with subsequent hepatocellular necrosis and swelling. The level of serum bilirubin may increase to 25 mg/100 ml or more, mostly of the conjugated variety. These findings may suggest biliary obstruction by a stone in the common duct, a diagnostic dilemma compounded by the finding of pigmentary cholelithiasis in many of these patients. As treatment for severe obstructive jaundice we recommend multiple transfusions of packed red cells. Gallbladder surgery is *not* performed unless the obstruction is chronic.

Central Nervous System Crises

Children with sickle cell disease may develop monoplegia or hemiplegia with other neurologic findings suggestive of upper motor neuron damage. The sequelae of these "strokes" are variable. Some patients recover rapidly and completely, even after apparent widespread involvement, indicating that there is a significant element of vasospasm and edema. Others are left with permanent neurologic deficits, showing that actual infarction may occur. Angiographic studies are not indicated in the early stages of these attacks. We have noted *in vitro* that the high tonicity of contrast media produces immediate sickling of the red cells suspended in them. This could aggravate the vaso-occlusive component. The treatment of central nervous system episodes includes prompt and vigorous hydration, administration of oxygen, and multiple transfusions of packed red cells.

Pulmonary Crises

Children with sickle cell disease often have severe and protracted episodes of pulmonary disease. Although the precipitating event may be bacterial infection due to the pneumococcus or even mycoplasma organisms, infarction may be a significant component. It may be very difficult to separate infection; in fact, both processes may be operative. After appropriate cultures are taken, antibiotic therapy, including penicillin, is given. Multiple transfusions of packed red cells are also indicated if the pulmonary involvement is extensive or protracted and is causing significant pulmonary insufficiency.

TREATMENT

There is no specific drug therapy for vaso-occlusive crises. Many medications of possible value have been proposed at various times. These include anticoagulants, low molecular weight dextran, alkalis, phenothiazines, and many others as well. Most recently, urea has been extolled (see below). Suitably controlled studies have not proved the efficacy of most of these.

Management of the vaso-occlusive crises must include therapy directed at reversal of the following conditions that are known to enhance sickling:

Dehydration. Hypertonicity enhances the sickling process *in vitro*. The expanded plasma volume may show a sharp constriction during painful crises or infection. In addition, these patients are hyposthenuric and may become dehydrated very easily; therefore, optimal hydration should be ensured. Oral fluids can be encouraged in the milder episodes, but if the pain is severe, and particularly when fever, vomiting, or other processes which contribute to dehydration are present, parenteral hydration is indicated. The use of a half and half mixture of normal saline in 5 per cent dextrose, infused at a rate of 2000 to 2500 ml/m²/day, is advised.

Acidosis. This also aggravates sickling, and pain can be produced by the infusion of acidifying compounds such as ammonium sulfate. Accordingly, alkali therapy is administered to rectify potential or actual acidosis. Although data to prove the effectiveness of such therapy are contradictory, in mild vaso-occlusive crises oral sodium bicarbonate is given in a dose of 3 to 4 gm/m²/day in four divided doses, or polycitrate (Shohl's solution) in a dose of 3 tablespoons four times a day. If intravenous therapy is used, sodium bicarbonate is added to the hydrating solution and the urine pH is maintained at 6.5 to 7.0.

Hypoxia. Since reduced oxygenation increases sickling, an atmosphere of well-humidified oxygen may be used so long as the child is experiencing severe pain; the modest increase in oxygenation attained with an oxygen tent is of uncertain value.

Besides attention to these three contributing factors, the possible uses of transfusion must be considered. Since the ordinary vaso-occlusive crisis is not associated with hematologic changes, blood is not routinely administered for anemia. The beneficial effects of a single blood transfusion of 10 to 15 ml/kg may be counterbalanced by the increased blood viscosity caused by an increase in hematocrit. But in severe or prolonged vaso-occlusive crises, more vigorous, multiple transfusion therapy to "dilute" the patient's sickle cells may be considered.

If the number of sickle cells in the circulation can be reduced effectively, many of the clinical manifestations of the disease will cease. The most effective way to accomplish this reduction is by transfusion of normal red blood cells from proved non-sickle-cell donors. When at least 50 per cent of the patient's circulating red blood cells are replaced by normal red cells, vaso-occlusive symptomatology will usually stop. Transfusions of fresh packed red blood cells, 10 to 15 ml/kg, are infused every 12 hours until the hemoglobin is increased to 12 to 13 gm/100 ml. At this point, simple dilution will have decreased the circulating complement of the patient's red blood cells and his erythropoiesis will be suppressed. Because of their 15-to-20 day survival, the patient's own red blood cells, which contain hemoglobin S, disappear rapidly. With small packed cell transfusions given as indicated, the proportion of circulating hemoglobin-S- containing cells will fall to very low levels, thus effectively producing an exchange transfusion in a few days. Packed cell transfusions every 2 to 3 weeks will ensure that the circulating blood will contain predominantly normal red blood cells. Although this "hypertransfusion regimen" is symptomatically effective, there are inherent risks of isoimmunization, hepatitis, and hemosiderosis. This type of program is usually used, therefore, only for specific indications, such as prolonged or very severe vaso-occlusive crises, preparation for anesthesia and surgery, management of pregnancy in sickle cell anemia, and as supportive therapy during complicating medical conditions.

Sedation and Analgesia

Considerable relief of pain and discomfort may be obtained with the judicious use of sedatives and analgesics. Aspirin in large doses should be avoided so as not to aggravate a tendency to metabolic acidosis. Acetaminophen (Tylenol) in a dose of 120 to 240 mg every 4 to 6 hours may provide some relief in mild painful crises and may act as an antipyretic. When pain is more severe, codeine sulfate (30 to 60 mg) may be necessary. Use of meperidine hydrochloride or morphine sulfate may lead to addiction, so these are not employed unless pain is extreme.

Compounds such as prochlorperazine and chlorpromazine are useful adjuncts for treatment of painful crises. Because of their sedative and tranquilizing action, 0.5 mg/kg of chlorpromazine every 6 to 8 hours or prochlorperazine in a dose of 2 to 5 mg every 8 hours may reduce the need for narcotics.

Urea Therapy

Considerable publicity in the lay press has extolled the possible benefit of intravenous urea in invert sugar for the painful crisis of sickle cell disease. The proposed action of this therapy is that high concentrations of urea disrupt the molecular bonds which may be the basis of the sickling phenomenon. The documentation of the possible efficacy of this therapy is sketchy, for as late as June, 1971, only 15 patients had been treated by Nalbandian,[10] its chief proponent, and his protocol had not been formally published.* To add to the confusion, another research group has indicated that the effect of urea in reversing sickling *in vitro* may be due to the presence of cyanate—an invariable contaminant of commercial urea preparations.[11] The use of urea increases the patient's BUN to 150 to 200 mg/100 ml and produces profound diuresis which must be vigorously treated if dehydration is to be avoided.

Smaller doses of oral urea have also been suggested as prophylactic therapy. A proportion of oral urea is ordinarily converted to ammonia by gut bacteria. It is possible that another mechanism rather than the proposed one could be responsible for any possible beneficial effect.

The history of sickle cell disease is studded with enthusiastic preliminary reports of effective therapies but, when these are subjected to test in larger controlled studies, no significant benefit can usually be shown. The problem of evaluation is compounded by the extreme variability of the sickle cell "crisis." Ultimately any beneficial therapy of sickle cell disease must be reflected in a decrease of *in vivo* sickling. Unless unequivocal proof is demonstrated, any sketchy evidence must be viewed with healthy skepticism, especially if very real hazards are involved, as in using urea.[12]

SUMMARY

This brief review, being limited in scope to the recognition and management of the life-threatening and painful crises in infants and children with sickle-cell disease, has not even touched on the intriguing mystery of the molecular basis for the sickling phenomenon—how one amino-acid substitution (gene-controlled) in the beta chain sequence of 146 amino acids can cause such serious disruption in form and function; or how this mutation occurred in the first place and why it has persisted in contrast to the rapid disappearance of many other deleterious mutants. Nor has there been even mention of the many milder symptoms, signs, and complications due to the presence of hemoglobin S, either in the homozygous (disease-producing) state or heterozygous form, when found in combination with other hereditary hemoglobin defects. The ac-

---

*Since submission of this manuscript, the book by R. M. Nalbandian gives a preliminary report on urea treatment of sickle cell disease.[13]

cumulated knowledge about this mutant gene, its biochemical effects, and geographic distribution is enormous. From a fundamental scientific standpoint, sickle cell disease is one of the best understood of human afflictions.

However, from a practical point of view treatment of the patient itself is often only symptomatic and palliative. Nevertheless, prompt and effective therapy of the myriad manifestations of sickle cell disease can effectively reduce morbidity and mortality. The pediatrician with black children in his practice should be familiar with the cardinal diagnostic and clinical aspects of sickle cell disease and its crises.

References

1. MacIver, J. E., and Parker-Williams, E. J.: The aplastic crisis in sickle cell anaemia. Lancet, *1*:1086, 1961.
2. Pearson, H. A., and Cobb, W. T.: Folic acid studies in sickle cell anemia. J. Lab. Clin. Med., *64*:913, 1964.
3. Oski, F. A., and Delevoria-Papadopoulos, M.: The red cell, 2-3 diphosphoglycerate and tissue oxygen release. J. Pediat., *77*:941, 1970.
4. Diggs, L. W.: Sickle cell crisis. Amer. J. Clin. Path., *44*:1, 1965.
5. Smits, H. L., Oski, F. A., and Brody, J. I.: The hemolytic crisis of sickle cell disease: the role of glucose-6-phosphate dehydrogenase deficiency. J. Pediat., *74*:544, 1969.
6. Jenkins, M. E., Scott, R. B., and Baird, R. L.: Studies in sickle cell anemia. XVI. Sudden death during sickle cell crises in young children. J. Pediat., *56*:30, 1960.
7. Pearson, H. A., Spencer, R. P., and Cornelius, E. A.: Functional asplenia in sickle-cell anemia. New Eng. J. Med., *281*:293, 1969.
8. Diamond, L. K., Price, D. C., and Young, E.: Functional asplenia, a newly recognized splenic disorder. Clin. Res., *18*:209, 1970.
9. Pearson, H. A., Cornelius, E. A., Schwartz, A. D., Zelson, J. H., Wolfson, S. L., and Spencer, R. P.: Transfusion-reversible functional asplenia in young children with sickle-cell anemia. New Eng. J. Med., *283*:334, 1970.
10. Nalbandian, R. M.: Urea for sickle-cell crises (Letter). New Eng. J. Med., *284*:1381, 1971.
11. Cerami, A., and Manning, J. M.: Potassium cyanate as an inhibitor of the sickling of erythrocytes, *in vitro.* Proc. Nat. Acad. Sci., *68*:1180, 1971.
12. Desforges, J. F.: Treatment of sickle crisis (Editorial). New Eng. J. Med., *284*:913, 1971.
13. Nalbandian, R. M.: Molecular Aspects of Sickle Cell Hemoglobin: Clinical Applications. Springfield, Ill., Charles C Thomas, 1971.

22

Anaphylaxis

C. Warren Bierman, M.D.

This additional chapter, published as a Committee report after the original series, is added as an obviously valuable inclusion.

The Editor

Anaphylaxis* is an acute reaction, which may range from mild self-limited symptoms to a grave medical emergency. It is caused by a variety of agents, usually occurs unexpectedly, frequently is iatrogenic, and can be fatal if not treated promptly and appropriately. Every physician's and dentist's office, pediatric outpatient clinic, hospital emergency room, allergy clinic, and radiology department should be equipped to treat this potential disaster.[1]

The Committee on Drugs of the American Academy of Pediatrics has reviewed the equipment and procedures necessary to treat this emergency, and offers this guide to physicians.

CLINICAL PICTURE

Anaphylaxis is usually characterized by the following sequence of signs and symptoms: generalized flush, urticaria, paroxysmal coughing, severe anxiety, dyspnea, wheezing, orthopnea, vomiting, cyanosis, and shock. The sooner symptoms develop after the initiating stimulus, the more intense the reaction. Symptoms beginning within 15 minutes after administration of the inciting agent require the most expedient management.

From the Department of Pediatrics, University of Washington School of Medicine, Seattle, Washington.

*In this chapter, anaphylactic reactions (which result from specific allergy, i.e., prior sensitization) and anaphylactoid reactions (which do not require prior sensitization and can occur on the first administration of a substance) are combined, since the clinical picture and management are identical.

260

The primary cause of death in the child is laryngeal edema. In the adult, cardiac arrhythmias may be superimposed on acute upper airway edema.[2]

MAJOR CAUSES OF ANAPHYLAXIS

Table 1 lists the most common agents associated with anaphylaxis in children. The severity and acuteness of onset depend upon both the type of agent and the route of administration. Generally, agents ad-

TABLE 1   MAJOR CAUSES OF ANAPHYLAXIS[3]

1. *Antibiotics*
   Penicillin and its semisynthetic derivatives
   Cephalosporins (Keflex, Kafocin, Loridine, Keflin)
   Chloramphenicol
   Colymycin
   Kanamycin
   Polymyxin B
   Streptomycin
   Tetracyclines
   Troleandomycin (Cyclamycin, TAO)
   Vancomycin (Vancocin)
   Amphotericin B (Fungizone)

2. *Biologicals*
   Foreign serums (Antitoxins, Antilymphocyte Globulins (A.L.G.))
   Chymotrypsin
   Gamma globulin
   Asparaginase
   Polypeptide hormones (ACTH, TSH, insulin)
   Influenza vaccine
   Tetanus toxoid
   Measles and other egg-based vaccines

3. *Injectable Medications*
   Iron dextran (Inferon)
   Dextran
   Methylergonovine maleate (Methergine)
   Nitrofurantoin

4. *Local Anesthetics*

5. *Aspirin (Acetylsalicylic acid)*

6. *Diagnostic Agents*
   Iodinated contrast media
   Sulfobromophthalein (B.S.P.)

7. *Hymenoptera Stings* (Bee, yellow-jacket, wasp, and hornet)

8. *Allergic Extracts* (Skin-testing and treatment solutions)

9. *Foods* (Especially eggs, nuts, cottonseed, and shellfish)

10. *Intravenous Narcotics* (Heroin)

ministered parenterally are more apt to result in severe life-threatening or fatal anaphylactic reactions than those ingested orally or administered topically to mucous membranes. Medications administered orally, such as aspirin or penicillin, however, have been associated with fatal reactions; therefore, the oral route cannot be utilized with impunity.

Before administration of substances such as are listed in Table 1, the physician should inquire carefully for a history of reactions. If the patient thinks he is allergic to a drug, it would be preferable to select an alternate drug if possible. If there is a possibility of sensitivity to foreign proteins, such as horse serum or egg-based vaccines, or to penicillin, skin testing for immediate hypersensitivity to the agent should be performed prior to its therapeutic administration. Since even skin testing may induce anaphylaxis, such testing should be done carefully with emergency equipment on hand. Vaccines containing foreign proteins should be diluted 1:100 with saline for skin testing and penicillin should be diluted to 1000 units per ml.[4] The intracutaneous injection of 0.01 ml of the material into the forearm should be preceded by a preliminary scratch test. A wheal 5 mm greater than the saline control should be considered evidence of allergy and an indication for an alternate preparation. Skin testing is of little value in predicting anaphylactic sensitivity to human gamma globulin, local anesthetics, aspirin, or to most diagnostic agents listed in Table 1.

MANAGEMENT OF ANAPHYLAXIS

Recognizing the early signs of anaphylaxis will save valuable minutes.[5] By initiating treatment early, the life-threatening stages of anaphylactic shock may be avoided or minimized. The physician should always have basic emergency equipment available to treat this condition. The quantity of equipment, and medication to be kept on hand for immediate therapy of anaphylaxis, will depend upon the location of the practice and the secondary support available to the physician. For example, the physician who is located miles from the nearest hospital, or the allergist who is more likely to encounter anaphylaxis, needs more equipment than the physician attending patients within a medical center who can summon an emergency team within minutes.

Principles of Therapy

In anaphylaxis there is a massive release into the cardiovascular system of allergic mediator substances, including histamine, slow reactive substance of anaphylaxis (SRS-A) and kinins as well as activated complement fractions such as anaphylatoxin. These substances cause generalized vasodilation and urticaria, and increased vascular permeability, induce bronchospasm, and produce glottid and subglottid edema. This results in upper and lower airway obstruction, a fall in blood pressure, and usually in vomiting, which may present an additional hazard of aspiration pneumonia.

Therapy designed to counter these factors may thus be divided into three stages:

Stage 1 — Immediate Therapy: To be initiated with any patient presenting the early signs of anaphylaxis.

Stage 2 — Supportive Therapy: For patients who have not responded to the immediate therapy.

Stage 3 — Therapy of Complication: For those few patients who have developed the most severe complications of anaphylaxis, occlusion of the upper airway, cardiac arrhythmias, or severe derangement of acid-base balance.

The physician should monitor the patient for the following manifestations:

1. *Upper Airway Obstruction.* One of the most dramatic aspects of acute anaphylaxis in the pediatric age group is frequently overlooked, though pharyngeal and uvular edema develops acutely in children and is readily visible. The pharynx should be observed frequently. At the first sign of upper airway obstruction an oral or endotracheal airway should be inserted.

2. *Lower Airway Obstruction.* Dyspnea, frequently without wheezing, accompanies anaphylaxis in children. Bronchospasm may be so severe that wheezing is not heard because of a markedly diminished tidal volume.

3. *Hypotension.* Frequent blood pressure determinations should be taken. Every effort should be made to keep pressure stable using plasma volume expanders and vasopressor medications if necessary.

4. *Aspiration of Gastric Contents.* Vomiting usually accompanies anaphylaxis in children. Aspiration of gastric contents should be anticipated.

Stage 1 — Immediate Therapy

All patients with early signs of anaphylaxis should receive the following therapy at once. Its prompt initiation may prevent subsequent complications which would require further therapy. Table 2 lists primary equipment and medications which should be present in an emergency kit.

TABLE 2 PRIMARY EQUIPMENT AND MEDICATIONS FOR ANAPHYLAXIS
(To be kept by all physicians in an emergency kit.)

A. Tourniquet
B. 1 ml and 5 ml disposable syringes
C. Oxygen tank and mask
D. Epinephrine Solution (Aqueous) 1:1000
E. Diphenhydramine (Benadryl), Injectable 50 mg/ml

TABLE 3 SUPPORTING EQUIPMENT AND MEDICATION FOR ANAPHYLAXIS
(These should be available within minutes though not necessarily in the
primary emergency unit.)

A. Intravenous infusion sets
B. Intravenous needles
C. Laryngoscope with interchangeable pediatric and adult blades
D. Oral airway—infant to adult
E. Apparatus to establish airway patency[8]
   1. #12 needles for temporary airway
   2. Endotracheal tubes (Numbers 18, 22, 26 and 30 French)
   3. Cricothyrotomy tube or tracheotomy setup
F. Suction apparatus
G. Bag resuscitator for assisted ventilation[9, 10] (Resusci-Folding
   bag, P.M.R. or Ambu bag)
H. Sterile surgical cutdown set
I. Aminophylline Solution (Injectable), 25 mg/ml
J. Hydrocortisone/hemisuccinate (Solu-Cortef) or equivalent
K. 5% glucose in isotonic saline (two 500 ml bottles)
L. Metaraminol bitartrate (Aramine), 1% for injection

1. *Tourniquet.* If subcutaneous or intramuscular injection has been given into an extremity, a tourniquet should immediately be applied proximal to the site to obstruct venous return from the injection.

2. *Epinephrine*—0.1 to 0.3 ml of 1:1000 aqueous epinephrine should be injected subcutaneously. An equal amount may be injected around the site of injection or sting to decrease absorption of antigen. If the patient is in shock, the physician may administer 1 or 2 ml 1:10,000 aqueous epinephrine, intravenously.

3. *Oxygen.* Since hypoxemia associated with hypotension or upper airway edema contributes to myocardial irritability and ventricular fibrillation as major causes of death, oxygen should be administered by mask early in the course of anaphylaxis.

4. *Antihistamines.* Diphenhydramine (Benadryl) may be administered intravenously (2 mg/kg) or orally (5 mg/kg/24 hours) for the therapy of urticaria. Such therapy should be considered of *secondary importance* and should not delay more therapeutic steps.

Stage 2—Supportive Therapy

If the patient fails to respond to initial therapy or is in shock when first seen, the following therapy should be given immediately after steps 1, 2, and 3 of initial therapy. Table 3 lists the necessary supporting equipment and medication, which need not be in the emergency kit but should be readily available to the physician.

1. *Intravenous fluids.* If the patient does not respond promptly to the initial therapy, intravenous fluids should be initiated immediately to support blood pressure to treat hypovolemia. In anaphylaxis, shock, resulting primarily from vasodilation and loss of plasma volume, should be treated by rapid infusion of saline or other plasma volume expanders. (See also pp. 11–13.)

TABLE 4   OPTIONAL EQUIPMENT AND SUPPLIES FOR ANAPHYLAXIS
(These items are desirable but may be available only in a well-equipped
emergency room or intensive care unit.)

A. EKG Monitor
B. Defribrillator
C. Calcium gluconate 10% (parenteral)
D. Digoxin (Lanoxin) 0.25 mg/ml
E. Diazepam (Valium), injectable 5 mg/ml
F. Lidocaine (Xylocaine) 2% with 1:1000 epinephrine for injection
G. Lidocaine (Xylocaine) 2% for injection
H. Sodium bicarbonate 3.75 gm in 500 ml

2. *Aminophylline solution* — 7 mg/kg diluted in 2 equal volumes of saline, given intravenously over a 5 to 10 minute period followed by 9 mg/kg/24 hours[6] aids in reversing bronchospasm and may inhibit further mediator release from mast cells.[7]

3. *Adrenocorticosteroids* have little effect during the initial crucial few minutes of anaphylaxis treatment and should be used only to supplement the major therapeutic steps. Hydrocortisone 7 mg/kg stat followed 7 mg/kg/24 hours administered intravenously may aid during the later recovery phase.

4. *Metaraminol bitartrate (Aramine).* If the blood pressure fails to respond to saline, Aramine 0.5 mg to 5 mg (0.4 mg/kg) may be added to the intravenous fluids, but cardiac side effects should be closely monitored.

Stage 3 — Therapy of Complications

Late complications of anaphylaxis include occlusion of the airway, cardiac arrhythmias, hypoxic seizures, and metabolic acidosis. For therapy of these conditions a hospital intensive care unit and blood gas laboratory are essential.[11] Table 4 lists equipment and supplies which are necessary in the therapy of these late complications.

Detailed description of this tertiary therapy is not included here, since therapy will vary greatly with the patient's clinical course, and will need to be individualized by the physician or his consultants. Basically an airway must be established, blood gas derangements must be corrected, aberrant cardiac rhythms corrected, seizures treated, and tissue hypoxemia corrected.

COMMENT

Since most anaphylaxis results from iatrogenic causes, it may be prevented or minimized by (1) obtaining an adequate history of drug reactions prior to their administration, (2) minimizing the use of foreign biological products, and (3) testing for hypersensitivity prior to administering such agents as penicillin to a patient with a history of penicillin allergy. No physician can afford to administer a drug which can induce an anaphylactic reaction without appropriate emergency equipment on hand. Finally, when an agent capable of inducing anaphylaxis, such as an allergy vaccine or penicillin, has been administered, the patient should be required to remain in the immediate vicinity of the physician's office or Emergency Room for at least 15 minutes so that appropriate therapy can be initiated at the first sign of a constitutional allergic reaction. Anaphylaxis occurs unexpectedly and suddenly and may occur in spite of extensive precautions. Appropriate and prompt therapy will increase the chances of a favorable outcome.

References

1. Van Arsdel, P. P., Jr.: Anaphylaxis and serum sickness. *In* Current Therapy, edited by H. L. Conn. W. B. Saunders Co., 1965, p. 415.
2. James, L. P. J., and Austen, K. F.: Fatal systemic anaphylaxis in man. New Eng. J. Med., *270*:597, 1961.
3. Siegel, S. C., and Heimlich, E. M.: Anaphylaxis. Pediat. Clin. N. Amer. *9*:29, 1962.
4. Bierman, C. W., and Van Arsdel, P. P., Jr.: Penicillin allergy in children. J. Allergy, *43*:267, 1969.
5. Frick, O. L.: Anaphylaxis. *In* Current Pediatric Therapy 4, edited by S. S. Gellis, and B. M. Kagan. W. B. Saunders Co., 1970, p. 934.
6. Pierson, W. E., Bierman, C. W., Stamm, S. J., and Van Arsdel, P. P., Jr.: Double blind trial of aminophylline in status asthmaticus. Pediatrics, *48*:642, 1971.
7. Orange, R. P., Austen, W. G., and Austen, K. F.: Immunologic release of histamine and slow reactive substance of anaphylaxis from human lung. J. Exp. Med., *134*:136 (Suppl.), 1971.
8. Safar, P.: Recognition and management of airway obstruction. J.A.M.A., *208*:1008, 1969.
9. Manually operated emergency ventilation devices. The Medical Letter, *11*:53, 1969.
10. Manually operated emergency ventilation devices. The Medical Letter, *13*:76, 1971.
11. Hanashiro, P. K., and Weil, M. H.: Anaphylactic shock in man. Arch. Int. Med., *119*:129, 1967.

INDEX

Page numbers in *italics* denote tables.

Abdomen, pain in, in diabetic acidosis, 174
  in sickle cell disease, 244
  trauma to, 15
  visceral infarction of, as sickle cell disease crises, 254
Accidents, burns, 46
  head injury, 62–75
Acetaminophen, for mild crises in sickle cell disease, 257
Acid phosphatase deficiency, *193–195*
Acidemia, correction of, in endotoxin shock, 38
  isovaleric, *191, 195*
  propionic, *192, 195*
Acidosis, diabetic, confusion with salicylate intoxication, 202
  in anaphylaxis, 263, 265
  in renal failure, 120
  in respiratory distress syndrome, 153, 154, 157–159
  metabolic, 188
    and respiratory acidosis, in cardiac failure, 100
      in respiratory distress of the newborn, 157
    in dehydration, 215
    in diabetic ketoacidosis, 172, 173
      treatment of, 175–178
    in shock, 16
  of salicylate intoxication, 200
  treatment of, in sickle cell disease crises, 256
Aciduria, argino-succinic, *190, 194*
Adrenal cortex, hypofunction of, and adrenal insufficiency, in newborn, 41

Adrenal hyperplasia, congenital, 42
Adrenal insufficiency, acute, 41–45
  causes, 41–42
  treatment, 42–44
Adrenalectomy, in relation to acute adrenal insufficiency, 73
Adrenocortical hormones, and regulation of blood sugar in fasting hypoglycemia, 184, 186
Adrenogenital syndrome, 42
Air flow, laminar, in isolation of burn patient, 55, *56*
Airway, adequacy of, following burns, 50
  maintenance of, in meningitis, 84
    in tracheostomy, 139–151
  obstruction of, in anaphylaxis, 263
Albumin, serum, in diagnosis of acute hepatic failure, 104
  transfusion of in burns, 59
Alimentation, intravenous. See Intravenous Alimentation.
Alkali therapy, contraindicated in dehydration secondary to diarrhea, 215
  in diabetes, 175, 177
  in respiratory distress syndrome of newborn, 157–160
Alkalosis, respiratory, in salicylate intoxication, 201
Allergic extracts, as cause of anaphylaxis, *261*
Amino acids, for intravenous alimentation, 226
  metabolic disorders of, 188–198
Aminophylline solutions, in therapy of anaphylaxis, 265

267

Ammonia salts, and avoidance in hepatic failure, 107
Amnesia, after head injury, 64
Ampicillin, in treatment of meningitis, 86
Anaphylaxis, *241*, 260–266
    acute reactions of, DIC as complicating mechanism, *241*
    causes of, 261, 262
    equipment and medication for treatment, *263–265*
    signs and symptoms of, 260
    therapy of, immediate, 263
        of complications, 265
        supportive, 264
Anemia, hemolytic, DIC as etiologic or complicating mechanism of, 240, *241*
    in renal failure, 120
    in sickle cell disease, 250
    therapy for, in cardiac failure, 101
Anesthesia, DIC as complicating factor of, *241*
    local, as cause of anaphylaxis, *261*
Antibiotics, as cause of anaphylaxis, *261*
    in treatment of cardiac failure, 101
    in treatment of endotoxin shock, 37
    in treatment of meningitis, 87
    in treatment of respiratory distress syndrome of newborn, 163
    in treatment of sickle cell disease, 252
Anticonvulsants, in head injury, 72
    intravenous, for status epilepticus, 77
Antifibrinolytic agents, contraindication of, in disseminated intravascular coagulation, 246
Antihistamines, in anaphylaxis therapy, 264
Anuria, calcium and phosphorus balance in, 122
    infections during, 122
    management of, in renal failure, 121, 122
    nutritional maintenance during, 121
    water and electrolyte balance in, 121
Apnea, in newborn, 152, 164
Aramine, for hypotension in anaphylaxis therapy, 265
Argininemia, *190, 194*
Arrhythmias, cardiac, in anaphylaxis, 263, 265
Arterial catheterization, 6
Arthritis, in meningitis, 82
Ascites, in liver disease, 108
Asparaginase, as cause of anaphylaxis, *261*
Asphyxia, of newborn, 152, 154, 159
Aspirin, as cause of anaphylaxis, *261, 262.* See also *Salicylate.*
    contraindicated in sickle cell disease crises, 257
Asplenia, functional, in sickle cell disease, 253
Atelectasis, of newborn, 152, 154, 156

Australia antigen, in diagnosis of hepatic failure, 105

Bacteria, of skin, control of after burns, 55
Bacterial meningitis, 80–91
Bacterial sepsis, with DIC as etiologic or complicating mechanism, *241*
Behavior, and change in self-image, after burns, 59, 60
Bicarbonate. See also Alkali Therapy.
    and emergency therapy in cardiac failure, 101
    sodium, in treatment of respiratory distress syndrome of newborn, 157–160
        in treatment of salicylate intoxication, 206
β-Alaninemia, *191, 194*
Blood
    acid-base disturbances of, and treatment, in dehydration secondary to diarrhea, *210,* 215–216
        in diabetic ketoacidosis, 173–176
        in renal failure, 114–117
        in respiratory distress syndrome of newborn, 154–155, 157–160
        in salicylate intoxication, 203–204
    replacement of, in trauma and shock, *12*
    volume and circulation of, in cardiac failure, 93
Blood cultures, in diagnosis of meningitis, 83
Blood gases, in respiratory distress syndrome, 154, 158–161
Blood glucose concentration, and hyperglycemia. See Diabetic Ketoacidosis and Coma.
    and hypoglycemia, 180, 181, 183
    physiologic regulation of, 183
Blood platelets, in DIC, 239
Blood pressure, in shock, 6–10
    monitoring and support of in meningitis, 84
Body surface, estimation of burned areas, 49
Brain, abscess of, in meningitis, 89
    edema of, and risk of rapid rehydration, 214
Branched-chain ketoaciduria, 189, *190, 191, 194, 195*
Breathing. See Respiration, Respiratory Arrest, Respiratory Distress.
Bronchospasm, in anaphylaxis, 262, 263
Burns, 46–61
    and family problems, 47
    first aid for, 47
    incidence of, 46
    prevention of, 46, 47

Burns (*Continued*)
  treatment of, 47–61
  with DIC as complicating factor, *241*

Calcium, homeostasis of, abnormalities
      of in dehydration, 216
  in status epilepticus, 78
Carbohydrate metabolism, disorders of,
      192
  in diabetic ketoacidosis, 169–173
  in salicylate poisoning, 199
Cardiac failure, diseases confused with,
      97
  etiology of, 94
  in infants, 92–103
  in renal failure, 120
  pathogenesis and pathophysiology of,
      92–94
  prognosis of, 97
  signs and symptoms of, 95–97
  treatment of, 97–101
    immediate, 98
Cardiac massage, as emergency therapy
      for cardiac failure, 101
  external, *128, 129*, 131
Cardiomegaly, in cardiac failure, 95
Cardiovascular system, and endotoxin
      shock, 23–30
  treatment of, 36
Carnosinemia, *191, 194, 195*
Catecholamines, relation to kinins in
      endotoxin shock, 27
Catheters and catheterization,
  arterial, 6
  cardiac, for diagnosis after acute car-
      diac failure, 102
  for suctioning in tracheostomy, 142
  superior vena caval, in intravenous
      alimentation, 227
    complications of, 237
  umbilical in management of respiratory
      distress syndrome of newborn, 154
Cellulitis, after burns, 54
Central nervous system, dysfunction of,
      as complication of burns, 55
  in salicylate intoxication, heat reg-
      ulation in, 202
    other dysfunctions in, 203
    stimulation of, and respiratory cen-
        ter, 200
Central venous pressure, in trauma and
      shock, 7–9
Cerebrospinal fluid, in head injury, 65, 70
  in meningitis, diagnostic use of, 83
    obstruction in, 83, *83*, 85
Chest, roentgenography of, 144
Chloride requirements, following burns,
      53
Chlorpromazine, in painful crises of sickle
      cell disease, 257

Chymotrypsin, as cause of anaphylaxis,
      261
Circulation. See also Blood and Cardio-
      vascular System.
  cross, in hepatic failure, 110
  in respiratory arrest, 128
  in shock, 6–12, 17
Cirrhosis, DIC as complicating factor of,
      241
Citrullinemia, 190, 194
Clotting factors, in disseminated intra-
      vascular coagulation, 243
Coagulation
  intravascular, as cause of renal failure,
      115
    diffuse, in meningitis, 85
    disseminated. See Disseminated Intra-
        vascular Coagulation (DIC).
  in endotoxin shock, 30
  tests for, in newborn infants, *244*
Coma, in acute metabolic disease, 188
  in diabetic ketoacidosis, 168–179
  in hepatic failure, 105, 107
  in hypoglycemia, 183
  in renal failure, 118, 119
  in salicylate intoxication, 203
Concussions, 63
Contracture, and scarring, following
      burns, 56
Contrast media, iodinated, as cause of
      anaphylaxis, *261*
Contusions and lacerations, of cerebral
      tissue, 64
Convulsions, hypoxic, as late complication
      of anaphylaxis, 264
  in acute metabolic disease, 188
  in hypoglycemia, 181
  in renal failure, 118, 119
  in salicylate intoxication, 203
  in status epilepticus, 76
Cord injury, cervical, in head injury, 69
Corticosteroids. See also Steroids.
  in treatment of adrenal insufficiency, 43
  in treatment of burns, 50
  in treatment of endotoxin shock, 37
  in treatment of shock, 16
  use of in anaphylaxis therapy, 264
  use of in meningitis, 84
  use of in tracheostomies, 147
Cross circulation, animal and human, in
      hepatic failure, 110
Cyanosis, as symptom of anaphylaxis, 260
  in cardiac failure, 97
  in respiratory distress syndrome, 160–
      161

Dactylitis, in sickle cell disease, 254
Dehydration
  clinical evaluation of, 209–216
  dangers and treatment of, in sickle cell
      disease, 256

Dehydration (*Continued*)
hyper-, hypo-, and iso-natremic, 213
in salicylate intoxication, 200, 202
treatment of, *205*
secondary to diarrhea, 208–219
therapy of, 216–219
emergency, 217
recovery, 218
repletion, 217
water volume repletion and maintenance of, 210
Dextran, as cause of anaphylaxis, *261*
Diabetic ketoacidosis and coma, 168–179
clinical and laboratory findings in, 173
incidence of, 168
metabolic derangements in, 169
onset of, 173
therapy of, 175–179
Dialysis, in hepatic failure, 109
in renal failure, 118, 120, 121
Diarrhea, use of intravenous alimentation to sustain life in, *224*
with secondary dehydration, 208–219
Diazepam (Valium), for status epilepticus,
78
DIC (Disseminated Intravascular Coagulation), 239–248
Diet, in diabetes, 179
Digitalis, difficulties of use in renal failure,
120
in treatment of cardiac failure, 98
Digoxin, in treatment of cardiac failure,
98
Diphenylhydantoin sodium (Dilantin), in
therapy of status epilepticus, 78
Disseminated intravascular coagulation
(DIC), 239–248
clinical conditions producing, 241–246
differential diagnosis of, 245–246
tests indicative of, *243*
treatment of, 246–247
Diuretics, in treatment of cardiac failure,
99
Doppler ultrasound, to monitor infants in
cardiac failure, 98
Drug reactions, history of, for avoiding
anaphylaxis, 265
and ingestion, with DIC as
complicating mechanism, *241*
Drugs, in trauma and shock, 5
intravenous, as cause of anaphylaxis,
261
sympathomimetic, in shock, 16
Dyspnea, as sign of anaphylaxis, 260,
263
in cardiac failure, 95

Edema, cerebral, in meningitis, 84
in anaphylaxis, 263, 265

Edema (*Continued*)
in cardiac failure in infants, 96
in head injury, 65, 68, 71, 72
pulmonary, in renal failure, 120
Effusions, chronic subdural, after head
injury, 74
Egg-based vaccines, as cause of anaphylaxis, *261*
Electrocardiography, to monitor therapy
of cardiac failure, 99
Electroencephalography, in diagnosis of
head injury, 70
value of in status epilepticus, 79
Electrolyte and water deficits, in diabetic acidosis, 172, 173
correction of, 175–178
in diarrhea, 208–219
Electrolytes, for intravenous alimentation, 226
replacement of, in acute adrenal insufficiency, 42
Emotional changes, in endotoxin shock,
36
Endothelium, vascular, in septic shock, 31
Endotoxemia, diagnosis of, in laboratory,
34–35
Endotoxin Shock. See Shock, Endotoxin.
Endotoxins, biologic effects, 22–23
structure of, 22
Epilepsy, after head injury, 73
recurrent. See Status Epilepticus.
Epinephrine, in treatment of anaphylaxis,
264
Erythrocytes, abnormal, in DIC, 244
Erythroid aplasia, in sickle cell disease,
251
Escharotomy, after burns, *51*
Ethosuximide, in therapy of petit mal
status epilepticus, 78
Exanthems, in meningitis, 82
Extracellular fluid volume (ECFV) re-
duction. See also Dehydration.
as cause of renal failure, 114
treatment of, 116

Fat embolism, DIC as complicating factor of, *241*
Fatty acids, in endotoxins, 21
Feeding, and caloric intake, of burn patient, 57–59
and fluids, in infants in respiratory
distress, 161–162
in dehydration, 209, 218
in infants in cardiac failure, 96, 100
intravenous. See Intravenous Alimentation.
Fever, after burns, 55
in hepatic failure, 106
persistent, in meningitis, 84

Fibrin abnormalities, in disseminated intravascular coagulation, 243, 245

Flow charts, in management of diabetic ketoacidosis, 175

Flowmeters, arterial, 7

Fluid, extracellular, expanders for treatment of renal failure, 116, 117

Fluid replacement, after burns, 52, 53
in acute adrenal insufficiency, 42
in dehydration secondary to diarrhea, 213–217
in trauma and shock, 11

Fluid therapy,
after head injury, 70
in salicylate intoxication, 201, 203–205

Foods, as cause of anaphylaxis, *261*

Formininotransferase deficiency, *192,194*

Fractures, after positive pressure ventilation or cardiac massage, 131
of skull. See Head injury.

Fructose intolerance, *193, 194*
in hypoglycemia, 184, 186

Galactosemia, *192, 194*, 196

Gallop rhythm, in cardiac failure, 96

Gamma globulin, as cause of anaphylaxis, *261*

Globulin, binding, in diagnosis of endotoxemia, 34

Glomerulonephritis, causing renal failure, 115

Glucagon, in hypoglycemia, 185

Glucose, for intravenous alimentation, 220
tolerance of, 236
hypertonic, in respiratory arrest, 130
in status epilepticus, 78
in treatment of diabetic ketoacidosis, 178
in treatment of hypoglycemia, 182, 186

Glucose-galactose malabsorption *192,194*

Glycogen storage disease, and hepatomegaly, 186

Green acyl dehydrogenase deficiency, *193,195*

Growth, failure, in infants with cardiac failure, 96

Hageman factor, activation in endotoxin shock, 26

"Hand-foot syndrome," in sickle cell disease, 254

Head injury
and shock, 15
complications of, 67, 73
diagnosis and management of, 62–75
pathology of, 63–66
prognosis of, 73, 74

Heart. See also Cardiac Failure, Cardiac massage.

Heart disease, cyanotic congenital, DIC as complicating mechanism of, *241*

Heat stroke, with DIC as complicating factor, 241

Hemangioma, giant, DIC as complicating factor, *241*

Hematoma, cerebral, and head injury, 74

Hemiplegia, in sickle cell disease, 255

Hemoglobin S, in sickle cell disease, 258

Hemoglobinuria, following burns, 53

Hemolytic transfusion reactions, with DIC as etiologic or complicating mechanism, *241*

Hemolytic uremic syndrome, as cause of renal failure, 115
DIC as etiologic or complicating mechanism of, *241*

Hemorrhage, after head injury, 64, 65, 68, 69
bilateral adrenal, in newborn, 41
in trauma and shock, 14

Heparin, in treatment of DIC, 244, 246
in treatment of intravascular coagulation in endotoxin shock, 38

Hepatic failure, acute, 104–112
causes and outcome of, 105
contraindicated drugs, 107
prevention and prognosis of, 106
treatment of, 107–110
tabulation, 111

Hepatic Failure Surveillance Study, 105

Hepatitis, infectious, as cause of hepatic failure, 105

Hepatomegaly, in cardiac failure, 96

Histamine, in endotoxin shock, 26, 27

Hormones, polypeptide, as cause of anaphylaxis, *261*
steroid, and adrenal insufficiency, 43

Hyaline membrane disease, clinical counterpart of respiratory distress syndrome, 153
diagnosis of, 153–156
treatment of, 156–166
prognosis of, 166

Hydration, and clinical appraisal of problems in dehydration, 209, *210*
calcium ion homeostasis in, 209, 216
hydrogen ion status in, 209, *210*, 215
intracellular ions in, 209, 216
osmolality in, 209, 213–215
volume replacement in, 209, *210*, 210–213

Hydrogen ion, excess in dehydration secondary to diarrhea, 215

Hyperalimentation, intravenous, in burns, 59

Hyperammonemia, *190, 194, 195*

Hyperbilirubinemia, in respiratory distress syndrome, 163

Hyperglycemia, in diabetic ketoacidosis, 174, 175

Hyperglycinemia, *191, 194*
Hyperkalemia, treatment of, in renal failure, 117
Hyperlysinemia, *191, 194*
Hypermetabolism, before reepithelialization in burn patient, 57
Hypernatremia, in dehydration secondary to diarrhea, 213–215, 218
in salicylate poisoning, 202
Hyperosmolar agents, to reduce cerebral pressure in head injuries, 71
Hyperosmolarity, dangers of, in respiratory distress syndrome, 159
Hyperprolinemia, *190, 194, 195*
Hyperpyrexia, in salicylate intoxication, 200–204
treatment of, 204
Hypertension, and ECFV overload in renal failure, 119
Hyperthermia. See also Hyperpyrexia. DIC as complicating factor, *241*
Hypertonic solutions, in status epilepticus, 78
Hyperuricacidemia, *193, 195*
Hypervalinemia, *191, 194*
Hyperventilation, as symptom of salicylate intoxication, 201
Hypoglycemia, 180–187
causes of, *184*
diagnosis of, 180, 183–186
in older infants and children, 182, 183
neonatal, 181
neurological sequelae of, 182
therapy of, 182, 186
with hepatic failure, 107
Hypomagnesemia, familial, *193, 194*
Hypotension, as result of anaphylaxis, 263
Hypothermia, questionable value of in meningitis, 85
Hypovolemia, in burns, 52, 54
in trauma and shock, 11–13
treatment in endotoxin shock, 36
Hypoxemia, differentiation of causes of in respiratory distress syndrome of newborn, *161*
Hypoxia, acute, tissue damage in, 131
in tracheostomy, 142
treatment of, in sickle cell disease crises, 256

Identification, personal, for adrenal crises and other medical emergencies, 43
Infant of diabetic mother, with DIC as complicating factor, *241*
of mother with abruptio placenta, DIC as etiologic or complicating factor in, *241*

Infant *(Continued)*
of toxemic mother, with DIC as etiologic or complicating factor, *241*
Infection
after skull fracture, 66
and acute adrenal insufficiency, 41
as complication of intravenous alimentation, 236
as complication of liver failure, 108
in acute bacterial meningitis, 81
in sickle cell crises, 252, 253
prevention of, in respirator care, 133
with DIC as complicating mechanism, *241, 245*
with gram-negative bacteria, as cause of endotoxin shock, 23
Inferon, as cause of anaphylaxis, *261*
Inflammation, from endotoxins, 22
Infusates, for intravenous alimentation, 226, 227
Injuries, 1. See also Trauma.
Insulin, deprivation of, causing diabetic ketoacidosis, 169
effects of, 170
in hypoglycemia, 184, 185
in treatment of ketoacidosis, 178
Intracranial pressure, after head injury, 68, 71
Intravenous alimentation, 220–238
central venous technique for, *228,* 228–235
complications of, 236–238
content of infusate in, *226*
indications for, 221–225
metabolic observation and responses of, 235–236
pump and filter for, 227, 228
statistics of, 238
Ischemia, and necrosis in DIC, 240
Isovaleric acidemia, *191, 195*
Isuprel, emergency therapy of cardiac failure, 101

Jaundice, in acute hepatic failure, 104, 106, See also Hyperbilirubinemia.
Joints, pain in, in sickle cell disease, 254

Kallikrein, in formation of kinins, 26
Ketoacidosis, diabetic, mechanisms and effects of, 171
Ketoaciduria, branched-chain, 189, 190, 191, *194, 195*
Kidneys, effects of hepatic failure on, 108 See also Renal Failure.
Kininogens, as precursors of kinins, 26

Kinins, in endotoxin shock, 24
Kussmaul breathing, in diabetic acidosis, 173

Lactic and pyruvic acidosis, *193–195*
Leukemia, DIC as complicating factor of, *241*
Leukocytosis, after burns, 55
Lifeline. See Intravenous Alimentation.
Limulus test, for endotoxemia, 35
Lipids, changes in, in diabetic keto-acidosis and coma, 169, *171*
  in hyperlipidemia, 174
  metabolism of, disorders of, *193*
Liver. See also Hepatic Failure.
  biopsy of, to diagnose hepatic failure, 105
  damage after endotoxin shock, 33
  glucose production (gluconeogenesis) in, 183–185
  in glycogen storage disease, 186
  involvement in sickle cell disease crises, 255
  regeneration after hepatic failure, 107
Lorfan, as narcotic antagonist, 130
Lumbar puncture, cautious use in head injury, 70
Lungs. See also Respiration, Respiratory Arrest, Respiratory Distress.
  in respiratory distress syndrome of newborn, 152–166
  involvement in sickle cell disease crises, 255
  lesions, from mechanical ventilation, 135

Malaria, with DIC, *241*
Malformations, circulatory, as cause of cardiac failure in infancy, 94
  renal, as cause of renal failure, 115
Malnutrition, after burns, 58, *58*
Meningitis, acute bacterial, 80–91
  acid fast and fungal, 83
  causes of, by age incidence, *81*
  clinical recognition of, 81–84
  differential and specific diagnosis of, 83
  H. influenzae, 81, 85
    relapse and resistance in, 88
  prophylaxis of, 88, 89
  questionable value of sulfonamides in treatment of, 87
  rehabilitation of, 90
  surgical considerations of, 89, 90
  therapy of, antimicrobial, 85–88
  underlying disease associated with, 82
  viral, 83

Metabolic disease, acute, 188–198
Metabolism, effects of endotoxin on, 32–34
  expenditure of, in dehydration, 211, 212
  in endotoxin shock, 32
    carbohydrate, 32, 33
    cellular, 33, 34
    protein, 33
  in infants in cardiac failure, 100
  inborn errors of, *190–193*
    screening for, *194, 195*
Methergine, as cause of anaphylaxis, *261*
Methylmalonic aciduria, 189, *191, 192, 195*
Microcirculation, in shock, 24
Monoplegia, in sickle cell disease, 255
Morphine, in treatment of cardiac failure, 100

Nalline, as narcotic antagonist, 130
Necrosis, hepatic, 104, 105
  renal cortical and tubular, causing renal failure, 115
Neoplasms, causing renal failure, 115
Nephritides, familial, causing renal failure, 115
Newborn infants, cardiac surgery and blood loss in, as cause of renal failure, 114
  hypoglycemia in, causes of, 181
    signs of, 181
    treatment of, 182
      with glucose, 182
      with hydrocortisone, 182
  resuscitation of, 130
  with DIC complicating other conditions, *241*
    diagnosis of, 244
  with respiratory distress syndrome, 152–167
Nitrofurantoin, as cause of anaphylaxis, *261*
Nitrogen balance, in intravenous alimentation, 236
Nocardiosis, of central nervous system, 87
Nursing care, for central venous alimentation, standing orders for, 228–235

Oast-hourse syndrome, *192, 194, 195*
Oliguria, following severe burns, 53, *53*
Orthopnea, as symptom of anaphylaxis, 260
Osmolality of body fluids, in dehydration secondary to diarrhea, 210, 213–215
Oxygen, for cardiac failure, 99

Oxygen (*Continued*)
  therapy and toxicity of, in respiratory distress syndrome, 159–161
  use and dangers of, in respiratory failure, 135
Oxygen consumption and affinity, in shock, 10, 13

Pancreatic tumors and hyperplasia, causing hypoglycemia, 184
Para-aminosalicylate, as cause of hepatic failure, 106
Paralysis, as result of status epilepticus, 76
  in salicylate intoxication, 203
Penicillin, as cause of anaphylaxis, *261, 262*
  in treatment of meningitis, 86
  sensitivity to, and prevention of anaphylaxis, 265
  to prevent cellulitis after burns, 54
Physiotherapy, chest, 146
Plasma, salicylate levels, in relation to intoxication, 201
  use in intravenous alimentation, 227
Pneumonia, aspiration, hazard of anaphylaxis in, 263
Poisoning, salicylate, 199–207
Positive pressure breathing, in therapy of respiratory distress syndrome of newborn, 126, 165
  intermittent, 143
Potassium, deficits, in dehydration secondary to diarrhea, 210, 216
  elevated, in serum, in renal failure, 117, 118. See also Hyperkalemia.
  in diabetic ketoacidosis and coma, depletion, 172
  replacement, 178
Prochlorperazine, for painful crises of sickle cell disease, 257
Propionic acidemia, *192, 195*
Protein, diet, avoidance and resumption of, in hepatic failure, 107, 108
  foreign, as cause of anaphylaxis, *261, 262*
  serum, maintenance of following burns, 52
Psychosis, as result of status epilepticus, 76
Purpura fulminans, or thrombotic thrombocytopenic purpura, DIC as etiologic or complicating factor, *241*
Pyelonephritis, chronic, causing renal failure, 115
Pyridoxine dependency, *192*
Pyruvic and lactic acidosis, *193–195*

Radiography, pulmonary, in differential diagnosis of respiratory distress syndrome, 155, *155*

Regression of behavior, after burns, 59
Rehabilitation, after acute bacterial meningitis, 90
  after head injury, 73
Renal failure, acute, 113–123
    causes and their treatment, 113–116
      postrenal, 116
      prerenal, 114
      renal, 114, 115
    treatment, 116–121
Respiration, following burns, 50, 55
  in salicylate intoxication, depression of, 204
  stimulation of, 200, 204
Respirators, negative *vs.* positive, in infants with respiratory distress, 164
Respiratory arrest, 124–138
  management, of emergency phase, 125–130
  of sequelae, 130–136
Respiratory distress, causes, 126, 127
  in tracheostomy patient, 143
Respiratory distress syndrome (RDS), DIC as etiologic or complicating factor of, *241*
  of newborn, 152–167
    diagnosis of, 153–156
    prognosis of, 166
    treatment of, 155–156
Resuscitation, equipment and drugs, 125, *125*
  in respiratory arrest, 125–130
  mouth-to-mouth, 128
  in trauma and shock, 5
  personnel availability for, 125, 126
Reye's syndrome, confusion with hepatic failure, 105
Rhinorrhea, after head injury, 71
Rickettsial infections, with DIC as complicating mechanism, *241*
Ringer's lactate solution, in treatment of burns, 52

Salicylate intoxication, 199–207
  acidosis, 203
  diagnosis and treatment, 200–206
    alkalosis, respiratory, 200
    dehydration, 202–205
    hyperpyrexia, 200–204
  excretion during, 205
  levels in plasma, 201
Scarring, and contracture, following burns, 55
Sedation, to treat burns, 50
Self image, after burns, 60
Septicemia, as complication of intravenous alimentation, 237

Serotonin, relation to endotoxin shock, 27
Serum, as cause of anaphylaxis, *261*
Shock, after head injury, 67
  as cause of renal failure, 115
  DIC as etiologic mechanism or complication, 240, *241*
  distinctions between cardiac, hypovolemic, and endotoxin, *30*
  endotoxin, 21–40
    treatment of, 35–39
  from acute adrenal insufficiency, 41–45
  hemorrhagic, 1–20
  in acute meningitis, 81
  in anaphylaxis, 260
    treatment of, 264
  in salicylate intoxication, 205
  septic, 29, 30
Sickle cell disease, crises and management of, 249–259
  aplastic, 250
  hyperhemolytic, 252
  laboratory values in blood, *250*
  splenic, 252–253
  transfusions in, 251, 256
  treatment of, 256–258
  vaso-occlusive, 253–256
Silver nitrate, in treatment of burns, 55, 59
Skin grafts, after burns, 56
Skull fracture, 65, 74
Snake bite, DIC as complicating factor of, *241*
Sodium, in therapy of diabetic ketoacidosis, *177*
  serum concentrations of, in dehydration, 213–215
Spleen, in sickle cell disease crises, 252–253
Status epilepticus, 76–79
  etiologic factors in, 79
Steroids. See also Corticosteroids.
  adrenal, 44
    withdrawal of, and acute adrenal insufficiency, 42
  questionable value of in acute hepatic failure, 108
Stimulants, respiratory, in respiratory arrest, 130
Stings, insect, as cause of anaphylaxis, *261*
Sulfite oxidase deficiency, *191, 196*
Sulfobromophthalein, as cause of anaphylaxis, *261*
Surfactants, pulmonary, in respiratory distress syndrome of newborn, 152, 165, 166

Tachycardia, after burns, 55
  in cardiac failure, 96

Tachypnea, in cardiac failure, 95
Tetanus toxoid, as cause of anaphylaxis, *261*
Tetany, control of in salicylate intoxication, 204
Tetracycline, as cause of hepatic failure, 106
Time-flow charts, in management of respirator care, 133
Trachea, intubation of, in respiratory arrest, 128, *129*, 131, 132
Tracheal tubes, nasal or oral, in prolonged respiratory failure, 132
Tracheostomy, aspects of care of, 139–150
  complications of, 149
  equipment for, 144
  home care of, 149–150
  in chronic respiratory failure, 132
  management of, 139–151
  weaning after, and removal of tube, 147–149
Transfusions, exchange, in hepatic failure, 109
  in sickle cell disease crises, 251, 256
Transplantation, organ, with DIC as complicating factor, *241*
Trauma, 1–20
  and blood loss, as cause of renal failure, 144
  with DIC as complicating mechanism, *241*
Tris hydroxymethyl aminomethane (Tham), to correct acidosis in respiratory distress, 159
Tumors, malignant, DIC as complicating factor of, *241*
Twin, with dead fetus, DIC as etiologic or complicating factor of, *241*
Tyrosyluria, *192, 195*

Unconsciousness, after head injury, 63
Urea nitrogen concentration, to assess volume depletion in dehydration, 212
Urea therapy, possible use of in treatment of sickle cell disease, 258
Uremia, as cause or result of renal failure, 115
  DIC as etiologic or complicating factor, *241*, 245
  treatment of, 119, 121
Urine, samples for diagnosing acute metabolic disease in infancy and childhood, 197
Urine output, after burns, 54
  in shock, 17
Urticaria, symptom of anaphylaxis, 260, 262

Vaccines, as cause of anaphylaxis, *261*, 266
Vasodilators, in treatment of endotoxin shock, 38
  pulmonary, as ineffective therapy in respiratory distress syndrome of newborn, 165
Vasopressors, in adrenal insufficiency, 43
Ventilation, assisted, in head injury, 72
  in respiratory arrest, 128
  in respiratory distress syndrome of newborn, 163–165
  mechanical, 132–135
    indications for, 133
  prolonged, in respiratory arrest, 132
Ventilator care, complications of, 134
  termination of in irreversible brain damage, 135
  unsuitable patients for, 135
Ventilators, in tracheostomy, 145
Virus infections, with DIC as complicating factor, *241*

Vitamin B_{12} responsive methylmalonic aciduria, *193, 195*
Vitamin B_{12} unresponsive methylmalonic aciduria, *193, 195*
Vitamins, for intravenous alimentation, 226
Vomiting, in anaphylaxis, 260, 263
  in diabetic ketoacidosis, 173

Water, normal requirements for in relation to age, weight, body surface, *212*
Water balance, in intravenous alimentation, 236
Weight gain, during intravenous alimentation, 236
Weight loss, in dehydration, 210, 211
Wheezing, as sign of anaphylaxis, 260
Wounds, stab, 15